Effective Leadership and Management in Nursing

FIFTH EDITION

Eleanor J. Sullivan, PhD, RN, FAAN
School of Nursing, University of Kansas
Kansas City, KS

Phillip J. Decker, PhD
University of Houston, Clear Lake
School of Business and Public Administration
Houston, TX

Consulting Editor
Patricia A. Jamerson, RNC, PhD
University of Missouri
Barnes College of Nursing
St. Louis, MO

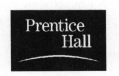 Prentice Hall

Upper Saddle River, New Jersey 07458

Library of Congress Cataloging-in-Publication Data

Sullivan, Eleanor J., 1938–
    Effective leadership and management in nursing / Eleanor J.
Sullivan, Phillip J. Decker.—5th ed.
        p.   cm.
    Includes index.
    ISBN 0-8053-2833-5
    1. Nursing services—Administration.   2. Leadership.
I. Decker, Phillip J.   II. Title.
RT89 .S85 2000
362.1′73′068—dc21   00-051490

Note: Care has been taken to confirm the accuracy of
information presented in this book. The authors, editors, and
the publisher, however, cannot accept any responsibility for
errors or omissions or for consequences from application of
the information in this book and make no warranty, express
or implied, with respect to its contents.

Publisher: *Julie Alexander*
Executive Editor: *Maura Connor*
Director of Production and Manufacturing: *Bruce Johnson*
Managing Production Editor: *Patrick Walsh*
Manufacturing Manager: *Ilene Sanford*
Production Liaison: *Julie Boddorf*
Production Editor: *Gretchen Miller*
Creative Director: *Marianne Frasco*
Cover Design Coordinator: *Maria Guglielmo*
Cover Designer: *Amy Rosen*
Cover Photo: *Otto Freundlich, 1878–1943*
Director of Marketing: *Leslie Cavaliere*
Marketing Coordinator: *Cindy Frederick*
Editorial Assistant: *Beth Romph*
Composition: *York Production Services*
Printing and Binding: *Courier Kendallville*

Prentice-Hall International (UK) Limited, *London*
Prentice-Hall of Australia Pty. Limited, *Sydney*
Prentice-Hall Canada Inc., *Toronto*
Prentice-Hall Hispanoamericana, S.A., *Mexico*
Prentice-Hall of India Private Limited, *New Delhi*
Prentice-Hall of Japan, Inc., *Tokyo*
Prentice-Hall Singapore Pte. Ltd.
Editora Prentice-Hall do Brasil, Ltda., *Rio de Janeiro*

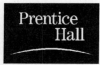

10 9 8 7 6 5 4 3 2

ISBN 0-8053-2833-5

This book is dedicated to my family for their continuing love and support.

Eleanor J. Sullivan

Preface

Leading and managing are essential skills for all nurses in today's rapidly changing health care arena. New graduates find themselves managing unlicensed assistive personnel, and experienced nurses are managing groups of health care providers from a variety of disciplines and educational levels. Declining revenues and increasing costs mandate that every organization use its resources efficiently; thus, nurses are challenged to manage effectively with fewer resources. Never has the information presented in *Effective Leadership and Management in Nursing*, Fifth Edition, been needed more. This textbook can help both student nurses and those with practice experience acquire the skills to ensure success in today's dynamic health care environment.

FEATURES OF THE FIFTH EDITION

Effective Leadership and Management in Nursing has made a significant and lasting contribution to the education of nurses and nurse managers in its four previous editions. Used worldwide, this award-winning textbook is now offered in an updated and revised edition to reflect changes in the current health care system and in response to suggestions from the book's users. The Fifth Edition builds upon the work of previous contributors to provide the most up-to-date and comprehensive learning package for today's busy students and professionals.

Two supplementary texts, the popular student workbook and the *Instructor's Resource Manual*, have been revised. In addition, we have added a few unique new supplements—a Companion Website and online course management systems—designed to enhance both student and faculty use of this textbook. Together this complete package facilitates rapid learning of essential content and skills.

Student-Friendly Learning Tools

Designed with the adult learner in mind, the book focuses on the application of the content presented and integrates clinical examples throughout each chap-

ter. To further illustrate and emphasize key points, each chapter in this edition includes these features:

- Chapter outline and content preview
- Key terms defined on the pages where they first appear
- "Leadership and Management in Action"—end-of-chapter critical thinking exercises that help students apply what they have learned
- A bulleted summary at the end of the chapter
- Up-to-date references

Plus, at the end of each chapter, the reader will find a link to the Companion Website at www.prenhall.com/sullivan_decker for additional exercises and research on the Web.

HALLMARK FEATURE: MULTIDISCIPLINARY AUTHORS

This book has been a success for many reasons. It combines practicality with conceptual understanding; is responsive to the needs of faculty, nurse managers, and students; and taps the expertise of contributors from a variety of disciplines, especially management professionals whose work has been adapted by nurses for current nursing practice. The expertise of management professors in schools of business and practicing nurse managers is seldom incorporated into nursing textbooks. This unique approach provides students with invaluable knowledge and skills and sets the book apart from others.

ORGANIZATION

The text is organized into three sections that address the essential information and key skills that nurses must learn to succeed in today's volatile health care environment.

Part I. Understanding Nursing Management and Organizations. Part I introduces the concepts of organizations and organizational theory and design with an emphasis on redesign, restructuring, reengineering, integrated care networks, and managed care. Leadership is presented within a theoretical framework, and management functions are explained. Also included in Part I is information about legal challenges, ethical dilemmas, power, and politics, all necessary for nurses to succeed and prosper.

Part II. Key Skills in Nursing Management. Essential skills for today's managers comprise Part II. These include creating and managing budgets, encouraging efficiency and productivity, promoting quality management, solving problems and making decisions, communicating with a variety of individuals and groups, resolving conflicts, using information technology effectively, managing time and stress, delegating, working in teams, and effecting change.

Part III. Human Resource Management. Human resources are the health care system's most valuable asset so nurses must be adept at recruiting and selecting staff, assigning staff, handling scheduling, managing turnover, appraising and enhancing performance, and handling the inevitable personnel problems. In addition, collective bargaining—a key issue today in many organizations—is included in Part III.

NEW EXPANDED TEACHING AND LEARNING PACKAGE

Effective Leadership and Management in Nursing has been designed for leadership and management courses for undergraduate students and for experienced nurses who are new managers. The book comes with a complete teaching/learning package, which includes the *Instructor's Resource Manual*; a student workbook, *Nursing Leadership and Management in Action*; a Companion Website; and online course companions available in WebCT and Blackboard.

Instructor's Resource Manual. The popular *Instructor's Resource Manual* provides instructors with a comprehensive outline of the entire book for syllabi and classroom lectures, a complete test bank, and overhead transparency masters. The *Instructor's Resource Manual* also guides instructors in how to get the most out of the other elements of the teaching/learning package, such as the student workbook, *Nursing Leadership and Management in Action*, and the Companion Website.

Nursing Leadership and Management in Action. The companion workbook, *Nursing Leadership and Management in Action*, has been designed for use with *Effective Leadership and Management in Nursing*, Fifth Edition. Developed to help students acquire practical management skills, the workbook consists of a series of modules, each focusing on a particular skill. Some modules are designed for individual student practice and others for use in the skills laboratory or classroom. This workbook provides the instructor with valuable teaching activities and gives students opportunities to practice the skills introduced in the textbook. Activities in the workbook cover important timely topics, including problem solving, critical thinking, leadership styles, budgeting, using the Internet, communication, conflict resolution, delegation, and sensitivity to multicultural issues.

Companion Website. New to this package is a free Companion Website at www.prenhall.com/sullivan_decker. This website serves as a text-specific, interactive online workbook to both *Effective Leadership and Management in Nursing* and *Nursing Leadership and Management in Action*. The Companion Website includes modules for objectives, chapter outlines, key terms and definitions, discussion questions with essay responses, NCLEX review questions with automatic grading, current event exercises with links to other sites for student research and essay responses, and more. Instructors adopting this textbook for their courses have free access to an online Syllabus Manager with a whole host of features that facilitate the students' use of this Companion Website.

Online Course Management. Also new to this package are online course companions available for schools using WebCT and Blackboard course management systems. For more information about adopting an online course management system to accompany *Effective Leadership and Management*, Fifth Edition, please contact your Prentice Hall Health sales representative.

ACKNOWLEDGMENTS

The success of previous editions of this book has been due to the expertise of many contributors. Nursing administrators, management professors, and faculty in schools of nursing all made significant contributions to earlier editions. I am enormously grateful to them for sharing their knowledge and experience to help nurses learn leadership and management skills. Without them, this book would not exist. A complete list of contributing authors to all the editions of *Effective Leadership and Management in Nursing* is found on page viii.

At Prentice Hall Health, Executive Editor, Maura Connor, and Beth Romph, Editorial Assistant, guided this revision throughout. Gretchen Miller provided editing services, Larry Purnell contributed advice about health care organizations, Carol Perry offered up-to-date information on employment law, and Karen Backus furnished information on the status of collective bargaining. I am grateful to all of them.

Because health care continues to change, reviewers who are using the book in their management practice and in their classes provided invaluable comments and suggestions. I am indebted to the reviewers listed on page viii.

A special thank you to Consulting Editor, Pat Jamerson. She managed the project throughout, updated content, wrote, and edited chapters. Her work was vital to this edition and is greatly appreciated.

To everyone who has contributed to this fine book over the years, I thank you.

Eleanor J. Sullivan, PhD, RN, FAAN

CONTRIBUTORS TO PREVIOUS EDITIONS

Larry D. Baker, DBA

Diane Bartels, RN, MA

Mary Ann Boyd, PhD, DNS, CS

Diane Boyle, RN, CS, BSN, MSN, PhD

James A. Breaugh, PhD, MA

Kenna J. Bridgmon, RN

Gabriel Buntzman, PhD

Rita Clifford, RN, PhD

Helen R. Connors, RN, PhD, FAAN

Donna Costello-Nickitas, RN, PhD

Susan Crissman, RN, MNEd

Tom S. DeCock, MBA

Dennis L. Dossett, PhD

Alejandra Dreisbach, RN, MBA

Pam Duchene, RN, DNSc

Sandra Edwardson, RN, BS, MN, PhD

Doris A. England, RN, MSN, FAAN

Brenda Ernst, RN, BSN, MA

David O. Evans, RN, MSN

Susan C. Fry, RN, MEd, CNAA

David P. Gustafson, PhD, deceased

Sherlyn Hailstone, RN, BSN

Helen E. Hansen, RN, PhD

Marlene Hartmann, RN, MSN

Janalee B. Heaton, RN

Judith M. Hibberd, RN, PhD, BScN, MHSA

Cynthia A. Hornberger, RN, MBA, PhD, ARNP-C

Pat Jamerson, RNC, PhD

Ruth Launius Jenkins, RN, PhD

Linda A. Knight, BS, MEd, DA

June Levine-Ariff, RN, MSN, CNA

David L. Martin, RN, MN

Diana J. Mason, RN, PhD

Elise McKenna, RN, MSEd, MPH

Rusti C. Moore-Greenlaw, RN, MEd

Patricia A. Muller-Smith, RN, EdD, RNC

Bill Mumford, RN, ADN, MSM

Steve Norton, PhD

Tim Porter-O'Grady, EdD, PhD, FAAN

Susan Reinhard, RN, PhD

Benjamin H. Rountree, DPA

Mona Ruddy-Wallace, RN, MSN, EdD

Vicki L. Sauter, PhD

Helen A. Schaag, RN, MSN, MA

Carolyn Hope Smeltzer, RN, EdD, FAAN

Donna Lynn Smith, RN, BScN, Prof.Dip., MEd

Robert J. Spaniol, RN, BSN, MBA

Marlene K. Strader, RN, PhD

Deborah E. Trautman, RN, MSN, CEN

Terri L. Wojcicki, MBA

Cynthia Woods, RN, PhD

REVIEWERS

Mary Jane Banks, RN, MNEd
Kent State University
College of Nursing
Kent, OH

Diane Forster Burke, RN, MS
Westminster College
School of Nursing
Salt Lake City, UT

Larry Purnell, RN, PhD
University of Delaware
School of Nursing
Newark, DE

Contents

PART II

KEY SKILLS IN NURSING MANAGEMENT   101

PART III

HUMAN RESOURCE MANAGEMENT   **263**

Contents **xv**

P A R T   1

Understanding Nursing Management and Organizations

Introduction to Nursing Management

Looking Ahead

Rapid changes in today's health care industry are reshaping the nurse's role. The emergence of new health care systems, the shift from a service orientation to a business orientation, and extensive redesign of the workplace directly affect where and how nursing care is delivered, as well as those who deliver the care. If we as nurses are to succeed and have our needs met in this new health care environment, we must learn how to manage ourselves and others effectively within the context of these changes and decreasing resources. This opening chapter introduces those challenges and the management education essential to all nurses.

Objectives

After reading this chapter, you will be able to:

- Describe how efforts to contain costs are changing today's health care industry.
- Compare and contrast today's health care system with that of the recent past.
- Discuss how changes in the health care system are affecting nursing.
- Delineate the changing roles of nurses in management and of managers.

Today, *all* nurses are managers. Whether they work on a medical floor in an acute care hospital, in a critical care unit, in an outpatient clinic, or in home care, they must deal with other staff (for example, other nurses and unlicensed assistive personnel) who work with them and for them, and they must use resources wisely. To manage well, nurses must understand the health care system and the organizations where they work. They need to recognize what external forces affect their work and how to influence those forces (for example, through political action). Nurses need to know what motivates people and how they can help create an environment that inspires and sustains the individuals who work in it. They need to be able to collaborate with others, both as leaders and as members of the team. They need to be confident in their ability to be leaders and managers.

This book is designed to provide new graduates or novice managers with the information they need to become effective managers and leaders in health care. More than ever before, today's rapidly changing health care environment demands highly refined management skills and superb leadership.

The Changing Health Care System

Today's health care system is undergoing significant changes. Lifesaving pharmaceutical products, innovations in imaging technologies and surgical procedures, telehealth and advances in research have combined to produce the most sophisticated and effective health care ever—and the most costly. Skyrocketing costs and inaccessibility to health care have become growing concerns for employers, health care providers, state legislatures, Congress, and the public at large.

Cost Containment

Although the United States spends more money on health care than any other country, millions of Americans have no access to basic health care. For some people, this is a temporary situation (due, for example, to changes in employment), but many others continue to go without health care because they work only part-time (and are thus often ineligible to participate in their employer's health care plan) or because they have a preexisting health condition. When the uninsured receive care, it is provided at great expense in emergency rooms, often after the condition has progressed and requires more complex and long-term care. Some of the costs of this unnecessarily expensive care are borne by the health care organization, and some

KEY TERMS

Diagnosis-related group A system of prospective payment used by Medicare that pays a provider a set amount for a specific condition.

Integrated health care systems Organizational health care structures that deliver a continuum of care, provide coverage for a group of individuals, and accept fixed payments for that group.

costs are passed on to other payers (such as Medicare and private insurance companies), who pass on their costs to their constituents (taxpayers, customers).

The government has made several attempts to contain health care costs. In the mid-1980s, a system of prospective, rather than retrospective, payment for health care was introduced for all Medicare recipients. Other third-party payers soon followed suit. This system, based on **diagnosis-related groups** (DRGs), pays a provider (physician or hospital) a set amount for a specific condition, stipulated ahead of time, instead of paying the bill after care is rendered. Hospitals have responded to these restrictions by instituting cost-cutting measures and by drastically reducing hospital stays.

Despite the change to a prospective payment system, health care costs have continued to rise. In 1997, the Balanced Budget Act was passed to attempt to control expenditures on Medicare. Medicare was targeted because of its impending bankruptcy and a projected 8.3 percent increase in spending over the next decade (Congressional Budget Office, 1997). The act provides defined federal contributions to health care and allows beneficiaries several provider options, including managed care, preferred provider organizations, and provider service organizations.

Individual states also have adopted or are considering plans to address these problems. Legislation varies from state to state, but the majority focuses on providing the uninsured access to care and on containing costs.

Besides legislation and government actions, marketplace changes are radically changing the way health care organizations operate. Competition has forced hospitals, physicians, and home care agencies into mergers, networks, and integrated systems of care. **Integrated health care systems** have emerged as organizations have struggled to find ways to survive in today's cost-conscious environment. Integrated systems encompass a variety of model organizational structures, but certain characteristics are common (Riley, 1994). For example, integrated systems are designed to deliver a whole continuum of care; to provide geographic coverage for the buyers of health care services; and to accept the risk inherent in taking a fixed payment in return for providing health care for all persons in the selected group (for example, all employees of one company). To provide such services, networks of providers encompassing hospitals and physician practices have emerged.

In integrated health care systems, the hospital is no longer the focal point; primary care is the focal point (Shortell, 1993). The goal is to keep patients healthy, treating them in the setting that incurs the lowest cost and thereby reducing expensive hospital treatments (Sovie, 1995). The former goal—to keep hospital beds filled—is replaced with a new goal: to keep patients out of them!

A variety of other arrangements have emerged, varying from loose affiliations between hospitals to complete mergers of hospitals, clinics, and physician practices. The movement away from independence and toward the formation of local, regional, and national systems is expected to continue throughout the 21st century.

Health care is now a competitive, market-based enterprise. This change has transformed health care from an industry with a service orientation to one with a business orientation. Scrutinizing costs is a way of life in health care today. Every expenditure, including supplies, equipment, and—most important—staff time, is closely examined (see Chapters 7 and 8). As a result, organizations are continuously restructuring and resizing, care systems are being reengineered, and nursing services redesigned (see Chapter 2).

In **redesign**, the distribution of activities, role overlap, excess specialization, and waste are examined. The goal is to design each job according to appropriate tasks and necessary qualifications and to have all jobs fit together so that the organization's work gets done in the most efficient and effective manner. Redesign usually focuses on the individual jobs in one clinical specialty area, although each area may be undergoing job redesign simultaneously or consecutively. (See also Chapter 2 on restructuring nursing care and job analysis in Chapter 17.)

Restructure means to change the structure of the organization. The administrative structure changes, as do reporting relationships and communication channels. Restructuring naturally follows organizational affiliations, mergers, and the establishment of integrated health care systems as efforts to reduce duplication among the network's various entities ensue.

Reengineering is an examination of job *processes*—of how the job is done, not just what tasks the job involves. Reengineering is collaborative, data-driven, and patient-focused. Reengineering usually involves the entire organization and results in major change to both the organization and its members.

Quality and Outcomes

In addition to cost containment, consumers are seeking quality care. The quality movement began in post–World War II Japan, when Japanese industries adopted a system that W. Edwards Deming designed to improve the quality of manufactured products. Its philosophy is that the consumer's needs should be the focus and that employees should be empowered to evaluate and improve quality. By acting on this philosophy, the Japanese quickly became able to produce goods superior in quality to those made in the United States. Japanese automobiles, television sets, copy machines, and other products required fewer repairs and lasted longer, often at a cost equal to or even less than comparable American-made products. The experiences of the U.S. auto makers, who refused to acknowledge consumer demands for fuel-efficient cars and subsequently saw their market share decline, taught American industry that focusing on the consumer's wants and needs is good business. The health care industry was slow to catch on, but competition has forced an emphasis on service to emerge.

Quality management is a preventive approach designed to address problems before they become crises. Built into the system is a mechanism for continuous improvement of products and services through constant evaluation of how well the consumer's needs are met and devising plans to perfect the process. Besides businesses in the United States and elsewhere, the health care industry also has adopted total quality management or variations on it. More recently, performance initiatives by the government and professional organizations have been instituted. These initiatives identify outcome indicators by which quality can be compared across disciplines or organizations rather than structures or processes. An example is the Health Employer Data and Information System (HEDIS) used to accredit managed care organizations (see Chapter 9).

Rural Health Care

Cost containment has had an especially deleterious effect on rural areas. A smaller population, a larger proportion of whom are elderly, makes it difficult to

KEY TERMS

Redesign A technique that examines the tasks within each job with the goal of combining appropriate tasks to improve efficiency.

Restructuring An examination of a health care organization's structure to improve the organization's productivity.

Reengineering A complex and often radical approach to the organization of patient care in which new relationships and expectations are adopted.

Quality management A preventive approach designed to address problems efficiently and quickly.

Telehealth The use of telecommunications technology to provide medical, nursing, and radiologic services.

maintain cost efficiency in isolated rural areas. Innovative methods of delivering care in rural areas are emerging, however. Bringing health care providers from cities to small towns on a rotating basis is one way of sharing physicians or physical therapists, for example, among several small communities. Rapid growth in nurse practitioner education, especially programs targeted to rural areas, represents another attempt to meet rural residents' needs for primary care.

Telehealth, the use of telecommunications technology to provide medical, nursing, and radiologic services, is growing. Besides video conferencing for consultation, this technology allows specialists to assess patients and view x-ray films from a distant location while interacting with the patient and the treating physician or nurse practitioner.

Cultural Diversity

While the United States is commonly referred to as the melting pot of the world, more than 8 percent, or 19.8 million people, are foreign-born residents (U.S. Census Bureau, 1993). Since 1972, the number of immigrants to this country has been steadily rising and the Census Bureau (1993) estimates that the United States will continue to attract two-thirds of the world's immigrants, with the majority coming from Central and South America. This influx of immigrants means that health care must assume a transcultural focus. Health care policy and provision of clinical services must

consider the values, beliefs, and lifestyles of a number of diverse cultures. To do so requires *awareness* of the differences and similarities between cultures, a *sensitivity* to other cultures' perspectives, and a resolution of health problems within the cultural belief system of the patient (Kozier, Erb, & Blais, 1997).

One obvious barrier to health care delivery to people of foreign-born cultures is language. The Census Bureau (1993) estimates that 14 percent, or 32 million people, in the United States speak a language other than English. Spanish is by far the most prevalent, but French, German, Italian, and Chinese also are common. To meet the needs of these individuals, health care providers need to be fluent in more than one language, or at least identify interpreters to facilitate assessment, education, and counseling of these individuals.

Another barrier is socioeconomic status. If you can pay for health care, access is not an issue; but for those who can't, health care may not be accessible. Again, health policy and health care providers need to identify ways to provide universal access regardless of race or ethnic origin.

Another barrier to health care delivery is *prejudice*, a strongly held opinion about a group of people that often leads to differential treatment (discrimination). Prejudice is not limited to people from other countries. Some maintain negative attitudes toward the elderly, others toward women, and still others toward lesbians and gay men.

Leninger (1991) suggests *culturally congruent care* is provided by (a) accepting and complying with an individual's beliefs, (b) planning, negotiating, and accommodating culturally specific practices, and (c) restructuring care based on knowledge about the culture.

Changes in Nursing

As an integral and vital component of health care, nursing is changing as part of, and in response to, other changes in the system, especially cost containment.

Cost containment has significantly affected the manner in which care is being delivered. Nursing has traditionally operated as if it were an isolated discipline, and the "nursing process" has been taught as if it were completely independent of the care given by other providers. Today's health care demands teamwork—from professionals and nonprofessionals alike. Collaborative teams consisting of nurses, physicians and other health care providers are developing clinical maps that define patient care needs and establish outcome measures.

The use of the most cost-effective provider also is the focus of change in the health care system. For example, if assistive personnel can do a nursing task (such as providing bed baths) at less cost and without adverse effects on the patient, it makes sense to use them wherever possible. By the same token, it is fiscally sound to allow a nurse practitioner to do certain tasks that were formerly performed only by physicians, such as taking medical histories and performing physical examinations. Thus, health care is moving toward multidisciplinary practice (health care providers from two or more disciplines working side by side) as well as interdisciplinary practice (health care providers from two or more disciplines working interdependently). The outcome of the cost containment measures is a restructuring of health care delivery. As a result, the numbers of registered nurses in acute care have diminished and further decline is projected from 63.8 percent in 1994 to 57.4 percent in 2005 (Malone & Marullo, 1997). Currently, 60 percent of registered nurses work in hospital settings, 17 percent in community or public health settings, 8.5 percent in ambulatory care settings, such as HMOs or clinics, and 8.1 percent in nursing homes or extended care facilities (HRSA, 1999).

Since there are fewer RNs in relation to assistive personnel, *all* nurses today are managers. They manage the care of a defined group of patients, doing some of the care themselves, directing others to provide care, and collaborating with still others. Nurses participate in teams of care providers and lead teams of professionals and nonprofessionals. Nurses therefore need new skills, especially management skills. Nurses must know how to delegate, supervise, evaluate, motivate, and communicate with practitioners of other disciplines, other nurses, and with unlicensed personnel. They must be skilled in negotiation, conflict resolution, and collaboration, and they must be able to participate in, as well as lead, teams.

Preparation for management must be an integral part of nursing education, and specific training in management skills is needed in nursing school and in the work setting. Most important, however, is that nurses transfer their newly acquired skills to the job itself. Thus, nurse managers must be experienced in management themselves and be able to assist their staff in developing adequate management skills. Management training for nurses at all levels is essential for any organization to be efficient and effective in today's cost-conscious and competitive environment.

The cultural diversity seen in the general population is also reflected in nursing. The Health Resources and Services Administration (1999) reports that about 10 percent of nurses come from racial or ethnic minorities, 4.2 percent of which are African-American, 3.4 percent Asian Pacific Islanders, 1.6 percent Hispanics, and 0.5 percent Native American/Alaskan Native. Nurse managers must develop sensitivity to cultural differences among their staff as well as their patients and be responsive to these differences within the context of the work environment.

Challenges for Nurse Managers

The system of health care in the United States continues to shift, change, and adjust to market forces, political pressures, and consumer demands. The radical changes in health care systems are still evolving. No one knows yet exactly how the system of the future will look. What seems certain is that it will be decidedly different from today's health care system; consequently, nursing services will be delivered in very different ways. Nurses and nurse managers will be key players in these changes.

The challenge for nurse managers and administrators is how to manage in this vastly different arena. Working with teams of administrators and providers to deliver quality health care in the most cost-effective manner offers opportunity as well. Nurses' unique skills in communication, negotiation, and collaboration position them well for the system of today and the system of the future.

The manager's integrity is crucial to the success of the work group and to the collaborative relationships with other providers. Integrity is defined as a quality or state of possessing sound moral principles: uprightness, honesty, and sincerity. Stephen Covey (1989) writes that integrity includes but goes beyond honesty. Honesty involves telling the truth, whereas integrity involves conforming reality to one's words. Kerfoot (1990) states that the most important positive influence on higher productivity in the workplace and employee satisfaction is the creation of a sense of trust. The manager develops trust by demonstrating behaviors that support established standards. If, for example, a standard has been established for patient education, the manager sees that quality assurance monitoring is in place to measure that goal. If patient education is a part of the orientation and performance evaluation plan for the staff, the manager might arrange to make additional written educational materials available in the work area to share with patients. The manager must take a proactive approach to confront all staff who fail to meet the standard. This consistency of purpose enhances both the manager's credibility and the effectiveness and morale of the work group.

Nurse managers today are challenged to manage with decreasing resources, to help design new systems of care, to supervise teams of professionals and non-professionals from a variety of cultures, and, finally, to teach personnel how to function well in the new system. This is no small task. It requires that nurses and their managers be committed, involved, enthusiastic, flexible, and innovative; above all else, it requires that they have good mental and physical health. Because the nurse manager of today is responsible for others' work, the nurse manager must also be a coach, a teacher, and a facilitator. The manager works through others to meet the goals of individuals, of the unit, and of the organization. Most of all, the manager must be a leader who can motivate and inspire.

Nurse managers must address the interests of both administrators and employees. Both want the same result—quality care. Administrators, however, must focus on cost and efficiency in order for the organization to compete and survive. Employees want to be supported in their work with adequate staffing, supplies, equipment, and, most of all, time. Therein lies the conflict. Between the two is the nurse manager, who must balance the needs of both. Being a nurse manager today is the most challenging opportunity in health care. This book is designed to prepare nurses to meet these challenges.

Summary

- Health care is radically changing today and is expected to continue to change in the foreseeable future.
- Health care structures have become integrated systems of care designed to maximize the organization's competitive advantage.
- To survive in a competitive environment, health care has adopted a market-based approach that includes a focus on customers, attention to cost, and quality improvement.
- Collaboration and cost-effectiveness are the keys to success for the health care organization now and in the future.
- Organizational restructuring and new models for delivery of nursing care are emerging as strategies to better manage resources.
- The nurse manager is an active participant and plays a key role in changing the organization and in implementing changes.

LEADERSHIP AND MANAGEMENT
in Action

1. How does today's health care system differ from the health care system of the recent past?
2. How has redesign, restructuring, and reengineering affected nursing?
3. Describe how cost-containment measures have affected health care in rural areas.
4. What effect does cultural diversity have on health care?

References

American Hospital Association (1994). *AHA Hospital Statistics*. Chicago: Author.

Balanced Budget Act of 1997, PL 105-33, Title IV.

Congressional Budget Office (February 12, 1997). *Testimony to the House Subcommittee on Health and the Environment.*

Covey, S. R. (1989). *The seven habits of highly effective people.* New York: Simon & Schuster.

Health Resources & Services Administration [HRSA](1999). Notes from the National Sample Survey of Registered Nurses 1996. http://158.72.83.3/bhpr/dn/survnote htmp accessed 6/20/2000.

Kerfoot, K. M. (1990). To manage by power or influence: The nurse manager's choice. *Nursing Economics, 8*(2), 117–119.

Kozier, B., Erb, G., & Blais, K. (1997). *Professional nursing practice concepts & perspectives,* 3rd ed. Menlo Park, CA: Addison-Wesley.

Leninger, M. M. (1991). *Culture care diversity and universality: A theory of nursing.* New York: National League for Nursing Press Publication 15-2402.

Malone, B. L. & Marullo, G. (1997). Workforce trends among U. S. Registered Nurses. A report for the International Council of Nurses (ICN) Workforce Forum. Stockholm, Sweden, http://www.ana.org/readroom/usworker.htm accessed June 20, 2000.

Riley, D. W. (1994). Integrated health care systems: Emerging models. *Nursing Economics, 12*(4), 201–206.

Shortell, S. M. (1993). Creating organized delivery systems: The barriers and facilitators. *Hospital & Health Services Administration, 38*(4), 46–47.

Sovie, M. D. (1995). Tailoring hospitals for managed care and integrated health systems. *Nursing Economics, 13*(2), 72–83.

U.S. Census Bureau (1993). *1990 census of population, social and economic characteristics.* Washington, DC: Government Printing Office.

Organizational Theory and Design

Organizational Theories

Classical Theory
Neoclassical Theory
Technological Theory
Systems Theory
Contingency Theory
Chaos Theory

Health Care Organizations

Types of Health Care Organizations
Interorganizational Relationships
Diversification

Organizational Structure

Functional Structure
Service-Integrated Structure
Hybrid Structure
Matrix Structure
Parallel Structure
Shared Governance
Self-Organizing Structures

Redesigning, Restructuring, and Reengineering

Strategic Planning

Values
Vision
Mission
Philosophy
Goals

Organizational Environment and Culture

Looking Ahead

Understanding the health care environment, a crucial element of management, begins with understanding organizational theory. These theories lay the foundation for the types of health care organizations in existence today. Hospitals, agencies, clinics, and other health care organizations are designed by integrating goals, size, technology, and environment. Chapter 2 outlines broad-based theories and discusses specific challenges nurses face in designing and implementing organizational structures.

Objectives

After reading this chapter, you will be able to:

- Compare and contrast organizational theories.
- Describe the different types of health care organizations.
- Discuss the various types of interorganizational relationships.
- Compare and contrast the different types of organizational structures.
- Discuss the advantages of shared governance.
- Explain how health care organizations are redesigning, restructuring, and reengineering.
- Describe the role of organizational environment and culture.

Within our society are numerous organizations—schools, churches, businesses, and so on. An **organization** is a collection of people working together under a defined structure for the purpose of achieving predetermined outcomes through the use of financial, human, and material resources. The justification for developing organizations is both rational and economic. Properly coordinated efforts capture more information and knowledge, purchase more technology, and produce more goods, services, opportunities, and securities than individual efforts (Anderson, 1992). This chapter discusses organizational theory, structures, and functions.

Organizational Theories

The earliest recorded example of organizational thinking comes from the ancient Sumerian civilization, around 5000 B.C. The early Egyptians, Babylonians, Greeks, and Romans also gave thought to how groups were organized. Later, Machiavelli in the 1500s and Adam Smith in 1776 established the management principles we know as specialization and division of labor (Cannon, 1925). Nevertheless, organizational theory remained largely unexplored until the Industrial Revolution. During the late 1800s and early 1900s, a number of approaches to the structure and management of organizations developed. These approaches, or schools of thought, are traditionally labeled classical theory, neoclassical theory, systems theory, contingency theory, and chaos theory.

Classical Theory

The *classical* approach to organizations focuses almost exclusively on the structure of the formal organization. The main premise is efficiency through design. People are seen as operating most productively within a rational and well-defined task or organizational design. Therefore, one designs an organization by subdividing work, specifying tasks to be done, and only then fitting people into the plan. Theorists who significantly contributed to this school of thought include Frederick Taylor, the founder of scientific management; Frank and Lillian Gilbreth; Henri Fayol; and Max Weber, the founder of organizational theory. Classical theory is built around four elements: division and specialization of labor, chain of command, organizational structure, and span of control.

Division and Specialization of Labor Dividing the work reduces the number of tasks that each employee

KEY TERMS

Organization A collection of people working together under a defined structure for the purpose of achieving predetermined outcomes.

Chain of command The hierarchy of authority and responsibility within the organization.

Line authority The linear hierarchy of supervisory responsibility and authority.

Staff authority The advisory relationship in which responsibility for actual work is assigned to others.

must carry out, thereby increasing efficiency and improving the organization's product. This concept lends itself to proficiency and specialization. Therefore, division of work and specialization are seen as economically beneficial. In addition, managers can standardize the work to be done, which in turn provides greater control.

Chain of Command The **chain of command** is the hierarchy of authority and responsibility within the organization. *Authority* is the right or power to direct activity, whereas *responsibility* is the obligation to attain objectives or perform certain functions. Both are derived from one's position within the organization and define accountability. The line of authority is such that higher levels of management delegate work to those below them in the organization.

There are two types of authority. Command or **line authority** is the linear hierarchy through which activity is directed. **Staff authority** is an advisory relationship; recommendations and advice are offered, but responsibility for the work is assigned to others. In Figure 2-1, the relationships among the chief nurse executive, nurse manager, and staff nurse are examples of line authority. The relationship between the clinical nurse specialist and the nurse manager illustrates staff authority. Neither the clinical nurse specialist nor the nurse manager is responsible for the work of the other; instead, they collaborate to improve the efficiency and productivity of the unit for which the nurse manager is responsible.

Organizational Structure Organizational structure describes the arrangement of the work group. It is a rational approach for designing an effective organization. Classical theorists developed the concept of *departmentation* as a means to maintain command and

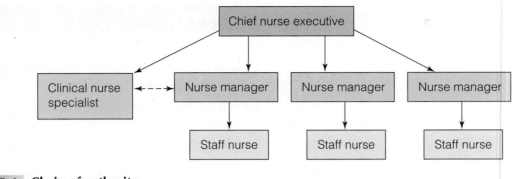

Figure 2-1   **Chain of authority.**

reinforce authority and provide a formal system for communication. The design of the organization is intended to foster the organization's survival and success. Characteristically, the structure takes shape as a set of differentiated but interrelated functions. Max Weber (1958) proposed the term **bureaucracy** to define the ideal, intentionally rational, most efficient form of organization. Today this word has a negative connotation, suggesting long waits, inefficiency, and red tape.

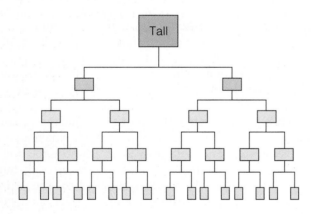

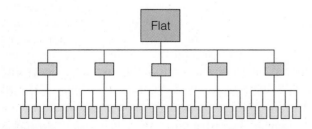

Figure 2-2   **Contrasting spans of control.** *Note: From* Managing health services organizations, *3rd ed. (p. 218) by J. S. Rakich, B. B. Longest, and K. Darr, 1992, Baltimore: Health Professions Press.*

Span of Control   **Span of control** is a concept related to organizational structure that addresses the pragmatic concern of how many employees a manager can effectively supervise. Complex organizations usually have numerous departments that are highly specialized and differentiated; authority is centralized, resulting in a *tall* organizational structure with many small work groups. Less complex organizations have *flat* structures; authority is decentralized, with several managers supervising large work groups. Figure 2-2 depicts the differences.

Using a classical perspective, Mintzberg (1989) described five organizational designs: simple structure, machine bureaucracy, professional bureaucracy, divisionalized form, and adhocracy. The designs differ in their executive-level management (strategic apex); the individuals responsible for doing the organizational work (operating core); the managers; individuals who help standardize and improve the work, such as accountants, inservice educators, and nurse recruiters (technostructure); and the support staff, individuals supporting others who provide the basic work, such as housekeepers and unit secretaries.

An organization with a *simple structure* design consists of only a strategic apex and an operating core. The private physician's office, in which the physician is the strategic apex and the staff are the operating core, is an example of a simple structure design.

The *machine bureaucracy* is representative of the bureaucracy described by Weber. A tall structure with centralized decision making and departmentalization is characteristic. Government-owned hospitals frequently are machine bureaucracies.

In the *professional bureaucracy*, the operating core of professionals is the dominant feature. Decision making is usually decentralized, and the technostructure is underdeveloped. The support staff, however, is well developed. Most hospitals are professional bureaucracies.

The *divisionalized form* is characterized by a number of independent divisions that are joined by a mutual administration. Decision making is decentralized; both technostructure and support staffs are minimal. A multiorganizational health system is an example of the divisionalized design.

Adhocracy represents a fluid structure in which management, staff, and experts work together on teams. Power, coordination, and control are constantly shifting. Health care organizations that use matrix structures exemplify this design. (Matrix structure is discussed later in this chapter.)

Neoclassical Theory

Criticism of classical theory led to the development of *neoclassical* or *humanistic theory*, an approach identified with the human relations movement of the 1930s. The neoclassical theorists had a common desire to humanize classical theory without totally rejecting the structural view. All recognized the need to design a rational organizational structure, but the neoclassicists proposed that it be done through cooperation and participation, tapping the motivation of the individual. A major assumption of this theory is that people desire social relationships, respond to group pressures, and search for personal fulfillment. This theory was developed as the result of a series of studies conducted by the Western Electric Company at their Hawthorne plant in Chicago. The first study was conducted to examine the effect of illumination on productivity. However, this study failed to find any relationship between the two. In most groups, productivity varied at random, while in one study productivity actually rose as illumination levels declined. The researchers concluded that unforeseen "psychological factors" were responsible for the findings. Further studies of working conditions, such as rest breaks and the length of the work week, still failed to reveal a relationship to productivity. The researchers concluded that the social setting created by the research itself—that is, the special attention given workers as part of the research—enhanced productivity. This tendency for people to perform as expected because of special attention became known as the **Hawthorne effect**. Although the findings are controversial, they led organizational theorists such as Maslow and McGregor to focus on the social aspects of work and organizational design. (See Chapter 19 for a description of their motivational theories.) One important assertion of this school of thought was that individuals cannot be coerced or bribed to do things they consider

unreasonable; formal authority does not work without willing participants (Barnard, 1938).

Systems Theory

Organizational theorists who maintain a systems perspective view productivity as a function of the interplay among structure, people, technology, and environment. Like nursing theories based on systems theory (such as those of Roy and Neuman), organizational theory defines *system* as a set of interrelated parts arranged in a unified whole (Robbins, 1983). Systems can be closed or open. Closed systems are self-contained and usually can be found only in the physical sciences. An open system, in contrast, interacts both internally and with its environment.

In organizational systems theory, an organization is defined as a complex, sociotechnical, open system. This theory provides a framework by which the interrelated parts of the system and their functions can be studied. According to Katz and Kahn (1978), resources, or **input**, such as employees, patients, materials, money, and equipment, are imported from the environment. Within the organization, energy and resources are utilized and transformed; work, a process called **throughput**, is performed to produce a product. The product, or **output**, is then exported to the environment. An organization, then, is a recurrent cycle of input, throughput, and output. Each health care organization—whether a hospital, outpatient clinic, home health care agency, and so on—requires human, financial, and material resources. Each also

---

KEY TERMS

Bureaucracy   A term proposed by Max Weber to define the ideal, intentionally rational, most efficient form of organization.

Span of control   The number of employees that can be effectively supervised by a single manager.

Hawthorne effect   The tendency for people to perform as expected because of special attention.

Input   Resources such as employees, patients, materials, money, and equipment.

Throughput   The work process to produce a product.

Output   The product of a work process.

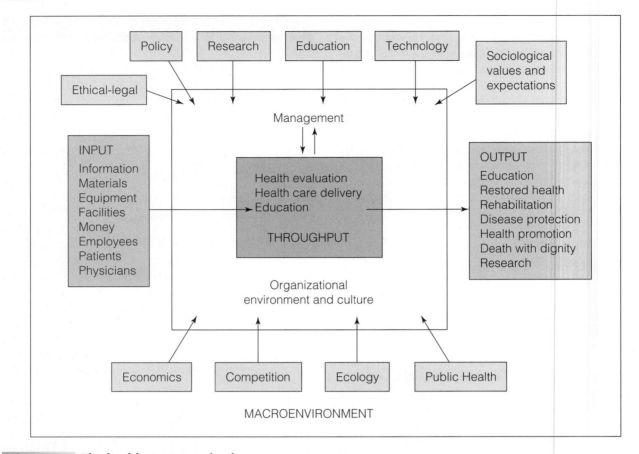

Figure 2-3 **The health care organization as an open system.**

provides a variety of services to treat illness, restore function, provide rehabilitation, and protect or promote wellness.

In this model, the manager is the catalyst for the input–throughput–output process. The manager is also the interface with the environment. Managers are responsible for integrating information and other stimuli from the environment, such as legislation or changes in health care delivery, to coordinate and facilitate the work of the organization. Figure 2-3 depicts a systems model of a health care organization.

Other systems theorists include March and Simon (1958), who view an organization as an information-processing network with many decision points for both individual members and the organization. Galbraith (1977) views the organization as a large communication system. He proposes a number of strategies for increasing capacity and decreasing uncertainty within the system. One such system is the *matrix organization*, which is discussed later in this chapter.

Systems theorists have provided great insight into important organizational and human variables. However, systems theory does not recognize the vast complexity of organizations or the interactive effects of many variables.

Contingency Theory

Contingency theorists believe organizational performance can be enhanced by matching an organization's structure to its environment. The *environment* is defined as the people, objects, and ideas outside the organization that influence the organization. The environment of a health care institution includes patients and potential patients; third-party payers, including managed-care companies; regulators; competitors; and suppliers of physical facilities, personnel (such as schools of nursing and medicine), equipment, and pharmaceuticals.

Health care organizations are unique with respect to the kinds of products and services they offer. However, like all other organizations, health care organizations are shaped by external and internal forces. These forces stem from the economic and social environment, the technologies used in patient care, organizational size, and the abilities and limitations of the personnel involved in the delivery of health care, including nurses, physicians, technicians, administrators, and, of course, patients.

Given the variety of health care services and patients served today, it should come as no surprise that organizations differ with respect to the environments they face, the levels of training and skills of their caregivers, and both the emotional and physical needs of patients. It is naive to think that the form of organization best for one type of patient in one type of environment is appropriate for another type of patient in a completely different environment. We would not expect to see the same staffing, rules and procedures, or chain of command in an inner-city substance abuse center as in a suburban women's health center. Thus, the optimal form of the organization is contingent on the circumstances faced by that organization.

Chaos Theory

The work of industrial theorists focused on linear cause-and-effect relationships. But as the proponents of chaos theory maintain, the universe is not an orderly place; instead, it is filled with chaos, unpredictability, and uncertainty (Kellert, 1994). This theory, which was inspired by the finding of quantum mechanics, challenges us to look at organizations and the nature of relationships and work from new perspectives. This theory challenges everything we know about organizations and how to manage them (Bergquist, 1993).

Chaos theory proposes that nature's work does not follow a straight line. The elements of nature often move in a circular, ebbing fashion; a stream destined for the ocean, for example, never takes a straight path. In fact, very little in life operates as a straight line; people's relationships to each other and to their work certainly do not. This notion challenges traditional thinking regarding the design of organizations. According to chaos theory, "Organizations are made up of intertwined links and diversified choices that generate unanticipated consequences." (Tetenbaum, 1998, p. 1.) Organizations are living, self-organizing systems, that are complex and self-adaptive (Tetenbaum, 1998).

The life cycle of an organization is fully dependent on its adaptability and response to changes in its environment. The tendency is for the organization to grow. When it becomes a large entity, it tends to stabilize and develop more formal standards. From that point, however, the organization tends to lose its

adaptability and responsiveness to its environment. Its new challenge is to avoid centralization, remain flexible, and redesign the structure to support the culture that provides the context for its purpose. The set of rules that guided the industrial notions of organizational function and integrity must be discarded, and newer principles that ensure flexibility, fluidity, speed of adaptability, and cultural sensitivity must emerge. Thus, the new definition of a system is a set of cyclic processes that are only temporarily manifested in stable structures that move between order and chaos as the demand on the system requires.

Chaos theory suggests that the drive to create permanent organizational structures is doomed to fail. The assumptions on which the work of the organization is built do not remain relevant. The role of leadership in these changing organizations is to build resilience in the midst of change, to maintain a balance between tension and order, which promotes creativity and prevents instability. Managers also are responsible for creating and maintaining a learning organization, one that tolerates conflict and supports experimentation, risk-taking, and trial-and-error modes of problem solving (Tetenbaum, 1998).

This theory requires us to abandon our attachment to any particular model of design and to reflect instead on creative and flexible formats that can be quickly adjusted and changed as the organization's realities shift. No one set of relationships is permanent or fundamental if it no longer sustains the organization and enables it to thrive (Drucker, 1994).

Health Care Organizations

Types of Health Care Organizations

The types of health care organizations in existence today vary from acute care hospitals to ambulatory care facilities to long-term care facilities. Today's health care organizations differ in ownership, role, activity, and size. Ownership can be either private or government, voluntary (not-for-profit) or investor-owned (for-profit), and sectarian or nonsectarian (Figure 2-4). Private organizations are usually owned by corporations or religious entities; whereas government organizations are operated by city, county, state or federal entities, such as the Indian Health Service. Voluntary organizations are usually not for profit, meaning that surplus monies are reinvested into the community. Investor-owned, or for-profit corporations, distribute surplus monies back to the investors,

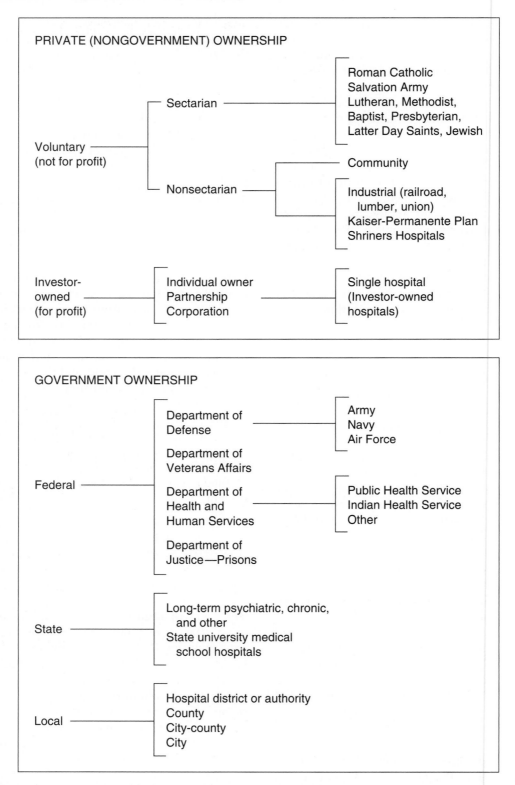

Figure 2-4 Types of ownership in health care organizations. *Note:* From *Managing health services organizations,* 3rd ed. (p. 263) by J. S. Rakich, B. B. Longest, and K. Darr, 1992, Baltimore: Health Professions Press.

who expect a profit. Sectarian agencies have religious affiliations.

Hospitals   Hospitals are frequently classified by length of stay and type of service. Most hospitals are acute (short-term or episodic) care facilities. The American Hospital Association (1995) defines an acute care hospital as a facility in which the average length of stay is less than 30 days; chronic or long-term hospitals are designed to care for patients whose average length of stay is longer than 30 days. In addition, hospitals may be classified as general or special care facilities, such as pediatric, rehabilitative, and psychiatric facilities. Many hospitals also serve as teaching institutions for nurses, physicians, and other health care professionals. The term *teaching hospital* commonly designates a hospital associated with a medical school that maintains a house staff of residents on call 24 hours a day. Nonteaching hospitals, in contrast, have only private physicians on staff. Because private physicians are less accessible than house staff, the medical supervision of patient care differs, as may the role of the nurse. This designation is changing dramatically as new forms of physician groups and allied practices emerge in partnerships with hospitals and medical schools. Some hospitals have adopted "hospitalists," physicians who provide care only to hospital inpatients.

Long-Term–Care Facilities   Long-term–care facilities provide skilled nursing or rehabilitative services. Currently two types of facilities, distinguished by the degree of nursing care provided, exist. *Nursing facilities* provide daily care; they may be free-standing or part of a hospital. *Residential care facilities* are sheltered environments in which no skilled care is provided.

Ambulatory Care Centers   A growing proportion of health care is delivered in ambulatory settings. Physician's offices, health maintenance organizations, emergency rooms, surgical centers, birthing centers, diagnostic imaging centers, and family planning clinics are just a few examples of the variety of ambulatory services available. Many hospitals offer both on- and off-campus outpatient sites to compete in this growing area of health care.

Home Health Care Agencies   Another growth area is in home health care. Home health care is the intermittent, temporary delivery of health care in the home by skilled or unskilled providers. With shortened lengths of hospital stay, more acutely ill patients are discharged to recuperate at home. Furthermore, more

---

KEY TERMS

Capitation   A fixed monthly fee for providing services to enrollees.

---

people are surviving life-threatening illnesses or trauma and require extended care. The primary service provided by home care agencies is nursing care; however, larger home care agencies also offer other professional services, such as physical or occupational therapy, and durable medical equipment, such as ventilators, hospital beds, home oxygen equipment, and other medical supplies.

Temporary Service Agencies   An outgrowth of the home health care industry is the temporary service agency. These agencies provide nurses and other health care workers to hospitals that are temporarily short-staffed; they also provide private duty nurses to individual patients.

Managed Health Care Organizations   The managed health care organization is the newest form of health care delivery. In this system, a group of providers is responsible for delivering services (that is, managing health care) through an organized arrangement with a group of individuals (for example, all employees of one company, all Medicaid patients in the state). Different types of managed care organizations exist: health maintenance organizations (HMOs), preferred provider organizations (PPOs), and point-of-service plans (POS). The HMO is a geographically organized system that provides an agreed-on package of health maintenance and treatment services. There are four different types of HMOs (ANA, 1997):

1. *Staff Model.* Physicians are HMO employees paid a salary.
2. *Independent Practice Association (IPA).* Physicians maintain individual or group practices, but contract with an HMO to serve enrollees for a negotiated fee.
3. *Group Model.* The HMO contracts with a multi-specialty group to provide enrollees' services for a negotiated fee.
4. *Network Model.* The HMO contracts with two or more IPAs, independent or group practices to provide enrollee services at a fixed monthly fee per enrollee, called **capitation**.

In a PPO, the managed care organization contracts with independent practitioners to provide enrollees

KEY TERMS

Horizontal integration   Arrangements between or among organizations that provide the same or similar services.

Vertical integration   An arrangement between or among dissimilar but related organizations to provide a continuum of services.

Diversification   The expansion of an organization into new arenas of service.

Joint venture   A partnership in which one partner finances and manages the venture, while the other provides a needed service.

with established discounted rates. If an enrollee obtains services from a nonparticipating provider significant copayments are usually required.

The POS is considered to be a HMO–PPO hybrid. In a POS, enrollees may use the network of managed care providers to go outside the network as they wish. However, use of a provider outside the network usually results in additional costs in copayments, deductibles, or premiums.

Interorganizational Relationships

With increased competition for resources and public and governmental pressures for better efficiency and effectiveness, organizations have been forced to establish relationships with one another for their continued survival. Multihospital systems and multiorganizational arrangements, both formal and informal, are mechanisms by which these relationships are forming. Arrangements between or among organizations that provide the same or similar services are examples of **horizontal integration**. For instance, Hospital X provides laundry services to Hospital Y, while Hospital Y provides dietary services to hospital X. **Vertical integration**, in contrast, is an arrangement between or among dissimilar but related organizations to provide a continuum of services. For example, an affiliation of a health maintenance organization with a hospital, pharmacy, and nursing facility represents vertical integration. Besides enhancing survival, vertical integration is thought to improve coordination of services, quality, cost effectiveness, efficiency, and bargaining power; promote continuity of care and improve

community service; expand services, which enhances competition; strengthen education and research opportunities; and use manpower more efficiently (Newhouse & Mills, 1999). Numerous arrangements using horizontal and vertical integration can be found. As health care becomes more unified, these models likely will become the common structure for delivery of health care. Some current arrangements include affiliations, consortia, alliances, mergers, and consolidations. Figure 2-5 illustrates these arrangements in greater detail.

A new form of integration is the virtual organization. A virtual organization is a time-delimited alliance of similar or dissimilar entities who agree to work together to achieve specific goals. VNA First is an example of such an alliance that was incorporated in 1987 to obtain managed-care contracts and develop critical pathways for home care (Craft & Spilotro, 1997).

Diversification

Diversification provides another strategy for survival in today's economy. **Diversification** is the expansion of an organization into new arenas. Two types of diversification are common: concentric and conglomerate.

Concentric diversification occurs when an organization complements its existing services by expanding into new markets or broadening the types of services it currently has available. For example, a children's hospital might open a day-care center for developmentally delayed children or offer drop-in facilities for sick child care.

Conglomerate diversification is the expansion into areas that differ from the original product or service. The purpose of conglomerate diversification is to obtain a source of income that will support the organization's product or service. For example, a long-term–care facility might develop real estate or purchase a company that produces durable medical equipment.

Another type of diversification common to health care is the joint venture. In a **joint venture**, one partner (general partner) finances and manages the venture, while the other partner (limited partner) provides a needed service. Joint ventures between health care organizations and physicians are becoming increasingly common. Integrated health care organizations, hospitals, and clinics seek physician and/or practitioner groups they can bond (capture) in order to obtain more referrals. The health care organization as financer and manager is the *general partner*, while physicians are *limited partners*.

PLURALISM

Informal affiliations	Joint undertaking without a written agreement
Formal affiliations	Formalized undertaking of limited activities
Shared or cooperative services	Common management; clinical service functions are used jointly or cooperatively by two or more organizations
Consortia and alliances	Limited voluntary associations for a specific purpose (e.g., management, consultants, purchasing)
Management contracts	One organization supplies senior management to another organization
Umbrella corporations	New corporation developed to span existing organizations
Mergers	One or more organizations dissolved and assumed by another organization that maintains its name and identity
Consolidations	One or more organizations dissolve and are unified into a new legal entity

FUSION

Figure 2-5 **Continuum of multiorganizational arrangements.** *Note:* **From** *Managing health services organizations,* **3rd ed. (pp. 361–362) by J. S. Rakich, B. B. Longest, and K. Darr, 1992, Baltimore: Health Professions Press.**

Organizational Structure

The optimal organizational structure integrates organizational goals, size, technology, and environment. When structure is not aligned with organizational needs, the organization's response to environmental change diminishes; decisions are delayed, overlooked, or poor; conflict results; and performance deteriorates (Porter-O'Grady, 1994). Organizational structure is an important tool through which managers can in-

crease organizational efficiency. Reorganization occurs in response to changes in organizational goals, size, technology, or environment.

Functional Structure

In *functional structures,* employees are grouped in departments by specialty, with similar tasks being performed by the same group, similar groups operating out of the same department, and similar departments reporting to the same manager (Figure 2-6). In a

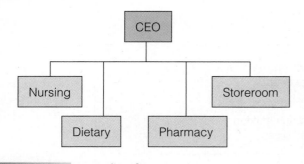

Figure 2-6 **Functional structure.**

functional structure, all nursing tasks fall under nursing service; the same is true of other functional areas. Functional structures tend to centralize decision making because the functions converge at the top of the organization.

Functional structures have several weaknesses. Coordination across functions is poor. Decision-making responsibilities can pile up at the top and overload senior managers, who may be uninformed regarding day-to-day operations. Responses to the external environment that require coordination across functions are slow. General management training is limited because most employees move up the organization within functional departments. Many health care organizations have a function-like structure.

Service-Integrated Structure

Service-integrated structures also are called *product-line* or *self-contained unit structures*. In a service-integrated structure, all functions needed to produce a product or service are grouped together in self-contained units (Figure 2-7). A large health care institution that acquires a smaller clinic may operate it as a self-contained unit. The service-integrated structure is decentralized; units are based on product, service, geographical location, or type of customer.

Integrated structures are preferred in large and complex organizations because the same activity (for example, hiring) is assigned to several self-contained units, which can respond rapidly to the unit's immediate needs. This is extremely appropriate when environmental uncertainty is high and the organization requires frequent adaptation and innovation.

One of the strengths of the service-integrated structure is its potential for rapid change in an unstable environment. Because each division is specialized and its outputs can be tailored to the situation, client satisfaction is high. Coordination across function (nursing, dietary, pharmacy, and so on) occurs easily; work partners identify with their own service and can compromise or collaborate with other service functions to meet service goals and reduce conflict. Service goals receive priority under this organizational structure because employees see

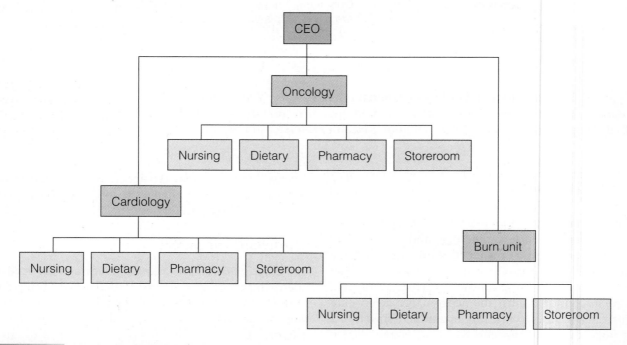

Figure 2-7 **Service-integrated structure.**

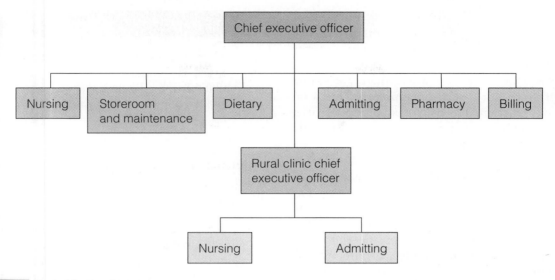

Hybrid structure.

the service outcomes as the primary purpose of their organization.

The major weaknesses of service-integrated structures include possible duplication of resources (such as ads for new positions) and lack of in-depth technical training and specialization. Coordination across service categories (oncology, cardiology, and the burn unit, for example) is difficult; services operate independently and often compete. Each service category, which is independent and autonomous, has separate and often duplicate staff and competes with other service areas for resources.

Hybrid Structure

When an organization grows, it typically organizes both self-contained units and functional units; the result is a hybrid organization (Figure 2-8). The strengths of the hybrid structure are that it (a) provides simultaneous coordination within product divisions while maintaining the quality of each function, (b) improves the alignment between corporate and service or product goals, and (c) fosters better adaptation to the environment while still maintaining efficiency.

The weakness of hybrid structures is conflict between top administration and managers. Managers often resent administrators' intrusions into what they see as their own area of responsibility. Over time, organizations tend to accumulate large corporate staffs to oversee divisions in an attempt to provide functional coordination across service or product structures.

Matrix Structure

The *matrix structure* is unique and complex (Figure 2-9); it integrates both product and functional structures into one overlapping structure. In a matrix structure, different managers are responsible for

Vice President outpatient services

	Oncology	Pediatrics	Family medicine
Vice President nursing services	Nurse manager	Nurse manager	Nurse manager

Matrix structure.

function and product. For example, the nurse manager for the oncology clinic may report to the vice president for nursing as well as the vice president for outpatient services.

Matrices tend to develop where there are strong outside pressures for a dual organizational focus on product and function. The matrix is appropriate in a highly uncertain environment that changes frequently but also requires organizational expertise.

A major weakness of the matrix structure is its dual authority, which can be frustrating and confusing for departmental managers and employees. Excellent interpersonal skills are required from the managers involved. A matrix organization is time-consuming because frequent meetings are required to resolve problems and conflicts; the structure will not work unless participants can see beyond their own functional area to the big organizational picture. Finally, if one side of the matrix is more closely aligned with organizational objectives, that side may become dominant.

Parallel Structure

Parallel structure is a structure unique to health care. It is the result of complex relationships that exist between the formal authority of the health care organization and the authority of its medical staff. In a parallel structure, the medical staff is separate and autonomous from the organization. The result is an organizational dilemma: two lines of authority. One line extends from the governing body to the chief executive officer and then to the managerial structure; the other line extends from the governing body to the medical staff. These two intersect in departments such as nursing, in which decision making involves both managerial and clinical elements. Parallel structures are found in health care institutions with a functional structure and separate medical governance structure (Figure 2-10). Parallel structures are becoming less successful as health care organizations integrate into newer models that incorporate physician practice under the organizational umbrella.

Shared Governance

A recent phenomenon in the structuring of nursing departments has evolved from the desire to build accountable decision making in hospitals, especially among the nursing staff. These innovations may simply take the form of participative decision making (which is discussed in Chapter 8) or more substantive systems known as **shared governance**. Shared

governance presents the values of interdependence and accountability as a basis for constructing a new organizational paradigm (Jenkins, 1991). Shared governance is based on a philosophy that nursing practice is best determined by nurses. It is a network of making nursing practice decisions in a decentralized environment. As a result, nurses gain significant control over their practice, efficiency and accountability are improved, and feelings of powerlessness are mitigated.

Over the past decade, more than 1000 hospitals in the United States have implemented a shared governance design for the nursing organization (Porter-O'Grady, 1992). Shared governance is by design and concept an invitational process. Because of its dynamic nature, it cannot be contained or owned in any exclusive framework and cannot be limited to any specific work group. If it is, it simply fails to maintain itself and eventually dissipates into parochialism, paternalism, and organizational isolation (Porter-O'Grady & Tornebini, 1993).

Shared governance allows staff nurses significant control over major decisions about nursing practice. These systems usually are built on a foundation of primary nursing, peer review, and some provision for clinical advancement. Most shared governance systems are similar to and reflect the principles often found in academic or medical governance models. For example, nurses may elect a council to represent the nursing staff collectively. Other councils may exist, such as a human resources council in charge of staffing levels, recruitment, and retention; a nursing council in charge of care standards, audit criteria, research, and staff education; and individual unit councils.

Some shared governance systems incorporate elected advisory boards for each service or clinical department. From these boards is elected a senate or congress that meets several times a year to decide larger policy issues.

The ultimate outcome of shared governance is that nurses participate in an accountable forum to control their own practice within the health care organization. The assumption is that nursing staffs, like medical staffs, will predetermine the clinical skills of staff

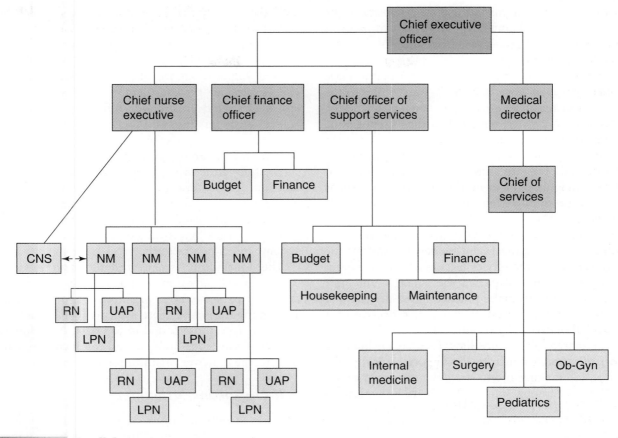

Parallel structure.

nurses and monitor the work of each through peer review while deciding on other practice issues through accountable forums or councils.

Such systems may improve efficiency as nurses take charge of their units, services, and practice and move away from relying on float pool or agency nurses to fill the gaps. When nurses control their own practice, patient care should improve. Many hospitals are examining such systems and weighing the costs and benefits. In a cost–benefit analysis conducted by Finkler and colleagues (1994), shared governance activities resulted in a more fiscally responsible and effective nursing organization. Nurse satisfaction and recruitment efforts improved, while personnel and unit costs decreased. Other researchers have noted similar findings (Jenkins, 1991; Lengacher, Kent, Mabe, Heinemann, VanCott, & Bowling, 1994; Ludeman & Brown, 1989). Jones, Stasiowski, Simons, Boyd, and Lucas (1993) noted that management styles became more consultative and job satisfaction improved, while turnover decreased. Such systems have been beneficial for nursing, allowing nurses to gain an

equal voice not only in nursing practice but also in health care.

Increasingly, shared governance principles integrate disciplines within newer service settings. As the continuum of care and the linkage of services become more important components of organizational design, shared governance provides a process and structure that supports decision making, quality imperatives, and collaboration among disciplines. Departmental and divisional structures are disappearing, and soon discipline-specific structures may give way to service configurations that address the continuum of care in a large health plan. Shared governance principles are increasingly being used as a framework for the models of structure that will integrate the organization's functions and structures.

The shared governance movement began purposefully with nursing. Major organizational transformation rarely succeeds if it exists only at the top of an organization or system (Drucker, 1992). Such change generally succeeds at the place closest to where the work gets done. In a service organization, that means that major change begins in the settings closest to the patient. Indeed, if the major purveyors of the organization's service, in this case nurses, are not fully invested in the change process, it doesn't matter where else it works (Drucker, 1993). Because of the large number of players and their varying proximity to the patient, it is reasonable to begin structural redesign with nurses and to create a milieu that supports the movement of such change to other parts of the patient care system. If successful, such movement is inevitable and essential. The literature is replete with information regarding its implementation and effectiveness as a process for empowering nurses (DeBaca, Jones, & Tornebini, 1993).

Much of this first-stage work in shared governance has focused on empowerment models for staff at the unit of service. At the service level in the organization, the expectation has been that the manager and staff collectively work to make practice-based decisions in the best interest of those they serve, reflective of a truly collaborative relationship. The second-stage efforts in shared governance have focused on building an organizational structure to support clinically driven decision making and to strengthen the partnership between and among staff and with the organization (McDonagh, 1991). Accountability has become a driving force for building structure to support practice and to involve staff actively in all decisions that affect their work.

The third stage of shared governance involves other service centers and disciplines related to the patient care functions in the health care system. Partners in care include all the professional and technical workers that operate within the patient care continuum. This group includes physicians, who have historically been viewed as working independently of the functional relationship of institutional providers. Because partnership is the driving theme of shared leadership and decision making, bringing the physician into the partnership creates the essential relationship necessary to initiate effective service arrangements, evaluate care, and build effective supporting structures (Goldsmith, 1993).

Integrative care models and multidisciplinary team approaches to care further facilitate the demand for an organizational structure more supportive of team members than that which is currently available in the more traditional hospital hierarchies. Creating more collateral structures that reflect the relationship of the players to each other acts more clearly in concert with interdisciplinary work than do more traditional structures (Peters, 1992).

These new shared governance models, which link nurses to the whole system in a much stronger partner orientation, are just beginning to take form as more partnered and integrated health care systems emerge. Implications for altering service, operations, and governance are considerable. The fact that principles of shared governance reflecting partnership, equity, accountability, and ownership form the basis for these newer approaches indicates the strong foundations that shared governance has established in successfully structuring an empowered nursing organization. It is natural to assume that these processes would expand as the health system moves to point-of-service design and constructs the empowerment processes necessary to make these more integrated systems function effectively.

The continuum of care and the structures that support it will have a major impact on nurses and the design of patient service organizations of the future. The configuration of these systems will be radically different from those found in the past. New foundations for knowledge-building and conducting research will emerge as newer organizational forms take shape.

Self-Organizing Structures

Wheatly (1992) describes a new adaptive organizational structure that evolves from organizational tasks. This self-organizing (self-renewing) structure is flexible and able to respond to both internal and external change. The only requirement of this structure is *self-reference*; that is, future structures are consistent with the previously established identity and its past. Rigid, permanent structures are avoided; the organizational structure changes when the need arises. Roles and structures are created out of need and interest; relationships, exchanges, and connections among employees are nurtured as the primary source of organizational creativity and success.

Redesigning, Restructuring, and Reengineering

To reduce the cost of delivering health care and maintain market positions, jobs are being redesigned, organizations restructured, and systems reengineered. In a study reported by Gellinas & Manthey (1997), 85 percent of health care organizations are involved in system redesign. In **redesign**, the distribution of activities, role overlap, excess specialization, and waste are examined. The goal is to design each job according to

KEY TERMS

Redesign   A technique that examines the tasks within each job with the goal of combining appropriate tasks to improve efficiency.

appropriate tasks and necessary qualifications and to have all jobs fit together so that the organization's work gets done in the most efficient and effective manner. Redesign usually focuses on the individual jobs in one clinical specialty area, although each area may be undergoing job redesign simultaneously or consecutively. (See job analysis in Chapter 17.)

Job redesign is intended to provide a high degree of internal motivation, leading to greater job satisfaction, higher-quality work, lower absenteeism, and less turnover (Hackman & Oldham, 1980). Job redesign attains these results by enabling staff to experience (a) greater meaningfulness in their work, (b) a sense of responsibility for the results of their work, and (c) feedback regarding the effectiveness of their work. However, many efforts at job redesign have resulted only in job enlargement—more work rather than better work, or work that entails greater responsibility and a higher level or different kinds of professional skills. Because professionals often have intrinsic needs to advance professionally, simply giving them more work does little to satisfy their needs, encourage job performance, or provide motivation. In many cases, it has the opposite effect, leading to resistance, job dissatisfaction, and minimal motivation.

Currently, job redesign is focused on using staff efficiently as downsizing and restructuring efforts continue (e.g., shared governance, differentiated practice). In the process, it is important that staff experience meaningful work, assume responsibility, and receive effective feedback.

Barriers to Job Redesign   The nurse manager should be aware of some common problems in the redesign of jobs. For example, the nurse manager's role may change from leader and director of unit staff to that of coordinator of staff activities. Somehow, the notion of coordinator seems inconsistent with our cultural stereotypes of leadership. We usually think of a leader as the person in charge, or the boss. That stereotype of leadership tends to include the unilateral and unquestioned use of power with objectives, strategies, and evaluation defined strictly from the leader's perspective.

A number of factors other than the power afforded by virtue of job title and reporting relationships are involved in effective leadership. Effective leadership is accepted leadership, and there are many ways to foster acceptance of the nurse manager's legitimate organizational power (see Chapter 4). The strategies and techniques described in this chapter are tools meant to help in achieving both individual and unit effectiveness through the management of staff motivation. If effectiveness means being a coordinator as opposed to being the boss, then the strategies and techniques involved in carrying out that role are what the nurse manager should use.

Another barrier to job redesign is that the values implicit in job redesign may be at odds with those of the organization's administration. The notion of providing autonomy, feedback, greater responsibility, and self-direction in the performance of jobs may not be in tune with the philosophy and history of the organizational hierarchy—matters that are not under the nurse manager's immediate discretion or control. However, different management areas afford different degrees of responsibility, and there may be a good deal of flexibility within the limits of the organization's rules, especially with the flux in today's environment. Job redesign is just another tool to use within the limits of the situation at hand.

In some cases, staff members are reluctant to engage in job redesign or other motivational efforts because they fear that increased productivity may have implications for their job security. They are concerned that if productivity increases sufficiently, some people may lose their jobs because they are no longer needed to accomplish the work. Increased productivity, however, not only eases the workload but also, if properly managed (for example, rewarded), is likely to result in greater satisfaction and organizational commitment as well as less absenteeism and turnover. Also, fears regarding job security usually focus solely on the quantity of work and ignore the quality of work as a separate, but equally important, dimension. Effective motivation of staff members involves both of these dimensions, but job enrichment most consistently increases job satisfaction and work quality rather than the quantity of work produced.

The fourth major barrier to job redesign is that not everyone desires change or growth in his or her job. Some people prefer to have their work clearly prescribed, unvarying in its content or procedure, and highly predictable from day to day. Job redesign is appropriate only for staff members whose jobs are too highly structured to suit their needs.

Still another major barrier to job redesign is the lack of exact specifications of what is to be accomplished by redesigning an individual's job. For that reason, organizations may restructure and reengineer systems.

Restructuring and Reengineering Job redesign focuses on individual jobs; restructuring and reengineering examine the entire health organization's structure with a goal of improving the organization's functioning and productivity (Greenberg, 1994). **Restructure** means to change the structure of the organization. The administrative structure changes, as do reporting relationships and communication channels. Restructuring naturally follows organizational affiliations, mergers, and the establishment of integrated health care systems as efforts to reduce duplication among the network's various entities ensue. In restructuring, coordination of work effort is stressed and interdependence valued. Organizationally based models, such as case management, total quality management, and product-line management, are used in system reorganization.

Another type of restructuring is downsizing. **Downsizing** or *right-sizing* simply means cutting the number of staff positions. The workload may or may not be the same as it was before the cuts; most often the degree of downsizing depends on the number of patients in the system, the care they need, and the mix of staff skills. With today's reduced hospital occupancy, cutting staff makes economic sense. For nurses, who are used to being always in demand, hospital downsizing is especially threatening.

Downsizing without job redesign encourages self-promotion, reduces trust, destroys morale, and consumes inordinate amounts of the time and energy of the staff and management. Mortality and malpractice exposure may increase. The organization operates in a continuous crisis mode, with those most affected assuming a bunker mentality in an attempt to protect their own turf. Although cost containment is the im-

petus for downsizing, the acuity of today's hospitalized patients makes downsizing imprudent. Similarly, reducing the number and qualifications of staff in outpatient settings may contribute to increased complications and concomitant higher costs.

Reengineering involves examining and improving the process by which health care is delivered. Reengineering is collaborative, data-driven, and patient-focused. Reengineering usually involves the entire organization and results in major change to both the organization and its members.

Reengineering is very complex and often radical. A new approach to the organization of patient care is adopted. Nurses, physicians, and other health care professionals develop different teams and the use of patient outcomes are integral parts of restructuring and reengineering. Working in collaborative teams and using a multidisciplinary approach requires open communication, the ability to accept and give criticism, clarity about responsibilities, and accountability by all. Adopting these behaviors is challenging and stressful, and some individuals resist it. The challenge for nurse managers is to help staff members understand the ultimate goal, participate in the process, and use their professional expertise to contribute to the well-being of the organization's patients, both now and in the future.

Restructuring and reengineering also may be used in system redesign. Common themes in system redesign are integration/coordination across department lines; critical path/protocol development; management restructuring; multiskilled worker development; implementation of patient-focused care and case management (Gellinas & Manthey, 1997).

Nurse managers are key players in the redesign efforts. Not only are they expected to initiate change while reducing costs, maintaining or improving quality of care, coaching and mentoring, and team building, but they are to do so in an ever changing environment full of ambiguities while their own responsibilities are expanded (Gellinas & Manthey, 1997).

Strategic Planning

Successful organizations, both for-profit and not-for-profit, have learned that they must focus their resources on a limited number of activities. Trying to be all things to all people only results in a dissipation of resources and ineffective outcomes in many areas. Health care organizations were slow to adopt such a focused approach, but cost constraints have forced them to reexamine their mission, vision, and goals. Comprehensive strategic planning, often using outside consultants, can produce a plan to guide the organization in the near future. **Strategic planning** is long-range planning by the organization for a 3- to 5-year period into the future. Strategic planning guides the direction the organization is to take. It is based on the values, philosophy, and mission of the organization and the vision of its leaders.

Values

Values are the beliefs or attitudes one has about people, ideas, objects or actions that form a basis for behavior (Kozier, Erb, & Blais, 1997). Organizations use **value statements** to identify those beliefs or attitudes esteemed by the organizational leaders.

Vision

A **vision statement** describes the goal to which the organization aspires. The vision statement is designed to inspire and motivate employees to achieve a desired state of affairs. "Our vision is to be a regional integrated healthcare delivery system providing premier healthcare services, professional and community education, and healthcare research," is a vision statement from the BJC Health System in St. Louis.

Mission

The **mission** of an organization is a broad, general statement of the organization's reason for existence. Developing the mission is the necessary first step to designing a strategic plan. "Our mission is to improve the health of the people and communities we serve," from BJC Health System in St. Louis, is an example of a mission statement that guides decision making for the organization. If, for example, a proposed activity does not promote the organization's stated mission, it probably would not be pursued. Purchasing a medical equipment company, for example, might not be considered an activity that helps meet the mission of improving the community's health.

Philosophy

The **philosophy** is a written statement that reflects the organizational values, vision, and mission.

Goals

Goals are specific statements of what is to be achieved. They follow the mission and vision of the organization. Goals are measurable and precise. "Every patient

KEY TERMS

Strategic planning   Long-range planning for the future.

Value statements   Statements about an organization's beliefs or attitudes.

Vision statement   A description of the goal to which an organization aspires.

Mission   A general statement of the purpose of an organization.

Philosophy   The mission, values, and vision of an organization.

Goals   Specific statements of achievement that provide direction.

Objectives   Statements of achievement specific to abilities within the organization.

Strategies   Actions by which objectives are to be achieved.

Organizational climate   The perceived characteristics of an organization.

will be satisfied with his or her care" is an example of a goal. Goals apply to the entire organization, whereas **objectives** are specific to an individual unit. A nursing objective to meet the above goal might be "Provide appropriate information and education to patients from pre-admission to discharge." **Strategies** follow objectives and specify what actions will be taken. "Implement patient education classes for prenatal patients" is an example of a strategy to meet the patient satisfaction objective.

Other categories often included in a strategic plan include the personnel responsible for each activity, the projected cost, criteria to establish that the goal has been met, expected date of completion, and the current status. Strategic planning is an ongoing process, not an end in itself. It requires a continual focus on the goal and meticulous attention to progress; the organization's mission and vision must always guide activities.

Organizational Environment and Culture

The environment within an organization can be defined in terms of its climate and culture. **Organizational climate** is the perceived characteristics of the organization — its physical attributes, organizational

KEY TERMS

Organizational culture   The norms and traditions within an organization.

structure, lines of communication, policies and procedures. For example, some aspects of an organization's climate are its benefits offered, staffing ratios, the location of employee parking, and the layout of the nursing unit. **Organizational culture**, however, is the norms and traditions maintained. Organizational culture affects the practices and procedures of the organization. For example, are uniforms or scrubs worn? When is report given? To whom? Is tardiness tolerated? How late is acceptable?

Like climate, organizational culture varies from one institution to the next and subcultures and countercultures may exist. A *subculture* is a group that has shared experiences or like interests and values. Nurses form a subculture within health care environments. They share a common language, rules, rituals, and dress (Suominen, Kovasin, & Ketola, 1997). Individual units also can become subcultures. *Countercultures* usually maintain beliefs and values that contradict those of the dominant culture. For example, nurses who abuse drugs might be part of a counterculture.

Besides organizational cultures differing between institutions, culture may differ between the organization and its subculture. If the subculture's norms and traditions are in agreement with the organization's, then *consonance* occurs, if not, *dissonance* occurs (Fleeger, 1993).

Cooke and Lafferty (1989) have identified three types of culture: (a) constructive or positive, where the focus is on self-actualization, humanism, affiliation, and achievement; (b) passive or defensive, where the focus is on approval, dependence, convention, and avoidance; and (c) aggressive or defensive, where the focus is on competition, perfectionism, power, and opposition.

The presence of a constructive culture promotes employee retention and decreases patient mortality (McDaniel & Stumpf, 1993). Similarly, Shortell and colleagues (1991) found a correlation between a constructive or positive work culture in the intensive care unit and a decrease in mortality for acutely ill patients. The classic magnet hospital study in the early 1980s indicated an increased ability to recruit and retain nurses, an increased level of work satisfaction for nurses, and an increased level of patient satisfaction in

hospitals that were categorized as having an "excellent culture" (McClure, Poulin, Sovie, & Wandelt, 1983).

Managers are considered to be a major factor in determining organizational culture. In fact, when a change in management occurs, the culture on the unit also changes. Schneider (1994) has described four types of culture that reflect a manager's style. The authoritarian creates a culture of *control*. Workers are systematic, task-driven, and conservative. The manager who comes as a coach and team leader creates a *collaborative* culture that is democratic, collegial, supportive, and trusting. The visionary manager who challenges his or her workers to grow creates a culture of *competence* and the workers are task-driven and efficient. The manager who inspires and motivates creates a culture of *cultivation* in which the workers are people-oriented and nurturing.

One way to assess the organizational environment or culture is to evaluate the hiring preferences for key positions in the organization. An organization in which nursing leaders are innovative, creative, and energetic will tend to operate in a fast-moving, goal-oriented fashion. If humanistic, interpersonal skills are sought in candidates for leadership positions, the organization will focus on human resources, employees, and patient advocacy (Hersey & Blanchard, 1988).

Organizations that require decision-making ability and empower nurses to participate in determining their practice environment will retain nurses who desire a substantial degree of autonomy. Systems involving participatory management and shared governance create organizational climates that reward decision making, creativity, independence, and autonomy. These organizations retain and recruit independent, accountable professionals. In addition, in response to consumer demands for fast attention to concerns and questions, organizations that empower nurses to make decisions will better meet consumer requests. As the health care environment continues to evolve, more and more organizations are adopting consumer-sensitive cultures that require accountability and decision making from nurses.

Summary

- In order to survive, organizations change resources (people, capital, supplies) into services.
- Many factors influence a health care organization's performance: patients, suppliers, competitors, governmental regulatory bodies, physicians, third-party payers, and the labor market.

- Organizations can be viewed as social systems consisting of people working in a predetermined pattern of relationships who strive toward a goal. The goal of health care organizations is to provide a particular mix of health services.

- The schools of organizational theory are classical theory, neoclassical theory, technological theory, systems theory, contingency theory, and chaos theory.

- The organizational structure determines the formal communication system and guides organizational activities. This structure can be either horizontal or vertical.

- Common types of departmentalization found in organizations are functional, service-integrated, hybrid, matrix, parallel, and self-organizing structures.

- There are many different types of health care organizations: acute care, long-term care, ambulatory or community care, home health care, and temporary services. They may be private or public, for-profit or not-for-profit.

- Concepts of shared governance provide the framework for empowerment and partnership and are leading nursing organizations into stronger partnerships with other disciplines and with the health care organization.

- Organizations develop strategic plans based on the values, philosophy, and mission of the organization and the vision of its leaders.

- Organizational climate and culture define the environment of the organization.

■ LEADERSHIP AND MANAGEMENT
in Action

1. List the advantages and disadvantages of the different types of organizational structures.

2. How do inputs, throughputs, and outputs differ among the various types of health care organizations?

3. How does organizational environment and culture affect the organization? How has shared governance affected organizational environment?

References

American Hospital Association (1995). *AHA guide to the health care field* (1995–1996 ed.). Chicago: Author.

American Nurses Association (1997). *Managed care: Challenges and opportunities for nursing*. Washington, DC: Author.

Anderson, H. (1992). Hospitals seek new ways to integrate health care. *Hospital & Health Networks, 66*(7), 26–36.

Barnard, C. I. (1938). *The functions of the executive*. Cambridge, MA: Harvard University Press.

Bergquist, W. (1993). *The postmodern organization: Mastering the art of irreversible change*. San Francisco: Jossey-Bass.

Cannon, E. (Ed.). (1925). *Adam Smith, an inquiry into the nature and causes of the wealth of nations*, 4th ed. London: Methuen. Originally published in 1776.

Cooke, R. A., & Lafferty, J. L. (1989). *Organizational culture inventory*. Plymouth, MI: Human Synergistics.

Craft, J. S., & Spilotro, S. L. (1997). Integration for the future: Forming a virtual organization. *Journal of Nursing Administration, 27*(4), 3, 20.

DeBaca, V., Jones, K., & Tornebini, J. (1993). A cost-benefit analysis of shared governance. *Journal of Nursing Administration, 23*(7/8), 50–57.

Drucker, P. (1992). *Managing for the future: The 1990's and beyond*. New York: Truman Tally Books/Dutton.

Drucker, P. (1993). *Post-capitalist society*. New York: HarperCollins.

Drucker, P. (1994). The theory of the business. *Harvard Business Review, 72*(5), 95–104.

Finkler, S. A., Kovner, C. T., Knickman, J. R., & Hendrickson, G. (1994). Innovation in nursing: A benefit/cost analysis. *Nursing Economics, 12*(1), 18–27.

Fleeger, M. E. (1993). Assessing organizational culture: A planning strategy. *Nursing Management, 24*(2), 39–41.

Galbraith, J. R. (1977). *Organizational design*. Reading, MA: Addison-Wesley.

Gellinas, L. S., & Manthey, M. (1997). The impact of organizational redesign on nurse executive leadership. *Journal of Nursing Administration, 27*(10), 35–42.

Goldsmith, J. (1993). Driving the nitroglycerin truck: The relationship between the hospital and physician. *Healthcare Forum Journal, 36*(2), 36–40.

Greenberg, L. (1994). Work redesign: An overview. *Journal of Emergency Nursing, 20*(3), 28a–32a.

Hackman, J. R., & Oldham, G. R. (1980). *Work design*. Reading, MA: Addison-Wesley.

Hersey, P., & Blanchard, P. (1988). *Management of organizational behavior: Utilizing human resources*, 5th ed. Englewood Cliffs, NJ: Prentice Hall.

Jenkins, J. (1991). Professional governance: The missing link. *Nursing Management, 22*(8), 26–30.

Jones, C. B., Stasiowski, S., Simons, B. J., Boyd, N. J., & Lucas, M. D. (1993). Shared governance and the nursing practice environment. *Nursing Economics, 11*(4), 208–214.

Katz, D., & Kahn, R. (1978). *The social psychology of organizations*. New York: Wiley.

Kellert, S. (1994). *In the wake of chaos.* Chicago: University of Chicago Press.

Kozier, B., Erb, G. & Blais, K. (1997). *Professional nursing practice: Concepts & perspectives.* Menlo Park, CA: Addison-Wesley.

Lengacher, C. A., Kent, K., Mabe, P. R., Heinemann, D., VanCott, M. L., & Bowling, C. D. (1994). Effects of the partners in care practice model on nursing outcomes. *Nursing Economics, 12*(6), 300–308.

Ludeman, R. S., & Brown, C. (1989). Staff perceptions of shared governance. *Nursing Administration Quarterly, 1*(4), 49–56.

March, J. G., & Simon, H. (1958). *Organizations.* New York: Wiley.

McClure, M. L., Poulin, M. A., Sovie, M. D., & Wandelt, M. A. (1983). *Magnet hospitals: Attention and retention of professional nurses.* Kansas City, MO: American Nurses Association.

McDaniel, C., & Stumpf, L. (1993). The organizational culture. *Journal of Nursing Administration, 23*(4), 54–60.

McDonagh, K. (1991). *Nursing shared governance.* Atlanta: K. J. McDonagh Associates.

Mintzberg, H. (1989). *Mintzberg on management: Inside our strange world of organizations.* New York: Free Press.

Newhouse, R. P., & Mills, M. E. (1999). Vertical systems integration. *Journal of Nursing Administration, 29*(10), 22–29.

Peters, T. (1992). *Liberation management.* New York: Harper & Row.

Porter-O'Grady, T. (1992). *Implementing shared governance.* St. Louis: Mosby.

Porter-O'Grady, T. (1994). Re-engineering the nursing profession. *Aspen's Advisor for the Nurse Executive, 9*(7), 7–8.

Porter-O'Grady, T., & Tornebini, J. (1993). Outcomes of shared governance: Impact on the organization. *Seminars for Nurse Managers, 1*(2), 63–73.

Rakich, J. S., Longest, B. B., & Darr, K. (1992). *Managing health services organizations,* 3rd ed. Baltimore: Health Professions Press.

Robbins, S. P. (1983). *Organizational theory.* Englewood Cliffs, NJ: Prentice-Hall.

Schneider, W. E. (1994). *The reengineering alternative: A plan for making your current culture work.* Burr Ridge, IL: Irwin.

Shortell, S., Rousseau, D., Gillies, R., Devers, K. J., & Simons, T. L. (1991). Organizational assessment in intensive care units (ICUs): Construction, development, reliability and validity of the ICU nurse-physician questionnaire. *Medical Care, 29*(8), 709–726.

Suominen, T., Kovesin, M., & Ketola, O. (1997). Nursing culture—some viewpoints. *Journal of Advanced Nursing, 25*(2), 186–190.

Tetenbaum, T. J. (1998). Shifting paradigims: From Newton to chaos. *Organizational Dynamics, 26*(4), 21–32.

Weber, M. (1958). *From Max Weber: Essays in sociology.* H. Gerth & C. W. Mills (Eds.). New York: Oxford University Press.

Wheatly, M. J. (1992). *Leadership and the new science: Learning about organization from an orderly universe.* San Francisco: Berrett-Koehler.

Woodward, J. (1965). *Industrial organization: Theory and practice.* London: Oxford University Press.

CHAPTER 3

Nursing Care Delivery Systems

Types of Nursing Care Delivery Systems

> Functional Nursing
> Team Nursing
> Total Patient Care
> Primary Nursing
> Practice Partnerships
> Case Management
> Differentiated Practice
> Patient-Centered Care

Looking Ahead

Previous chapters have focused on understanding the environment in which nurses work, from the fundamental infrastructure of organizations to the effects of changes in health care on the roles of nurses and nurse managers. This chapter focuses on the way nursing care is delivered. Different types of nursing care delivery systems exist to provide structure to nursing care delivery. As the health care industry changes and restructuring occurs, nurses face the challenge of modifying existing methods to use fewer resources effectively.

Objectives

After reading this chapter, you will be able to:

- Compare and contrast the different types of nursing care delivery systems.

One of the significant issues challenging nursing is the way in which nursing care is delivered. An American Nurses Association survey indicates that the top three concerns of staff nurses are their ability to (a) provide quality patient care, (b) act in patients' best interests, and (c) be treated as professionals (Yeast, 1991). The essence of providing nursing care that meets these concerns revolves around the work environment and culture, the type of nursing care delivery system, and staffing and scheduling practices, especially as they relate to the results of workload calculations from patient classification systems. Pressures from many sources, all centered on an overall expectation to reduce the cost of care, enhance efficiency, and maintain quality, affect the organization of nursing care. This chapter describes how nursing care is organized to ensure quality care in an era of cost containment.

Types of Nursing Care Delivery Systems

The purpose of a nursing care delivery system is to provide a structure that enables nurses to deliver nursing care to a specified group of patients. The delivery of care includes assessing care needs, formulating a plan of care, implementing the plan, and evaluating the patient's responses to interventions.

Since World War II, nursing care delivery systems have undergone continuous and significant changes (Box 3-1). Over the years, various nursing care delivery systems have been critiqued. Debates regarding the pros and cons of each method have focused on identifying the perfect delivery system for providing nursing care to patients with varying needs of intensity of care. This ongoing evaluation has been spurred by changes in availability of nursing personnel, reductions in reimbursement for patient care and hospital revenue, changes in acuity levels of patients, shorter lengths of stay, demands by health care consumers for quality care at a reduced rate, and demands by nurses, physicians, and other health care professionals for more effective delivery systems. The major challenges of any nursing care delivery system include effectiveness, cost efficiency, quality, and the needs of consumers and practitioners.

No delivery system is perfect. Most organizations use a combination or modification of various nursing care delivery systems to meet the unique demands of different patient care units. The American Hospital Association (1991) surveyed hospitals in the United States to identify the types of nursing care delivery systems being used and the percentage of hospitals using each type of system. Team nursing was the most frequently used system, followed by total patient care and primary nursing (Table 3-1). Before adopting any

Box 3-1   Job Description of a Floor Nurse (1887)

Developed in 1887 and published in a magazine of Cleveland Lutheran Hospital.

In addition to caring for your 50 patients, each nurse will follow these regulations:

1. Daily sweep and mop the floors of your ward, dust the patients' furniture and window sills.
2. Maintain an even temperature in your ward by bringing in a scuttle of coal for the day's business.
3. Light is important to observe the patient's condition. Therefore, each day fill kerosene lamps, clean chimneys, and trim wicks. Wash windows once a week.
4. The nurse's notes are important to aiding the physician's work. Make your pens carefully. You may whittle nibs to your individual taste.
5. Each Nurse on day duty will report every day at 7 A.M. and leave at 8 P.M., except on the Sabbath, on which you will be off from 12 noon to 2 P.M.

6. Graduate Nurses in good standing with the Director of Nurses will be given an evening off each week for courting purposes, or two evenings a week if you go regularly to church.
7. Each nurse should lay aside from each pay a goodly sum of her earnings for her benefits during her declining years, so that she will not become a burden. For example, if you earn $30 a month you should set aside $15.
8. Any nurse who smokes, uses liquor in any form, gets her hair done at a beauty shop, or frequents dance halls will give the Director of Nurses good reason to suspect her worth, intentions, and integrity.
9. The nurse who performs her labor, serves her patients and doctors faithfully and without fault for a period of five years will be given an increase by the hospital administration of five cents a day providing there are no hospital debts that are outstanding.

| Table 3-1 | Nursing Care Delivery Systems Utilization—1991 |

Systems	Percentage
Team	39.9
Total patient care	22.8
Primary	14.4
Modular	10.6
Functional	4.9
Case management	2.5
Other	4.9

Note: From *AHA Hospital Nursing Personnel Surveys* by the American Hospital Association, 1991, Chicago: Author.

KEY TERMS

Functional nursing   A nursing care delivery system in which the needs of patients are broken down into tasks and assigned to caregivers.

Team nursing   The most common delivery system; nursing staff are divided into teams, which are responsible for the care of a group of patients.

nursing care delivery system, the nursing organization must consider its goals, characteristics, needs, and the demands placed on it and the cost of the nursing care delivery system.

Functional Nursing

Functional nursing, also called *task nursing* (Figure 3-1), began in hospitals in the mid-1940s in response to a national nursing shortage. The number of registered nurses serving in the armed forces during World War II depleted the supply of nurses at home. As a result of this loss of RNs, the composition of nursing staffs in hospitals changed; staffs composed almost entirely of RNs gave way to widespread use of LPNs and unlicensed assistive personnel (UAPs) to deliver nursing care.

In functional nursing, the needs of a group of patients are broken down into tasks. Tasks are assigned to RNs, LPNs, or UAPs so that the skill and licensure

of each caregiver is used to the best advantage. An RN assesses patients, while others give baths, make beds, take vital signs, administer treatments, and so forth.

The advantage of this system is that all employees, even UAPs, become very efficient and effective at performing their regular assigned tasks. However, these personnel are likely to be less effective and efficient if assigned to another task. Other disadvantages of functional nursing include (a) uneven continuity of care, (b) absence of a holistic view of the patient, (c) time-consuming communications, and (d) problems with follow-up. Today, functional nursing care is used infrequently in acute care facilities and only occasionally in long-term–care facilities.

Team Nursing

Team nursing (Figure 3-2) remains the most common nursing care delivery system in the United States in acute as well as long-term–care settings. Historically, team nursing evolved from functional nursing and has remained popular since the mid- to late 1940s. Under this system, a team of nursing personnel provides total patient care to a group of patients. In some instances, a team may be assigned a certain number of

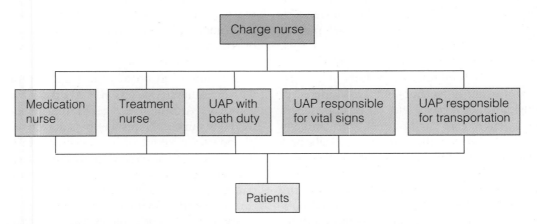

Figure 3-1 **Functional nursing.**

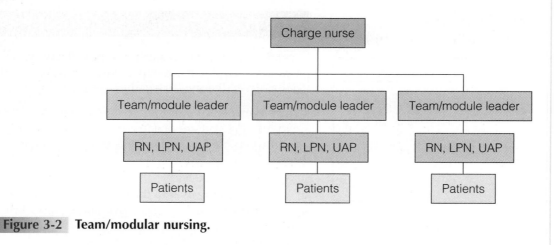

Figure 3-2   **Team/modular nursing.**

patients; in others, the assigned patients may be grouped by diagnoses or provider services.

Modular nursing is a modification of team nursing that tries to enhance the effectiveness of the team concept by assigning a module that is confined to a limited geographic area. The size of the module varies according to physical layout of the unit, patient acuity, and nursing skill mix (Magargal, 1987). The team or module is led by an RN and may include other RNs, LPNs, and UAPs. Team members provide patient care under the direction of the team (module) leader. The team, acting as a unified whole, has a holistic perspective of the needs of each patient. The team speaks for each patient through the team (module) leader. Typically, the team (module) leader's time is spent in indirect patient care activities such as (a) developing or updating nursing care plans, (b) resolving problems encountered by team (module) members, (c) conducting nursing care conferences, and (d) communicating with physicians and other health care personnel.

With team or modular nursing, the unit nurse manager consults with team leaders, supervises patient care teams, and may make rounds with all physicians. To be effective, team nursing requires that all team members have good communication skills. A key aspect of team nursing is the nursing care conference, where the team leader reviews with all team members each patient's plan of care and progress. An advantage of team nursing is that it allows the use of less prepared staff members (LPNs and UAPs) to carry out some functions (e.g., making beds, transporting patients, collecting some data) that do not require the expertise of an RN. Another advantage of team nursing is that it allows patient care needs requiring more

than one staff member, such as patient transfers from bed to chair, to be easily coordinated.

There are several negative features of team or modular nursing. First, a large amount of time is required for the team leader to maintain effective communication for team planning, supervising, and coordinating the care provided by all team members. Second, continuity of care may be diminished because of day-to-day changes in team members and leaders, as well as the group of patients assigned to the team. Third, because each member of the team is assigned specific tasks for the patient and no one considers the total patient, team or modular nursing does not allow for a holistic view of the patient. Role confusion and resentment are other potential problems. The UAPs and licensed team members may view the role of the team leader as more focused toward paperwork and less directed at the physical or real needs of the patient.

Skills in delegating, communicating, and problem solving are essential for a team leader to be effective. Open communication between team leaders and the nurse manager also is important to avoid duplication of effort, overriding of delegated assignments, or competition for control or power. Problems in delegation and communication are the most common reasons why team nursing is less effective than it theoretically could be. Although the geographical boundaries of modular nursing help save steps and time, these same boundaries pose an additional problem: Nurses have decreased control over their assignments; as a result, the assignments may be unequal if they are based on patient acuity or monotonous if nurses continuously care for patients with similar conditions (e.g., all patients with hip replacements).

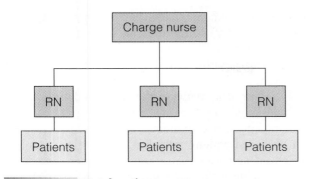

Figure 3-3 **Total patient care.**

Total Patient Care

The original model of nursing care delivery was **total patient care**, also called *case method* (Figure 3-3), in which a registered nurse was responsible for all aspects of the care of one or more patients. During the 1920s, total patient care was the typical nursing care delivery system. Student nurses often staffed hospitals, while RNs provided total care to the patient at home. In total patient care, RNs work directly with the patient, family, physician, and other health care staff in implementing a plan of care.

The goal of this delivery system is to have one nurse give all care to the same patient(s) for the entire shift. Currently, total patient care delivery systems are typically used in areas requiring a high level of nursing expertise, such as in critical care units or postanesthesia recovery areas.

The advantages of a total patient care system include (a) continuous, holistic, expert nursing care; (b) total accountability for the nursing care of the assigned patient(s) for that shift; and (c) continuity of communication with the patient, family, physician(s), and staff from other departments. The disadvantage of this system is that RNs spend some time doing tasks

that could be done more cost-effectively by less skilled persons. This inefficiency adds to the expense of using a total patient care delivery system.

Primary Nursing

Conceptualized by Marie Manthey and implemented during the late 1960s after two decades of team nursing, **primary nursing** (Figure 3-4) was designed to place the registered nurse back at the patient's bedside (Manthey, 1980). Decentralized decision making by staff nurses is the core principle of primary nursing, with responsibility and authority for nursing care allocated to staff nurses at the bedside. Primary nursing recognized that nursing was a knowledge-based professional practice, not just a task-based activity. The RN maintains a patient load of primary patients. A primary nurse designs, implements, and is accountable for the nursing care of patients in the patient load for the duration of the patient's stay on the unit. Actual care is given by the primary nurse and/or associate nurses (other RNs).

Primary nursing advanced the professional practice of nursing significantly because it provided (a) a knowledge-based practice model; (b) decentralization of nursing care decisions, authority, and responsibility

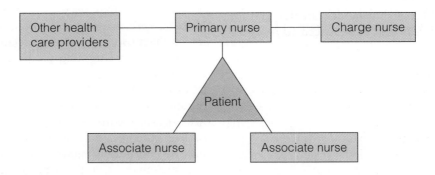

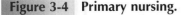

Figure 3-4 **Primary nursing.**

to the staff nurse; (c) 24-hour accountability for nursing care activities by one nurse; (d) improved continuity and coordination of care; and (e) increased nurse, patient, and physician satisfaction.

Disadvantages also exist. Primary nursing requires excellent communication between the primary nurse and associate nurses. Primary nurses must be able to hold associate nurses accountable for implementing the nursing care as prescribed. Because of transfers to different units, critically ill patients may have several primary care nurses, disrupting the continuity of care inherent in the model. Although the concept of 24-hour accountability is worthwhile, it is a fallacy. Staff nurses are neither compensated nor legally responsible for patient care outside their hours of work. Another difficulty is the unwillingness of associates to take direction from the primary nurse. Lastly, when primary nursing was first implemented, many organizations perceived that it required an all RN staff. This practice was viewed as not only expensive but also ineffective because many tasks could be done by less skilled persons. As a result, many hospitals discontinued the use of primary nursing. Other hospitals successfully implemented primary nursing by identifying one nurse who was assigned to coordinate care and with whom the family and physician could communicate, while other nurses or unlicensed assistive personnel assisted this nurse in providing care.

Practice Partnerships

The **practice partnership** (Figure 3-5) is a more recent concept also introduced by Marie Manthey (1989). Practice partnerships can be applied to primary nursing and used in other nursing care delivery systems, such as team nursing, modular nursing, and total patient care. As organizations downsize and reduce salary budgets, practice partnerships offer an efficient way of using the skills of a mix of professional and nonprofessional staff with differing levels of expertise.

In the practice partnership model, an RN and an assistant—UAP, LPN, or less experienced RN—agree

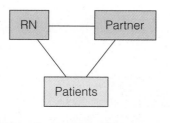

Figure 3-5   **Practice partnerships.**

to be practice partners. The partners work together with the same schedule and the same group of patients. The senior RN partner directs the work of the junior partner within the limits of each state's nurse practice act.

The relationship between the senior and junior partner is designed to create synergistic energy as the two work in concert with patients. The senior partner performs selected patient care activities but delegates less specialized activities to the junior partner. The partners can achieve the workload or outcomes that previously were achieved by two RNs (Manthey, 1989).

When compared to team or modular nursing, practice partnerships offer more continuity of care and accountability for patient care. When compared to total patient care or primary nursing, partnerships are less expensive for the organization and more satisfying professionally for the partners.

One disadvantage of this model is that organizations tend to increase the number of UAPs and decrease the ratio of professional nurses to nonprofessional staff. If, for example, one UAP is assigned to more than one RN, the UAP must follow the instructions of several people, making a synergistic relationship with any one of them difficult. Another problem is the potential for the junior member of the team to assume more responsibility than appropriate. Senior partners must take caution not to delegate inappropriate tasks to junior partners.

Case Management

Following the introduction and impact of prospective payment, nursing **case management**, used for decades in community and psychiatric settings, has been adopted for acute inpatient care. Nursing case management (Figure 3-6) is a model for identifying, coordinating, and monitoring the implementation of services needed to achieve desired patient care outcomes within a specified period of time (Zander, 1988). Nursing case management organizes patient care by major diagnoses or diagnosis-related groups (DRGs) and focuses on attaining predetermined patient outcomes within specific time frames and resources (Zander, 1988; 1992). The essential elements of nursing case management are (a) collaboration of all health care members, (b) identification of expected patient outcomes with time frames, (c) use of principles of continuous quality improvement (CQI) and variance analysis, and (d) promotion of professional practice.

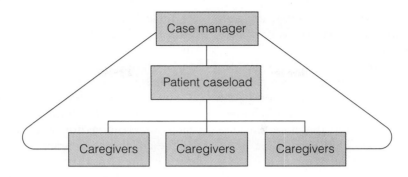

Figure 3-6 **Case management.**

On a patient care unit there may be one or more nursing case managers who coordinate, communicate, collaborate, problem solve, and facilitate patient care for a group of patients. Ideally, nursing case managers are nurses with advanced degrees and considerable experience. Typically, the case manager has a caseload of 10 to 15 patients and follows patients' progress through the system from admission to discharge, accounting for variances from expected progress. Some case managers, often called continuing care coordinators, also supervise the care of their patients in the outpatient setting. The case manager usually does not provide direct patient care but rather supervises the care provided by licensed and unlicensed nursing personnel. The system has contributed to a reduction in complications (Taunton, Kleinbeck, Stafford, Woods, & Bott, 1994; Hofmann, 1993), reduced cost (Cohen, 1991; Mahn, 1993), increased collaboration (Baggs, Ryan, Phelps, Richeson, & Johnson, 1992; Kimball, 1993), and improved quality of care (Outcome Management Department of St. Luke's Episcopal Hospital, 1994; Lumsdon & Hagland, 1993).

After a specific patient population is selected to be "case managed," a collaborative practice team is established. A collaborative practice team, made up of clinical experts from appropriate disciplines (e.g., nursing, medicine, physical therapy) needed for the selected patient population, defines the expected outcomes of care for the patient population. Based on expected patient outcomes, each member of the practice team, using his or her discipline's contribution, helps determine appropriate interventions within a specified time frame.

To initiate case management, specific patient diagnoses that represent high-volume, high-cost, and high-risk cases are selected. For example, high-risk cases include patients or case types who have complications, stay in a critical care unit longer than two days, or

require ventilatory support. High-volume cases are those that occur frequently, such as total hip replacements on an orthopedic floor. Patients also may be selected because they are treated by one particular physician who supports case management. Whatever patient population is selected, base-line data must be collected and analyzed before case management is initiated. These data provide bases for comparison of the effects of case management. Essential base-line data include length of stay, cost of care, and high-risk/complication information.

Five elements are essential to successful implementation of case management. These elements are (a) support by key members of the organization (administrators, physicians, nurses), (b) selection of a qualified nurse case manager, (c) collaborative practice teams, (d) a quality management system, and (e) established critical pathways.

Critical paths are tools or guidelines that provide direction for care. The term *critical path* refers to the expected outcomes and care strategies developed by the collaborative practice team. Other common terms are *care protocols, practice guidelines, clinical guidelines,*

KEY TERMS

Practice partnership A nursing care delivery system in which senior and junior staff members share patient care responsibilities.

Case management A model for identifying, coordinating, and monitoring the implementation of services needed to achieve desired patient care outcomes within a specified period of time.

Critical paths Tools or guidelines that direct care by identifying expected outcomes.

clinical outcomes, care maps, clinical paths, and *collaborative paths.* Each organization determines how specific these guidelines will be.

A critical path quickly orients the staff to the outcomes that should be achieved for the patient for that day. Nursing diagnoses facilitate identification of the outcomes needed. If patient outcomes are not achieved, the case manager is notified and the situation analyzed to determine how to modify the critical path. An alteration in time frames or interventions is categorized as a variance, and the case manager tracks all variances. After a time, the appropriate collaborative practice teams analyze the variances, note trends, and decide how to manage them. The critical pathway may need to be revised or additional data may be needed before changes are made.

Some features are included on all critical paths, such as specific medical diagnosis, the expected length of stay, patient identification data, appropriate time frames (in days, hours, minutes, or visits) for interventions, and patient outcomes. Interventions are presented in modality groups (medications, nursing activity, and so on). The critical path must include a means to identify variances easily and to determine whether the outcome has been met or not.

Table 3-2 is an example of a collaborative critical path for patients having a total hip replacement. Normally a patient would be expected to be discharged on the sixth day after surgery. This path describes expectations for days 1 through 3.

In case management, all professionals are equal members of the team; thus, one group does not determine interventions for other disciplines. All members of the collaborative practice team agree on the final draft of the critical pathways, take ownership of patient outcomes, and accept responsibility and accountability for the interventions and patient outcomes associated with their discipline. The nurse case manager may serve as both the clinical nurse expert and coordinator of the case management process.

A recent evolution of critical paths is the incorporation of actual and potential nursing diagnoses with specific time frames into the critical pathway (the lower section of Table 3-2). Education paths are also excellent tools for planning patient and family education (Table 3-3). A copy of this form is given to the patient and the family, and the nurse reviews the information with them. Thus, both the patient and the family know what to expect during an anticipated, uncomplicated hospitalization.

Table 3-2   Critical Path with Actual/Potential Nursing Diagnoses for Total Hip Replacement

Collaborative Critical Path
Case Type: Total Hip Replacement

Patient Name: _____   DRG: <u>209</u>
Record Number: _____   Expected LOS: <u>6 days</u>

	Day 1 / OR	Y/N	Day 2 / Postoperative Day 1	Y/N	Day 3 / Postoperative Day 2	Y/N
Patient Activity	Bed rest	___	Begin mobility plan;	___	Cont mobility plan	___
	T-DB q2h	___	T-DB q2h	___	T-DB q2h	___
	Initiate skin protection protocol	___	Cont skin protection protocol	___	Cont skin protection protocol	___
Nursing	VS qh × 4, then q4h	___	VS q4h	___	VS q8h	___
	Assess cir/neuro legs qh × 4, then q4h	___	Assess cir/neuro q4h	___	D/C assessment	___
					D/C Hemovac;	___
	Check drainage/ Hemovac qh × 4, then q4h;	___	Check drainage/ Hemovac q4h	___	Check drainage q8h	___
	I & O (Foley/ Hemovac) q8h;	___	I & O (Foley/ Hemovac) q8h	___	I & O q8h D/C Foley; urinates within 8h	___
	Thigh-hi elastic hose	___	Cont elastic hose	___	Cont elastic hose	___

Table 3-2	Continued

Medications	Antibiotic Pain control: PCA pump Stool softener Cont home Rx; IVs	___ ___ ___ ___ ___	Cont antibiotic Cont pain control Cont stool softener Cont home Rx IVs cont Coumadin Sleeping Rx	___ ___ ___ ___ ___ ___ ___	Cont antibiotic PO pain control Cont stool softener Cont home Rx IV to heparin lock Cont coumadin Sleeping Rx	___ ___ ___ ___ ___ ___ ___
Physical Therapy	Preop instructions	___	Evaluate mobility progress	___	Evaluate mobility progress	___
Diagnostic Tests	H & H 2h postop	___	H & H Prothrombin time	___ ___	Prothrombin time	___
Nutrition	NPO—Cl liq as tol	___	Diet as tolerated	___	Diet as tolerated	___
Teaching	*Preop:* Pain control Use of assist devices Gait control Incentive spirometry Mobility plan Pt/family crit plan given & reviewed	___ ___ ___ ___ ___ ___	Repeat teaching if nec Review pt/family crit plan if nec	___ ___	Repeat teaching if nec Review pt/family crit plan if nec	___ ___
Discharge Plan	SNU evaluation Home Health evaluation	___ ___			Review transfer discharge needs	___

Patient Problems and Outcomes for Total Hip Replacement

Nursing Diagnosis	Day 1 / OR	Y/N	Day 2 / Postoperative Day 1	Y/N	Day 3 / Postoperative Day 2	Y/N
Knowledge deficit: medications; use of assistive devices; treatments	Appropriately uses: PCA pump, incentive spirometry, assistive devices; Verbalizes mobility plan	___ ___ ___ ___	Uses all devices appropriately	___	Verbalizes additions to care	___
Pain related to surgery, physical injury	Pain managed	___	Pain managed	___	Pain managed	___
Risk for infection related to invasive procedures, immobility	Remains afebrile No skin breakdown	___ ___	Remains afebrile No skin breakdown	___ ___	Remains afebrile	___
Impaired physical mobility related to surgery, prosthesis	Verbalizes mobility plan Verbalizes role of staff providing assistance	___ ___	Meeting mobility expectations	___	Participates in transfer/discharge plans, decisions	___
Risk for injury related to altered tissue perfusion, altered mobiity, and prosthesis	Explains need for frequent assessments Verbalizes need for early mobility and hose	___ ___	Circulation to extremities good Leg maintained in proper alignment	___ ___	Circulation to extremities normal; Leg in proper alignment	___

| Table 3-3 | Patient/Family Education Path for Total Hip Replacement |

	Day 1 / OR	Day 2 / Postoperative Day 1	Day 3 / Postoperative Day 2
Unit	Admission process; surgery & recovery areas; then Orthopedic Unit	Orthopedic Unit	Orthopedic Unit (Possible transfer next day to SNU or Rehab Unit)
Patient Activity and Safety Issues	Bed rest first 24 h; leg exercises qh (q4h); T-DB q2h; explain skin protection plan; give copy of mobility plan; assist c̄ bath; thigh-hi elastic support hose	Up in chair c̄ help; Leg exercises q2h; T-DB q2h; cont skin protect plan; cont mobility plan; assist c̄ bath; cont thigh-hi elastic support hose	Up in chair and walking as outlined in mobility plan; T-DB q2h; cont skin protection plan; assist c̄ bath; cont thigh-hi elastic support hose
Nursing Care	Frequency of taking vital signs (BP-P-R-T); check drainage on dressing; check circulation and sensations to legs; intake & output measured q8h; Foley and Hemovac in for 48 h	Vital sign checks q4h; dressing, circulation, and sensation checks to legs q4h; I & O (Foley and Hemovac) measured q8h	Vital sign checks q8h; D/C Foley and Hemovac; I & O q8h; urinate within 8 h; D/C dressing, circulation, and sensation checks to legs
Medications	Verify list of home Rx so physician can order; pain medication and PCA pump; IVs and need for arm restraint; other drugs that will be ordered (e.g., antibiotics; stool softener)	Cont pain management c̄ PCA pump; IVs; cont arm restraint; cont antibiotic and other drugs (sleeping assistance)	Oral pain management; IV to heparin lock; cont antibiotic and other drugs
Diet	NPO before OR; clear liquids, ice chips	Diet as tolerated	Diet as tolerated
Tests	Blood test: Hemoglobin and hematocrit 2 h after OR	Blood tests: H & H and prothrombin time	Blood test: prothrombin time
Teaching	Pain management; use of assistive devices (trapeze, walker) and incentive spirometry; mobility plan reviewed: how to transfer from bed to chair, and so on	Clarify questions	Clarify questions
Discharge Plan	Discuss purpose of Skilled Nursing Unit and Rehab Unit; identify need for Home Health Service after discharge	Cont with discussion of SNU, Rehab, and Home Health Services	Clarify questions and needs with transfer/discharge plans

Differentiated Practice

Differentiated practice is a method that maximizes nursing resources by focusing on the structure of roles and functions of nurses according to their education, experience, and competence (Boston, 1990). Differentiated practice is designed to identify distinct levels of nursing practice based on defined abilities that are incorporated into job descriptions (Ehrat, 1991). In differentiated practice, the responsibilities of RNs (mainly those with bachelor's and associate degrees)

differ according to the competence and training associated with the two education levels as well as the nurses' experience and preferences. The scope of nursing practice and level of responsibility are specifically defined for each level.

Some organizations differentiate roles, responsibilities, and tasks for professional nurses, licensed practical nurses (LPNs), and unlicensed assistive personnel (UAPs), which are incorporated into their respective job descriptions. Differentiated practice improves patient care and contributes to patient safety, allows

KEY TERMS

Differentiated practice A nursing care delivery system that maximizes nursing resources by focusing on the structure of nursing roles according to education, experience, and competency.

Patient-centered care A nursing care delivery system that is unit-based and consists of patient care coordinators, patient care associates, unit support assistants, administrative support personnel, and a nurse manager.

for the most effective and efficient use of scarce resources, offers increased satisfaction for nurses, and provides opportunity to compensate nurses fairly based on their expertise, contributions, and productivity (McClure, 1991). Differentiated practice will become more important as quality of care, patient outcomes, and personnel budget concerns become more prominent.

Patient-Centered Care

Patient-centered care is a new model of nursing care delivery in which the role of the nurse is broadened to coordinate a team of multifunctional unit-based caregivers (Redman & Jones, 1998). In patient-centered care, all patient care services are unit-based, including admission and discharge, diagnostic and treatment services, and support services, such as environmental and nutrition services and medical records. The focus of patient-centered care is decentralization, the promotion of efficiency and quality, and cost control. In this model of care the number of caregivers at the bedside is reduced, but their responsibilities are increased so that service and waiting times are decreased. A typical team in a unit providing patient-centered care consists of patient care coordinators (RNs); patient care associates or technicians who are able to perform delegated patient care tasks; unit support assistants who provide environmental services and can assist with hygiene and ambulation needs; administrative support personnel who maintain patient records, transcribe orders, coordinate admission and discharge, and assist with general office duties; and, a nurse manager (Redman & Jones, 1998).

This model greatly affects the role of the nurse manager. Staff and management issues consume a greater proportion of the manager's time. No longer is the manager doing rounds and assisting with patient

care. Instead, being responsible for a staff that is more diverse with fewer professional RN staff demands a strong leader proficient in interviewing, hiring, training, and motivating. Some organizations share assistive staff between units, also increasing the need for more communication and coordination with other managers (Redman & Jones, 1998).

Summary

- Nursing care delivery systems provide a structure for nursing care. Most organizations use a combination of nursing care delivery systems or modify one or more systems to meet their own needs.
- The most commonly used nursing care delivery systems are team nursing, total patient care, and primary nursing.
- Case management is a collaborative patient care system that uses case managers (RNs) who are responsible for facilitating patient interventions and achieving patient outcomes from admission to discharge. Critical paths are used to designate specific patient outcomes within specified time frames.
- Differentiated practice and patient-centered care are two systems that use nurses and support personnel based on expertise of staff and needs of patients.

■ LEADERSHIP AND MANAGEMENT
in Action

1. What are the different types of nursing care delivery systems?
2. How do nursing roles and responsibilities change in each system?
3. How is responsibility of the manager different in each?

References

American Hospital Association. (1991). *AHA hospital nursing personnel surveys*. Chicago: Author.

Baggs, J. G., Ryan, S. A., Phelps, C. E., Richeson, J. F., & Johnson, J. E. (1992). The association between interdisciplinary collaboration and patient outcomes in a medical intensive care unit. *Heart & Lung, 21*(1), 18–24.

Boston, C. M. (1990). Introduction. In American Hospital Association. *Current issues and perspectives on differentiated practice*. Chicago: Author.

Cohen, E. L. (1991). Nursing case management: Does it pay? *Journal of Nursing Administration, 21*(4), 20–25.

Curtin, L. L. (1988). Fatal availability. *Nursing Management, 19*(12), 9–10.

Ehrat, K. S. (1991). The value of differentiated practices. *Journal of Nursing Administration, 21*(4), 9–10.

Hofmann, P. A. (1993). Critical path method: An important tool for coordinating clinical care. *Journal on Quality Improvement, 19*(7), 235–246.

Kimball, L. (1993). Collaborative care: A quality improvement and cost reduction tool. *Journal of Hospital Quarterly, 15*(4), 6–9.

Lumsdon, K., & Hagland, M. (1993). Mapping care. *Hospitals & Health Networks, 67*(20), 34–40.

Magargal, P. (1987). Modular nursing: Nursing rediscovers nursing. *Nursing Management, 18*(11), 98–104.

Mahn, V. A. (1993). Clinical nurse case management: A service line approach. *Nursing Management, 24*(9), 48–50.

Manthey, M. (1980). *The practice of primary nursing.* St. Louis: Mosby.

Manthey, M. (1989). Practice partnerships: The newest concept in care delivery. *Journal of Nursing Association, 19*(2), 33–35.

McClure, M. L. (1991). Differentiated nursing practice: Concepts and considerations. *Nursing Outlook, 39*(3), 106–110.

Outcome Management Department of St. Luke's Episcopal Hospital in Houston (1994). Focusing on outcomes. *RN, 54*(5), 57–60.

Redman, R., & Jones, K. (1998). Effects of implementing patient-centered care models on nurse and non-nurse managers. *Journal of Nursing Administration, 28*(11), 46–53.

Taunton, R. L., Kleinbeck, S. V. M., Stafford, R., Woods, C. Q., & Bott, M. J. (1994). Patient outcomes: Are they linked to registered nurse absenteeism, separation, or work load? *Journal of Nursing Administration, 24*(4S), 48–55.

Yeast, C. (1991). Who are we and what motivates us? *American Nurse, 23*(9), 14.

Zander, K. (1988). Nursing case management. *Nursing Clinics of North America, 23*(3), 503–520.

Zander, K. (1992). Focusing on patient outcome: Case management in the 90's. *Dimensions of Critical Care Nursing, 11*(3), 127–129.

Additional on-line resources for this chapter can be found on the World Wide Web at http://www.prenhall.com/sullivan_decker. Select Chapter 3 from the drop-down menu.

CHAPTER 4

Leading and Managing

Looking Ahead

What is the relationship between leaders and managers? What are the differences and similarities? How does leadership fit into these roles? This chapter completes Part I of the book with an in-depth look at theories of leadership and general management functions. Building on these concepts, the chapter explores the roles and functions of nurses in management and describes the various levels of management.

Objectives

After reading this chapter, you will be able to:

- Describe the different types of power that leaders use.
- Compare and contrast different leadership theories.
- Differentiate the roles of manager and leader.
- Compare and contrast the various levels of management.
- Describe the classical functions of management.
- Compare Mintzberg's behavioral description of management roles with his contemporary model.
- Discuss ways to become a more effective leader.

Managers are essential to any organization. A manager's functions are vital, complex, and frequently difficult. They must be directed toward balancing the needs of patients, the health care organization, employees, physicians, and self. Nurse managers need a body of knowledge and skills distinctly different from those needed for nursing practice, yet few nurses have the education or training necessary to be managers (Block, 1991). Frequently, managers depend on experiences with former supervisors, who also learned supervisory techniques "in the trenches." Often a gap exists between what managers know and what they need to know.

Today, all nurses are managers, not in the formal organizational sense but in practice. They direct the work of nonprofessionals and professionals in order to achieve desired outcomes in patient care. As such, all nurses need to learn leadership and management skills to be more efficient and effective. This chapter delineates the difference between leaders and managers, explains leadership and management theories, describes management levels in nursing, and discusses the roles and functions of nursing management.

Leaders and Managers

Manager, leader, supervisor, and *administrator* are often used interchangeably, yet they are not the same. A **leader** is anyone who uses interpersonal skills to influence others to accomplish a specific goal. The leader exerts influence by using a flexible repertoire of personal behaviors and strategies. The leader is important in forging links—creating connections— among an organization's members to promote high levels of performance and quality outcomes. Antrobus and Kitson (1999) found that leaders are skilled in empowering others, creating meaning and facilitating learning, developing knowledge, reflective thinking, communication, problem solving, decision making, and working with others. Leaders generate excitement; they clearly define their purpose and mission. Leaders understand people and their needs; they recognize and appreciate differences in people, individualizing their approach as needed. Leaders also have the capacity to earn and hold trust. They have a genuine concern for others and help others achieve their potential (Kerfoot, 1997).

The functions of a leader are to achieve a consensus within the group about its goals, maintain a structure that facilitates accomplishing the goals, supply necessary information that helps provide direction and clarification, and maintain group satisfaction, cohesion, and performance.

A **manager**, in contrast, is an individual employed by an organization who is responsible and accountable for efficiently accomplishing the goals of the organization. Managers focus on coordinating and integrating resources, using the functions of planning, organizing, supervising, staffing, evaluating, negotiating, and representing. Interpersonal skill is important, but a manager also has authority, responsibility, accountability, and power defined by the organization. Managers define the mission and goals of the organization; clarify the organizational structure; choose the means by which to achieve goals; assign and coordinate tasks, developing and motivating as needed; and evaluate outcomes and provide feedback.

All good managers are also good leaders—the two go hand in hand. However, one may be a good manager of resources and not be much of a leader of people. Likewise, a person who is a good leader may not manage well. Both roles can be learned; skills gained can enhance either role.

Leadership

Leadership may be formal or informal. Leadership is **formal** when practiced by a nurse with legitimate authority conferred by the organization and described in a job description (e.g., nurse manager, supervisor, coordinator, case manager). Formal leadership also depends on personal skills, but it may be reinforced by organizational authority and position. Thoughtful formal leaders recognize the importance of their own informal leadership activities and the informal leadership of others who affect the work in their areas of responsibility. Leadership is **informal** when exercised by a staff member who does not have a specified management role. A nurse whose thoughtful and convincing ideas substantially influence the efficiency of work flow is exercising leadership skills. Informal leadership depends primarily on one's knowledge, status (e.g., advanced practice nurse, quality improvement coordinator, education specialist, medical director), and personal skills in persuading and guiding others.

Power: How Managers and Leaders Get Things Done

Classically, managers in health care institutions relied on authority to rouse employees to perform tasks and accomplish goals. In contemporary health care organizations, managers use persuasion, enticement, and inspiration to mobilize the energy and talent of a work group and to overcome resistance to change.

Power may be defined as the capacity to produce or prevent change. A leader's use of power alters attitudes and behavior by addressing individual needs and motivations. There are seven generally accepted types of interpersonal power used in organizations to influence others (French & Raven, 1959; Hersey, Blanchard, & Natemeyer, 1979).

1. **Reward power** is based on the inducements the manager can offer group members in exchange for cooperation and contributions that advance the manager's objectives. The degree of compliance depends on how much the follower values the expected benefits. For example, a nurse manager may grant paid educational leave as a way of rewarding staff nurses for implementing a new patient database system. Reward power often is used in relation to a manager's formal job responsibilities.

2. **Punishment**, or coercive, **power** is based on the penalties a manager might impose on an individual or a group. Motivation to comply is based on fear of punishment or withholding of rewards. For example, the nurse manager might make undesirable job assignments, mete out a formal reprimand, or recommend termination for a nurse who engages in disruptive behavior. Punishment or coercion is used in relation to a manager's perceived authority to determine employment status.

3. **Legitimate power** stems from the manager's right to make a request because of the authority associated with job and rank in an organizational hierarchy. Followers comply because they accept a manager's prerogative to imp____ sanctions, and rewards in keeping w___ nization's mission and aims. For instanc___ nurses will comply with a nurse manager's dire___ tive to take time off without pay when the workload has dropped below projected levels because they know that the manager is charged with maintaining unit expenses within budget limitations.

4. **Expert power** is based on possession of unique skills, knowledge, and competence. Nurse managers, by virtue of experience and advanced education, often are the best qualified to determine what to do in a given situation. Employees are motivated to comply because they respect the manager's expertise. Expert power relates to the development of personal abilities through education and experience. Newly graduated nurses might ask the nurse manager for advice in learning clinical procedures or how to resolve conflicts with co-workers or other health professionals.

5. **Referent power** is based on admiration and respect for an individual. Followers comply because they like and identify with the manager. Referent power relates to the manager's likability and success. For example, a new graduate might ask the

KEY TERMS

Informal leadership   Leadership that is exercised by an individual who does not have a specified management role.

Power   The capacity to produce or prevent change.

Reward power   Power based on inducements offered by the manager in exchange for contributions that advance the manager's objectives.

Punishment (coercive) power   Power based on penalties a manager might impose if the individual or group does not comply with authority.

Legitimate power   A manager's right to make requests because of authority within an organizational hierarchy.

Expert power   Power based on the manager's possession of unique skills, knowledge, and competence.

Referent power   Power based on the admiration and respect for an individual.

admired nurse

on access to valued
cause they are moti-
ormation that will meet
and facilitate decision making.
tion power depends on a manager's organizational position, connections, and communication skills. For example, the nurse manager is frequently privy to information obtained at meetings
with administrators about pending organizational
changes that affect employees' work situations. A
nurse manager may exercise information power
by sharing significant information at staff meetings, thereby improving attendance.

7. **Connection power** is based on an individual's
formal and informal links to influential or presti-
gious persons within and outside an area or organization. Followers comply because they want
to be linked to influential individuals. Connection
power also relates to the status and visibility of

the individual as well as the position. In some
cases, nurse managers have personal relationships
with an organization's board members that followers believe will protect or advance their work
situation.

These power bases are available to managers and
may be classified more simply as personal or position
power (Table 4-1). **Position power** is determined by
the job description, assigned responsibilities, recognition, advancement, authority, the ability to withhold
money, and decision-making. Legitimate, coercive,
and reward power are positional because they relate
to the "right" to influence others based on rank or
role. The extent to which managers mete out rewards
and punishment usually is dictated by organizational
policy. Information and legitimate power are directly
related to the manager's role in the organizational
structure.

Expert, referent, information, and connection power
are based, for the most part, on personal traits. **Personal**

Table 4-1 Effects of Managerial Power

Type of Power	Overuse, Abuse, Misuse	Underuse	Proper Use
Position			
Reward	Jealousy	Lack of decision making	Commitment is possible if request is polite, reasonable, and nonthreatening.
Punishment/coercive	Distrust	Failure to achieve goals and objectives	
Legitimate	Fear	Loss of credibility	Compliance is likely if request is legitimate and impersonal; compliance is possible if coercion is used in a motivational way.
Information	Avoidance	Perception of incompetence	
	Filtered information		
	Stifled creativity		
	Undermining activities		
Personal			
Expert	Perception of manipu- lation, overstepping bounds, and inter- ference	Perception of unapproachability	Commitment is likely if request is persuasive or important to the leader and shared.
Referent		Lack of concern	
Connection		Being out of touch	Compliance is likely if leader is credible; compliance is possible if request is persuasive and perceived to be important to the leader.
Information	Appearance of indecisiveness		
	Accusations of unfairness		
	Lack of objectivity		
	Supervisor hostility		
	Loss of confidence		

Note: Developed from *Leadership in organizations*, 2nd ed., by G. A. Yukl, 1989, Englewood Cliffs, NJ: Prentice-Hall.

power refers to one's credibility, reputation, expertise, experience, control of resources or information, and ability to build trust. The extent to which one may exercise expert, referent, information, and connection power relates to personal skills and positive interpersonal relationships, as well as employees' needs and motivations.

Leaders and managers often exercise power differently. Leaders tend to rely primarily on personal power sources to provoke interest, inspire commitment, and instill confidence. Managers tend to use position power to ensure adherence to policies and standards and to complete work assignments. Managers also use position power to ensure orderly operation of their areas of responsibility. On the other hand, managers may use personal power to resolve conflicts among members of the work group, to develop an innovative approach to care delivery, or to improve working relationships with other professionals, clients, or organizational decision makers. Managers also rely on personal power to sustain commitment and interest in highly routinized jobs, as well as to maintain an esprit de corps among co-workers.

A manager must exercise power judiciously, which is effective because of the dependency that is inherent in a power relationship. For power to be used successfully, subjects of the applied power must be dependent on another, such as the manager. The manager is in a position to make decisions that affect the subject's welfare. The dependency relationship between manager and subject can result in vulnerability and exploitation, as well as benefit.

Improper use of power can de effectiveness (see Table 4-1). Power ca underused, or abused. A manager usually u positional and personal power, and both must used appropriately. The most effective combination depends on the manager's personality, the situation, the needs of followers, and balance in the power–dependency relationship. Box 4-1 provides guidelines for use of power in organizations.

Nurse managers in contemporary health care organizations must recognize that the use of power helps them influence actions and decisions that will benefit staff as well as patients, families, and communities. Nurse managers should view power as a valuable resource that they must acquire, conserve, and invest carefully. Power is used best to support organizational priorities, facilitate important activities and decisions, and to manage differences among interdependent organization members (Shortell & Kaluzny, 1994).

Table 4-1 depicts the likelihood that different power bases will result in staff members' genuine commitment to manager's requests or unit objectives, minimal compliance with requests and objectives, or active or passive rejection of the manager's leadership. Interpersonal skills and technical and managerial competence are far more likely to generate genuine commitment than the use of rewards and punishment.

A manager's desire for power is an important and necessary part of managerial motivation (Kouzes & Posner, 1987). Managers use power to motivate others, to strengthen their abilities, and to create alliances among diverse parties. Through the effective use of legitimate and expert power, a manager might require staff to improve skills and change personal behavior in anticipation of new technology or services. A manager also may use connection and referent power to bring conflicting parties together to solve problems or develop new programs. When the manager seeks power only to enhance his or her status, however, failures in performance, standoffs, or breakdowns in working relationships result. On the other hand, power used in the service of others—clients, employees, the community, the organization—increases the status and confidence of both the manager and employees. In fast-paced, contemporary organizations, power flows to individuals who have the ability to help the organization deal with complex, difficult tasks (Kanter, 1982). Nurse managers should consider how to demonstrate these principles and further develop their power bases.

...arrogant demands.

...clear, simple language, check for ...erstanding.

3. Explain reasons for requests.

4. Follow up to check for compliance.

Using Rewards

1. Don't overemphasize incentives; staff will expect rewards for every request. Emphasize mutual loyalty and teamwork.

2. Rewards are unlikely to produce commitment.

3. Reinforce past behavior; don't bribe for future performance.

4. The size of rewards should reflect total performance.

5. Money is not the only (and is often the least effective) reward.

6. Avoid appearing manipulative at all costs.

Using Coercive Power

1. Avoid coercion and punishment except when absolutely necessary.

2. Punish only to deter extremely detrimental behavior.

3. Try to determine genuine responsibility or liability before taking corrective action.

4. Discipline promptly and consistently without favoritism. Fit the punishment to the seriousness of the infraction.

5. State consequences without hostility; remain calm and express desire to help subordinate comply with requirements and avoid discipline.

6. Invite subordinate to share in responsibility for correcting disciplinary problems; set improvement goals and develop improvement plans.

7. Warn before punishing; don't issue idle or exaggerated warnings you are not prepared to carry out.

Using Expert Power

1. Preserve credibility by avoiding careless statements and rash decisions.

2. Keep informed about technical developments affecting the group's work.

3. In a crisis, remain calm; act confidently and decisively.

4. Avoid arrogance or talking down to staff; show respect for staff ideas and suggestions and incorporate them whenever feasible.

5. Do not threaten subordinates' self-esteem.

6. Recognize subordinates' concerns; explain why a proposed plan of action is best and what steps will be taken to minimize risk to them.

Using Referent Power

1. Be considerate, show concern for staff needs and feelings, treat them fairly, and defend their interests to superiors and outsiders.

2. Avoid expressing hostility, distrust, rejection, or indifference toward subordinates. Actions speak louder than words.

3. Explain the personal importance of requests and your reliance on staff support and cooperation.

4. Don't make requests too often; make requests reasonable.

5. Be a good role model.

Using Connection Power

1. Consider carefully the appropriate use of the connection or relationship.

2. Avoid name dropping.

3. Provide sound rationale for using the relationship.

4. Recognize the likelihood of being expected to reciprocate in return for favors provided in a relationship.

5. Recognize the reasonable limits of the connection. Don't overuse or exploit.

Note: Adapted from "The effective use of managerial power" by G. A. Yukl and T. Tabor, 1983, *Personnel* (March/April).

Leadership Theories

Most students of leadership find the search for definitive explanations of leadership effectiveness both fascinating and puzzling. Research on leadership has a long history, but the focus has shifted over time from personal traits to behavior and style, to the leadership situation, to change agency (the capacity to transform), and to other aspects of leadership. Each phase and focus of research has contributed to managers' insights and understandings about leadership and its development. This chapter discusses four categories of leadership theories: trait theories, behavioral theories, contingency theories, and contemporary theories.

Trait Theories

Studies conducted during the first seven decades of the 1900s were leader-centered and focused on defining *what leaders are.* Researchers sought to identify inborn traits of successful leaders. Attempts to specify a universal set of leadership characteristics produced ambiguous results. However, Stogdill (1974) developed a profile of successful leaders and traits. These traits are listed in Box 4-2.

Bass (1990) added more traits, which he classified into three categories: intelligence, personality, abilities (see Box 4-2). Gilbert (1975), in examining the personalities of nursing graduate students, found that potential leaders were more likely to exhibit traits such as dominance, aggressiveness, ambition, high capacity to attain status, poise, self-confidence, tolerance for others' views, high need to achieve, orderly thinking, sensitivity to others, and flexibility. Although inconclusive, these early attempts to specify unique leadership traits provided benchmarks by which most leaders continue to be judged.

Behavioral Theories

Research on leadership in the early 1930s focused on the abilities and behaviors of leaders, that is, *what leaders do.* In the behavioral view of leadership, personal traits provide only a foundation for leadership; real leaders are made through education, training, and life experiences.

Leadership Styles   Behavior-based theories assume that effective leaders acquire a pattern of learned behaviors. Initial studies of teams of teenage boys identified three patterns or *styles* of leadership: autocratic,

---

Box 4-2 | Traits of Successful Leaders

Stogdill Profile

- Drive for task completion and responsibility
- Vigor and persistence
- Creativity in problem-solving
- Social initiative
- Self-confidence
- Acceptance of consequences of actions
- Stress resistance
- Tolerance of frustration
- Ability to influence the behavior of others
- Ability to structure situations of social interaction

Bass Profile

Intelligence

- Judgment
- Decisiveness
- Knowledge
- Fluency

Personality

- Adaptability
- Alertness
- Integrity
- Nonconformity

Abilities

- Cooperativeness
- Popularity
- Tact

Note: Adapted from *Handbook of leadership: A survey of the literature* by R. M. Stogdill, 1974, New York: Free Press; and *Bass and Stogdill's handbook of leadership: Theory, research, and managerial applications,* 3rd ed., by B. Bass, 1990, New York: Free Press.

KEY TERMS

Autocratic leadership   A leadership style that assumes individuals are motivated by external forces; therefore, the leader makes all the decisions and directs the followers' behavior.

Democratic leadership   A leadership style that assumes individuals are motivated by internal forces; leader uses participation and majority rule to get work done.

Laissez-faire leadership   A leadership style that assumes individuals are motivated by internal forces and should be left alone to complete work; leader provides no direction or facilitation.

Bureaucratic leadership   A leadership style that assumes individuals are motivated by external forces; leader trusts neither followers nor self to make decisions and therefore relies on organizational policies and rules.

democratic, and laissez-faire (Lewin & Lippit, 1938; Lewin, Lippit, & White, 1939). The **autocratic leader** assumes that individuals are motivated by external forces, such as power, authority, and need for approval; the leader makes all the decisions and uses coercion, punishment, and direction to change followers' behavior and achieve results. The **democratic leader** assumes that individuals are motivated by internal drives and impulses, want active participation in decisions, and want to get the task done; the leader uses participation and majority rule in setting goals and working toward achievement. The **laissez-faire leader** also assumes that individuals are motivated by internal drives and impulses and that they need to be left alone to make decisions about how to complete the work; the leader provides no direction or facilitation. Jenkins and Henderson (1984) added a fourth style, the **bureaucrat** (Table 4-2). The bureaucrat assumes that employees are motivated by external forces. This leader trusts neither followers nor self to make decisions and therefore relies on organizational policies and rules to identify goals and direct work processes.

Table 4-2   **Comparison of Leadership Styles**

Leadership Style	Assumed Employee Motivators	Leader Characteristics
Authoritarian (autocratic)	External forces, e.g., power and authority, needs for approval	• Concerned with task accomplishment rather than relationships • Uses directive behavior • Makes decisions alone • Expects respect and obedience of staff • Lacks group support generated by participation • Exercises power with coercion • Proves useful (even necessary) in crisis situations
Democratic (participative)	Internal drives and impulses	• Is primarily concerned with human relations and teamwork • Fosters communication that is open and usually two-way • Creates a spirit of collaboration and joint effort that results in staff satisfaction
Permissive (laissez-faire)	Internal drives and impulses	• Tends to have few established policies; abstains from leading • Is not generally useful in highly structured organizations (e.g., health care institutions)
Bureaucratic	External forces	• Lacks a sense of security and depends on established policies and rules • Exercises power by applying fixed, relatively inflexible rules • Tends to relate impersonally to staff • Avoids decision-making without standards or norms for guidance

By the early 1950s, leadership styles in work settings began to be explored (Katz & Kahn, 1952; Stogdill & Coons, 1957). Two major dimensions of behavioral style were identified: initiating structure and consideration. *Initiating structure* refers to the behaviors that managers use to organize and define the goals of work, work patterns and methods, channels of communication, and roles. For example, administration develops a manual of job descriptions, personnel policies, and procedures for granting time off, implementing a new policy on intravenous tubing changes, or family visiting. *Consideration*, the employee-centered dimension, refers to behavior that conveys mutual trust, respect, friendship, warmth, and rapport between the manager and the staff. When the leader is considerate, the employee learns to expect that the manager will hear a concern openly and without reprisal, will involve employees in decision making, and will attend to the needs of the work group as a whole. The manager is alert to employees' responses to stress, the effects of personal crises on their work, and the social dynamics of the work group. To learn how structure and consideration apply to the effectiveness of nurse managers, Jenkins and Henderson (1984) studied staff nurses' responses to charge nurses' behaviors. The researchers found that charge nurses who showed that they recognized staff nurses' needs for belonging, love, social activity, self-respect, status, dignity, appreciation, and involvement were successful in motivating staff to provide quality patient care.

Despite the substantial contributions of the structure/consideration concepts to the development of leadership theory, research has produced confounding results. For example, followers' and managers' perceptions of managers' leadership style often differ; attempts to enhance a manager's style in one area or the other do not necessarily result in higher employee performance or improved goal achievement; equally effective leaders might possess strength in consideration or structure or both.

With the realization that different combinations of leader behaviors might produce different effects, researchers began searching for an optimal mix of behaviors that would produce optimal employee performance. As these models evolved, researchers began to recognize the complexity and range of the approaches managers use to produce results in organizations.

System 4 Management   Likert (1967) developed the System 4 model of management based on the premise that involving employees in decisions about work is central to effective leadership. The model is composed of four dimensions based on increasing levels of employee involvement. *Autocratic leaders* have little trust in employees and systematically exclude them from decision making. *Benevolent leaders* are kind to employees but still do not involve them in decision making. *Consultative leaders* seek employees' advice about decisions. *Participative* or *democratic leaders* value employee involvement, teamwork, and team-building; they also have high levels of confidence in employees and seek consensus in decision making. In doing so, the participative leader shares power.

Research on System 4 leadership demonstrates some key advantages (Miller & Monge, 1986). Employees are (a) more likely to be committed to the organization and its objectives, (b) less resistant to change, (c) more likely to grow and learn new process skills, (d) more likely to generate a variety of relevant strategies to solve problems, and (e) more likely to support organizational flexibility.

The Managerial Grid   Another model for depicting leadership along a continuum is the managerial grid (Figure 4-1). Five leadership styles are plotted in four quadrants of a two-dimensional grid. The grid depicts various degrees of leader concern for production (structure) and concern for people (consideration). Leadership styles are labeled "impoverished" (low concern for both production and people), "authority compliance" (high concern for production, low concern for people), "country club" (high concern for people, low concern for production), "middle-of-the-road" (moderate concern for both production and people), and "team" (high concern for both production and people).

Continuum of Leadership Behavior   Leadership behavior also is depicted as occurring along a continuum. This model focuses specifically on the decision-making style of managers. As displayed in Figure 4-2, the left end of the continuum reflects a manager-centered style. Managers are autocratic and directive and simply make and announce decisions. At the right end of the continuum, managers are employee-centered; they use a laissez-faire style and permit employees to set their own goals and function within established parameters. No single leadership style is correct or appropriate for every management situation.

The numerous variations of the multidimensional, behavioral approach have contributed significantly to our understanding of managers' performance and

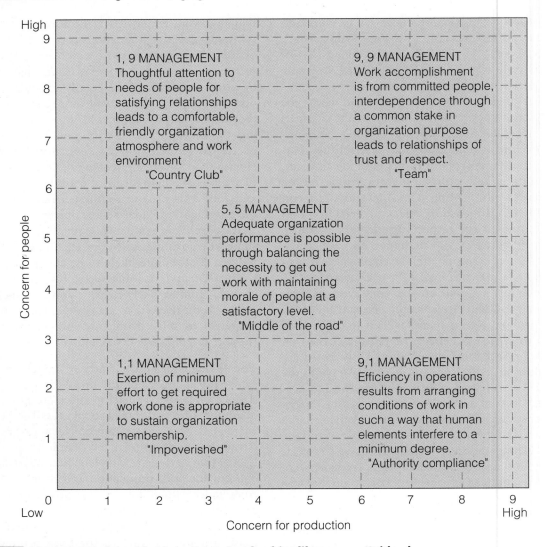

Figure 4-1 The managerial grid. *Note:* From *Leadership dilemmas—Grid solutions* by R. R. Blake and A. A. McCanse, 1991, Houston: Gulf Publishing.

effectiveness. Nurse managers may use these perspectives as a basis for analyzing the leadership styles of others and analyzing and developing their own styles.

Contingency Theories

Contingency approaches suggest managers adapt their leadership styles in relation to changing situations. According to contingency theory, leadership behaviors range from authoritarian to permissive and vary in relation to current needs and future probabilities. For example, a nurse manager may use an authoritarian style when responding to an emergency situation such as a cardiac arrest and use a participative style

to encourage development of a team strategy to care for patients with multiple system failure. The manager might delegate to a highly competent and eager follower group decision-making and task-completion in designing a new patient intake form. Therefore, the most effective leadership style for a nurse manager is the one that best complements the organizational environment, the tasks to be accomplished, and the personal characteristics of the people involved in each situation. Numerous contingency models have been developed. Four are discussed in this chapter: Fiedler's contingency theory, situational leadership theory, Vroom–Yetton expectancy model, and House–Mitchell path–goal theory.

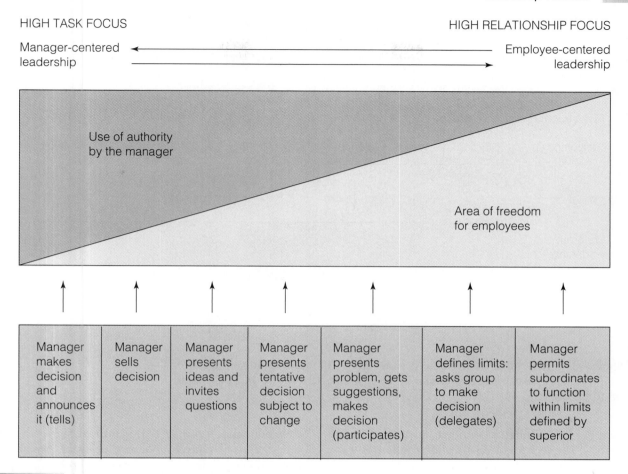

HIGH TASK FOCUS

Manager-centered
leadership

HIGH RELATIONSHIP FOCUS

Employee-centered
leadership

Use of authority
by the manager

Area of freedom
for employees

| Manager makes decision and announces it (tells) | Manager sells decision | Manager presents ideas and invites questions | Manager presents tentative decision subject to change | Manager presents problem, gets suggestions, makes decision (participates) | Manager defines limits: asks group to make decision (delegates) | Manager permits subordinates to function within limits defined by superior |

Figure 4-2 **Continuum of leadership behavior. *Note:* From "How to choose a leadership pattern" by R. Tannenbaum and W. H. Schmidt, 1973, *Harvard Business Review, 51,* p. 164.**

Fiedler's Contingency Theory Fiedler (1967) proposed that a leader is most effective when he or she matches leadership style (relationship-oriented or task-oriented) to situational factors. Fiedler described three situational factors of leadership, which are listed in decreasing order of importance: manager–follower relationship (good to poor); task structure (high to low); and manager power (strong to weak). *Manager–follower relations* reflect the degree to which the leader enjoys the loyalty and support of subordinates. *Task structure* is the degree to which the task or result is clearly described and/or standard operating procedures guarantee successful completion and evaluation of the quality of the task. *Position power* is the degree to which leaders are able to administer rewards and punishment by virtue of their positions (that is, legitimate power).

Various combinations of these three factors result in situations that are favorable, moderately favorable,

or unfavorable for manager effectiveness. Figure 4-3 illustrates the preferred leadership styles given different combinations of situational characteristics. For example, when leader–member relations are good, the task is highly structured, and the leader has strong position power, the leader can easily influence the group to accomplish organizational objectives.

Situational Leadership Theory Hersey and Blanchard (1988) expanded Fiedler's Contingency Model by considering the followers' readiness and willingness to perform the assigned tasks. In their theory of situational leadership, four distinct leadership styles (S) are prescribed according to the readiness and ability of followers (R) (Figure 4-4). Leaders use a *telling style* (S1—high task, low relationship) with followers who are unable and unwilling or insecure about performing the task (R1). Leaders use a *selling style* (S2—high task, high relationship) with followers who are

Combination of situational characteristics

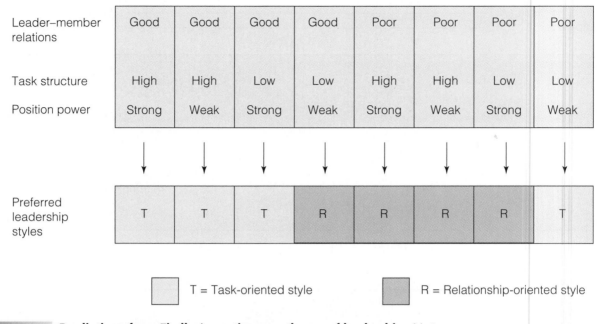

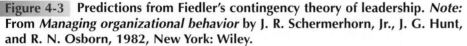

Figure 4-3 **Predictions from Fiedler's contingency theory of leadership.** *Note:* From *Managing organizational behavior* **by J. R. Schermerhorn, Jr., J. G. Hunt, and R. N. Osborn, 1982, New York: Wiley.**

unable but are willing or confident in performing the task (R2). Leaders use a *participating style* (S3—low task, high relationship) with followers who are able but unwilling or lacking in confidence in performing the task (R3). Finally, leaders use a *delegating style* (S4—low task, low relationship) with followers who are both able and willing and have confidence in performing the task (R4).

Vroom–Yetton Expectancy Model Vroom and Yetton (1973) developed a prescriptive model for determining the amount of participation leaders should seek from employees in decision making. This model, depicted in Figure 4-5, helps managers decide how to make a decision contingent on the task to be accomplished and needs of both managers and employees.

Three questions guide the manager's selection of an appropriate leadership style and the extent of participation employees should have in decision making. Is all the information available to make the decision? Is the staff's acceptance of the decision required for effective implementation? Would the group make a decision the leader could live with? Figure 4-6 depicts the factors and process a manager uses to select a leadership style. Less participative styles usually take less of the manager's and staff's time, but decisions may not be widely accepted.

Vroom and Yetton (1973) identified five leadership styles: tell, sell, consult, join, and delegate. A manager who uses a telling style assesses the problem, makes the decision independently, and informs followers; a manager who uses a selling style gathers information from followers about the problem, then makes the decision independently and persuades followers to implement it; a manager who uses a consultative style seeks advice from followers individually and then makes the decision independently and informs followers; a manager who joins the group, seeks suggestions, and then independently makes a decision and informs followers; and a manager who uses delegation works with followers in developing solutions to the problem and facilitates consensus-building toward a group solution, which generally is accepted and implemented as the group wishes.

Consider the following example. Administration wants to pilot a model of self-directed teams on one unit in the hospital. One of the nurse managers, Mary, volunteers. She analyzes the staff's responses. Using Figure 4-6, Mary addresses the following questions:

1. *Is the information needed to make the decision available?* The manager needs to know, for example, how much the staff know about self-directed teams, how they feel about them, and what they

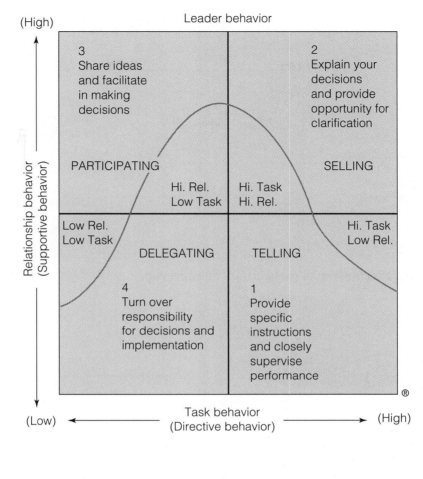

Leader behavior

(High)

3
Share ideas
and facilitate
in making
decisions

2
Explain your
decisions
and provide
opportunity for
clarification

PARTICIPATING

SELLING

Hi. Rel.
Low Task

Hi. Task
Hi. Rel.

Low Rel.
Low Task

Hi. Task
Low Rel.

DELEGATING

TELLING

4
Turn over
responsibility
for decisions and
implementation

1
Provide
specific
instructions
and closely
supervise
performance

Relationship behavior
(Supportive behavior)

(Low) ← Task behavior (High) →
(Directive behavior)

Follower readiness

High	Moderate		Low
← R4	R3	R2	R1
Able and willing or motivated	Able but unwilling or insecure	Unable but willing or motivated	Unable and unwilling or insecure

Figure 4-4 **Situational leadership.** *Note:* **Reprinted with permission from Hersey, Paul, (1988).** ***The management of organizational behavior: Utilizing human resources,*** **5th ed., Hersey and Blanchard, The Center for Leadership Studies, Escondido, California. All rights reserved.**

would need by way of training and development to implement them. The answer to question 1 is no.

2. *Is the staff's acceptance required for implementation?* In this case, the answer to question 2 is clearly yes.

3. *If the decision to adopt self-directed work teams is delegated to the staff, will they make a decision*

acceptable to Mary? She thinks not and realizes that it is the manager's responsibility to make a final decision with extensive staff involvement. Therefore, the answer to question 3 is no.

According to Figure 4-6, the leadership styles applicable in this case are either join or consult. Mary could participate with the staff in a meeting to consider the

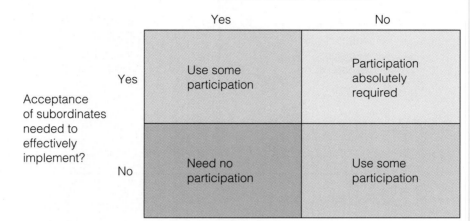

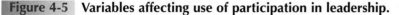

Figure 4-5 **Variables affecting use of participation in leadership.**

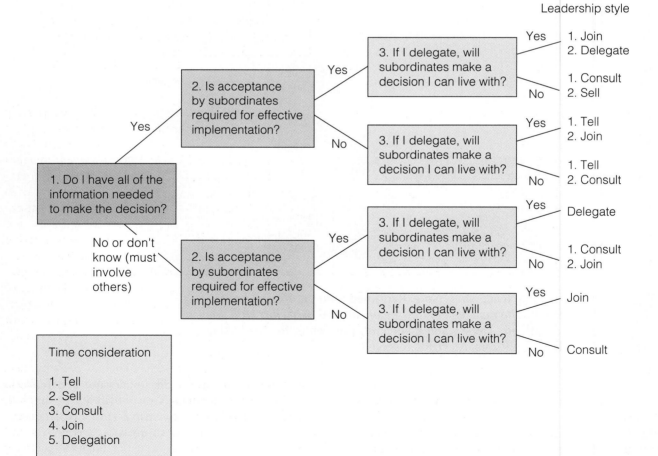

Figure 4-6 **Use of participative leadership styles. *Note:* Developed by P. J. Decker and J. Breaugh.**

costs and benefits of moving to self-directed teams, facilitate group decision making about what might be required to implement them, and create an implementation plan. Alternatively, she could discuss the pros and cons of implementing self-directed teams with individual staff members, gather information, analyze potential costs and other possible consequences to the unit, seek staff recommendations, and then make a decision.

The manner in which managers make decisions directly reflects their leadership style. A model or framework that addresses the many contingencies in a decision-making situation helps managers analyze how to make decisions successfully. It also helps managers demonstrate a consistent, predictable decision-making style, which enables co-workers to anticipate the manager's expectations and perform accordingly.

House–Mitchell Path–Goal Theory   Path–goal theory applies a theory of human motivation and task performance to leadership effectiveness (House & Mitchell, 1974). Because a primary function of leadership is to motivate others to attain goals, path–goal theory proposes that removing obstacles to goal attainment, coaching, and providing personal rewards for achievement will result in high levels of performance and productivity. The leader affects performance by influencing employees' perceptions of their work and personal goals and facilitating the process by which employees achieve goals.

The motivational functions of leadership derive directly from the expectancy theory of motivation (Porter & Lawler, 1968; Vroom, 1964.) (Also see Chapter 20.) Employees work for rewards they find attractive and that result from successful performance. Three concepts are central to expectancy theory: **Expectancy** is the perceived probability that effort will result in successful performance. **Instrumentality** is the perceived probability that performance will lead to desired outcomes. **Valence** is the probability that the desired outcomes will lead to a valued reward. The manager exercises leadership by defining and clarifying expectancies, instrumentalities, and valences associated with specific tasks and employees' personal goals.

Path–goal theory specifies four leader behaviors (House, 1971): **Directive leadership** involves telling employees what is expected, giving specific guidance, ensuring adherence to rules and procedures, and scheduling and coordinating work efforts. This type of leadership is most effective for employees who are marginally trained or prepared and are performing

---

KEY TERMS

Expectancy   The perceived probability that effort will result in successful performance.

Instrumentality   The perceived probability that performance will lead to desired outcomes.

Valence   The probability that desired outcomes will lead to a valued reward.

Directive leadership   A leadership style that involves telling employees expectations, giving guidance, ensuring adherence to rules, and scheduling work efforts.

Supportive leadership   A leadership style that focuses on the needs of employees.

Participative leadership   A leadership style that involves consultation with subordinates in decision making.

Achievement-oriented leadership   A leadership style that includes goal setting and maintaining high levels of performance in order to motivate employees.

---

partially routine and ambiguous tasks. Supportive leadership focuses on the needs of employees, displays concern for their well-being, and creates a friendly climate in the work environment. **Supportive leadership** behavior is most effective for employees who are performing routine work or are very experienced with the work. **Participative leadership** involves consultation with subordinates and requests for opinions and suggestions, which the leader takes into consideration when making decisions. This style works best for employees who have moderate skill levels and are performing somewhat ambiguous work. Involvement of employees encourages mutual clarification of objectives and specification of mutually helpful work processes. **Achievement-oriented leadership** includes setting challenging goals, seeking performance improvements, emphasizing excellence in performance, and showing confidence that employees will attain high levels of performance. It is indicated for employees who are skilled and perform highly innovative and ambiguous work. By setting challenging goals and pointing out valued rewards, managers fulfill a strong motivating role.

Staff members interpret and respond to leader behavior in different ways, depending on personal

characteristics and characteristics of the task and environment. Specifically, employees' needs for achievement, affiliation, power, competence, autonomy, and
personality traits form a context within which leaders
function. As in situational leadership, the effect of
leadership behavior on employee satisfaction and effort depends on the nature of the task and the work
situation.

Path–goal theory is interesting because it suggests
that there are substitutes for direct leader–follower
interaction. On one hand, the manager can influence
employee performance directly by clarifying the route
to desired goals. On the other hand, actions that clarify objectives, specify roles, increase the value of rewards, provide needed support to complete tasks successfully, and facilitate performance might be viewed
as substitutes for direct leadership activity.

The application of any contingency theory to leadership practice requires continuous monitoring of employees' expectancies, abilities, and motivations and
an understanding of the task and options for completing it. Managers must also thoroughly consider
the consequences of their actions on employee performance. For every leader's action, a predictable employee reaction is likely to occur. A nurse manager
must carefully observe the cause-and-effect relationships that exist between leader behavior and employee
response and continuously take into account the multitude of environmental factors that influence leader–
employee interactions.

Contemporary Theories: Quantum Leadership

Trait, behavioral, and contingency theories represent
conventional approaches to leadership and have provided important foundations for leadership. Current
views of leadership are neither complete reformula-
tions nor simple refinements of conventional perspectives. Evolved from the principles of quantum
mechanics, effective leadership today reflects a re-
markable fusion of trait, behavior, and contingency
approaches. Quantum leadership is based on the
concept that reality is a set of relationships expressed
at varying and continuously changing levels of complexity (Zohar, 1990). Within this framework, organizations are viewed as whole systems in which work
requirements and roles are fluid and change to effect
purposeful work that is outcome oriented. To this
end, the workers become directly involved in decision
making as equitable and accountable partners, while
managers assume more of an influential facilitative

role, rather than one of control (Porter-O'Grady, 1997,
1999). Following is a discussion of six perspectives
of quantum leadership—charismatic, transactional,
transformational, connective, shared, and servant—
and the contributions these conceptualizations have
made to the evolution of successful leadership.

Charismatic Leadership Charismatic leadership is
based on personal qualities such as charm, persua-
siveness, personal power, self-confidence, extraordinary ideas, and strong (often unconventional) convictions. The leader's personality arouses great affection
and emotional commitment, first to the leader and
secondarily to the beliefs and causes the leader es-
pouses. Few leaders possess genuine charisma. Those
who do often use their powerful personalities to advance revolutionary goals.

Transactional and Transformational Leadership
Transactional leadership is similar to the path–goal
view of leadership and is based on the principles of
social exchange theory (Homans, 1958; Thibaut &
Kelley, 1959). The primary premise of social exchange
theory is that individuals engage in social interactions
expecting to give and receive social, political, and psychological benefits or rewards. The exchange process
between leaders and followers is viewed as essentially
economic. Once initiated, a sequence of exchange behavior continues until one or both parties finds that
the exchange of performance and rewards is no longer
valuable. The nature of these transactions is determined by the participating parties' assessments of
what is in their best interests; for example, staff respond affirmatively to a nurse manager's request to
work overtime in exchange for granting special requests for time off. Leaders are successful to the extent that they understand and meet the needs of followers and use incentives to enhance employee loyalty
and performance. Transactional leadership is aimed at
maintaining equilibrium, or the status quo, by performing work according to policy and procedures,
maximizing self-interests and personal rewards, emphasizing interpersonal dependence, and routinizing
performance.

Transformational leadership, in contrast, moves
people beyond transactions and interpersonal exchanges to performance beyond basic expectations
(Bass, 1985). Transformational leadership is not concerned with the status quo, but with effecting revolutionary change in organizations and human service.
Whereas traditional views of leadership emphasize
the differences between employees and managers,
transformational leadership focuses on merging the

motives, desires, values, and goals of leaders and followers into a common cause. The goal of the transformational leader is to generate employees' commitment to the vision or ideal rather than to themselves.

Transformational leaders appeal to individuals' better selves rather than these individuals' self-interests. They foster followers' inborn desires to pursue higher values, humanitarian ideals, moral missions, and causes. Transformational leaders also encourage others to exercise leadership. The transformational leader inspires followers and uses power to instill a belief that followers also have the ability to do exceptional things (Burns, 1978). The effectiveness of this leadership style depends on the leader's ability to stimulate the growth and development of others and discourage dependence.

Transformational leaders may be a natural model for nursing managers, because nursing has traditionally been driven by its social mandate and its ethic of human service. Transformational leadership can be used effectively by nurses with clients or co-workers at the bedside, in the home, in the community health center, and in the health care organization.

Connective Leadership   Leaders in today's health care environment place increasing value on collaboration and teamwork in all aspects of the organization. They recognize that as health systems become more complex and require integration, personnel who perform the managerial and clinical work must cooperate, coordinate their efforts, and produce joint results. Leaders must use additional skills, especially group and political leadership skills, to create collegial work environments.

Recognizing the role of leaders in fostering collaborative intraorganizational and interorganizational relationships, Klakovich (1994) proposed a **connective leadership** paradigm for nursing. This paradigm acknowledges the need for more flexible systems in health care that empower employees, their interdisciplinary colleagues, clients, and families. Klakovich explains that contemporary nursing leadership skills should include the ability to create interconnections between and across caregiving settings and among multiple constituencies. The purpose of connective leadership is to better coordinate and integrate patient care services in a caring, noncompetitive manner. The focus of leadership is to link professionals, communities, governing groups, and voluntary agencies to improve patient-centered care. Connective leaders use their interpersonal skills to broker alliances, encourage collaboration, and integrate systems. Klakovich

stresses the importance of collegiality among health care professionals in achieving patient care and organizational goals.

The nurse manager applies connective leadership principles when convening a group of physicians, administrators, nursing staff, and representatives of other disciplines to plan a new patient care program, bringing nursing staff members together to develop a staff orientation program, or seeking the assistance of an external expert to help in the professional development of the nursing staff. Connective leadership, according to Klakovich, functions to break down hierarchical relationships and develop leadership skills at all levels in the organization.

Connective and integrative leaders apply unique skills. According to Charns and Tewksbury (1993), these leaders must use both content and process skills (such as the task and relationship skills discussed earlier). Use of both power and political tactics may be needed (see Chapter 6). The ability to manage groups and team interactions is essential. (Teams and team-building are discussed in Chapter 15.) In addition, leaders must recognize that integrating the activities of diverse participants in health care involves creating connections that extend beyond well-defined groups. The process of creating connections and fostering integration requires that the leader (a) identify actual and potential collaborators; (b) communicate and sell a potential shared vision to those in varied settings and under disparate conditions; (c) describe the value each collaborator could bring to the endeavor, both to the individual and others; (d) facilitate communication by sharing information, preparing for interactions, and following up on communications exchanges; (e) build and maintain social interaction and comfort; (f) define and sell roles and assignments; (g) track and reward contributions; and (h) formalize an integrated effort at the right time.

Shared Leadership   Reorganization, decentralization, and the increasing complexity of problem solving in health care have forced administrators to recognize the value of **shared leadership**, which is based on the empowerment principles of participative and transformational leadership. Essential elements of shared leadership are relationships, dialogues, partnerships and understanding boundaries (McCrea, 1998). The application of shared leadership assumes that a well-educated, highly professional, dedicated workforce is comprised of many leaders. It also assumes that the notion of a single nurse as the wise and heroic leader is unrealistic and that many individuals at various levels in the organization must be responsible for the organization's fate and performance. Different issues call for different leaders, or experts, to guide the problem-solving process. A single leader is not expected always to have knowledge and ability beyond that of other members of the work group. Appropriate leadership emerges in relation to the current challenges of the work unit or the organization. Individuals in formal leadership positions and their colleagues are expected to participate in a pattern of reciprocal influence processes. Examples of shared leadership in nursing include the following:

- *Self-directed work teams.* Work groups manage their own planning, organizing, scheduling, and day-to-day work activities.
- *Shared governance.* The nursing staff are formally organized at the service area and organizational levels to make key decisions about clinical practice standards, quality assurance and improvement, staff development, professional development, aspects of unit operations, and research. Decision making is conducted by representatives of the nursing staff who have been authorized by the administrative hierarchy and their colleagues to make decisions about important matters.
- *Co-leadership.* Two people work together to execute a leadership role. This kind of leadership has become more common in service-line management, where the skills of both a clinical and administrative leader are needed to successfully

direct the operations of a multidisciplinary service. For example, a nurse manager provides administrative leadership in collaboration with a clinical nurse specialist, who provides clinical leadership. The development of co-leadership roles depends on the flexibility and maturity of both individuals, and such arrangements usually require a third party to provide ongoing consultation and guidance to the pair.

Current health care environments require innovations in care delivery and therefore innovative leadership approaches. Clearly, the principles of participative, transformational, shared governance, and shared leadership have arisen in response to the leadership challenges of complex health care environments.

Servant Leadership   **Servant leadership** is based on the premise that leadership originates from a desire to serve and that in the course of serving, one may be called to lead. According to Greenleaf (1991, p. 7), servant leadership occurs when other people's needs take priority, when those being served "become healthier, wiser, freer, more autonomous, and more likely themselves to become servants." The servant leader must address the question of whether the least advantaged in society benefit from the leader's service. The concept of servant leadership may have some substantive appeal for nursing leadership because nursing is founded on principles of caring, service, and the growth and health of others. Nurse leaders serve many constituencies, often quite selflessly, and consequently bring about change in individuals, systems, and organizations.

The concepts of charismatic, transactional, transformational, connective, shared, and servant leadership comprise a new generation of leadership styles that have emerged in response to the need to humanize working environments and improve organizational performance. Traditional perspectives, especially participative leadership, also offer nurse managers leadership concepts that may be emulated, learned, modeled, and refined in management practice.

Management Functions

Classical Description

In 1916, French industrialist Henri Fayol first described the functions of management as planning, organizing, directing, and controlling. These are still relevant today.

Planning Planning is a four-stage process to (a) establish objectives (goals), (b) evaluate the present situation and predict future trends and events, (c) formulate a planning statement (means), and (d) convert the plan into an action statement. Planning is important on both an organizational and a personal level and may be an individual or group process that addresses the questions of *what, why, where, when, how,* and *by whom.* Decision making and problem solving are inherent in planning. Numerous computer software programs and databases are available to help facilitate planning.

Organization-level plans, such as determining organizational structure and staffing or operational budgets, evolve from the mission, philosophy, and goals of the organization. The nurse manager plans and develops specific goals and objectives for her or his area of responsibility. For example, if part of the mission of a home care agency is to meet the health care needs of the childrearing family, Tom, the nurse manager, might plan to establish an in-home phototherapy program. To effectively implement this program, he would need to address (a) how the program supported the organization's mission, (b) why the service would benefit the community and the organization, (c) who

would be candidates for the program, (d) who would provide the service, (e) how staffing would be accomplished, (f) how charges would be generated, and (g) what those charges should be.

Planning can be contingent or strategic. **Contingency planning** refers to the identification and management of the many problems that interfere with getting work done. Contingency planning may be *reactive*, in response to a crisis, or *proactive*, in anticipation of problems or in response to opportunities. For example, what would you do if two registered nurses called in sick for the 12-hour night shift? What if you were a manager for a specialty unit and received a call for an admission, but had no more beds? Or what if you were a pediatric oncology clinic manager and a patient's sibling exposes a number of immunocompromised patients to chickenpox? Planning for crises such as these are examples of contingency planning.

Strategic planning refers to defining and prioritizing long-term objectives of the organization and developing strategies for implementation. Strategic planning is future-oriented, focusing on plans for the next 2 to 5 years. Its purpose is to create an image of the desired future and design ways to make those plans a reality (Johnson, 1992). To do so involves a systematic process of assessing the internal and external environment, identifying strengths, recognizing demands, acknowledging sources of competition, and assessing available means by which to achieve the desired end. Strategic planning is a proactive process and is described in more detail in Chapter 2. Examples of strategic plans might include an acute care hospital's addition of home health care services or a health department's initiative to provide public health nurses with notebook computers.

Organizing Organizing is the process of coordinating the work to be done. Formally, it involves identifying the work of the organization, dividing the labor, developing the chain of command, and assigning authority. It is an ongoing process that systematically reviews the use of human and material resources. In health care, the mission, formal organizational structure, delivery systems, job descriptions, skill mix, and staffing patterns form the basis for the organization. For example, in organizing the home phototherapy project, Tom develops job descriptions and protocols, determines how many positions are required, selects a vendor, and orders supplies.

Directing Directing involves the process of getting the organization's work done. Power, authority, and

KEY TERMS

Controlling The process of establishing standards of performance, determining the means to be used in measuring performance, evaluating performance, and providing feedback.

leadership style are intimately related to a manager's ability to direct. Communication abilities, motivational techniques, and delegation skills also are important. In today's health care organization, professional staff are autonomous, requiring guidance rather than direction. Today's manager is more likely to sell the idea, proposal, or new project to staff rather than tell them what to do. The manager coaches and counsels to achieve the organization's objectives. In fact, it may be the nurse who assumes the traditional directing role when working with unlicensed personnel. For example, in directing the home phototherapy project, Tom assembles the team of nurses to provide the service, explains the purpose and constraints of the program, and allows the team to decide how they will staff the project, giving guidance and direction when needed.

Controlling **Controlling** functions involve establishing standards of performance, determining the means to be used in measuring performance, evaluating performance, and providing feedback. The efficient manager constantly attempts to improve productivity by incorporating techniques of quality management,

evaluating outcomes and performance, and instituting change as necessary.

Today, managers share many of the control functions with the staff. In organizations using a formal quality improvement process, such as continuous quality improvement (CQI), staff participate in and lead the teams. Some organizations use peer review to control quality of care. When Tom introduces the home phototherapy program, for example, the team of nurses involved in the program identify standards regarding phototherapy and their individual performances. A subgroup of the team routinely reviews monitors designed for the program and identifies ways to improve the program.

Planning, organizing, directing, and controlling reflect a systematic, proactive approach to management. This approach is used widely in all types of organizations, health care included. A newer model is based on a behavioral approach to management.

Mintzberg's Behavioral Description

Mintzberg (1973) believed that much of a manager's activity involves human relations, a premise that would seem to be supported in nursing. A study of nurse managers in community agencies and hospitals (Dienemann & Shaffer, 1992) found that managers reported devoting more than half their time to human resource management and nursing services (Figure 4-7). Mintzberg also believed managers were more reactive than proactive. As a result of these two premises, he identified ten management roles, which he placed in

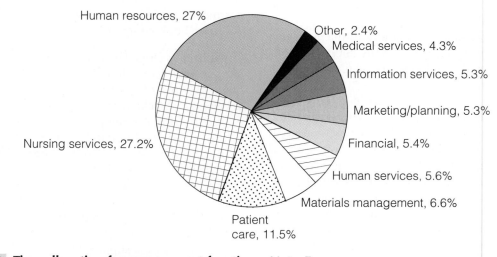

Human resources, 27%
Other, 2.4%
Medical services, 4.3%
Information services, 5.3%
Marketing/planning, 5.3%
Financial, 5.4%
Human services, 5.6%
Materials management, 6.6%
Patient care, 11.5%
Nursing services, 27.2%

Figure 4-7 **Time allocation for management functions.** *Note:* **From "Management Responsibilities in Community Agencies and Hospitals" by J. Dienemann and C. Shaffer, 1992,** *Journal of Nursing Administration, 22,* **p. 43.**

| Table 4-3 | Mintzberg's Managerial Roles and Functions |

Roles	Functions
Interpersonal roles	
Figurehead	Performs ceremonial duties.
Leader	Defines work environment and is responsible for subordinate's work.
Liaison	Expands outside information sources and networks.
Informational roles	
Monitor	Internally seeks information about organization.
Disseminator	Shares information within organization.
Spokesperson	Shares information outside organization.
Decisional roles	
Entrepreneur	Seeks ways to solve problems/improve organization.
Disturbance handler	Responds to problems.
Resource allocator	Manages time and coordinates efforts.
Negotiator	Mediates resources/decisions with outside forces.

Note: Developed from *The nature of managerial work* by H. Mintzberg, 1973, New York: Harper & Row.

three categories: interpersonal roles, informational roles, and decisional roles (Table 4-3).

Interpersonal Roles Mintzberg describes three interpersonal roles that reflect the formal authority inherent in the manager's position: the figurehead, the leader, and the liaison. The *figurehead* role reflects the ceremonial performance of duties, such as welcoming new employees at orientation or attending social events. As a *leader*, the manager defines the work environment of the organization and is responsible for the work of associates—motivating, training, and disciplining as needed. The manager, as a leader, determines the mission and objectives of the organization and sees that they are accomplished efficiently. The third interpersonal role, *liaison*, deals with expanding the manager's information sources and networks outside the organization. National conferences, local coalitions, and professional meetings are valuable resources for obtaining information and expanding networks.

Informational Roles Mintzberg also describes three informational roles. As a *monitor*, the manager informally seeks information about the organization through internal networks, gossip, and observations. Tours of the organization, as well as formal and informal meetings, provide the manager with information about the needs and functions of the organization. In the *disseminator* role, managers either share information between work units or share information from outside the organization. Information is a source of power; sharing information empowers employees and improves job satisfaction. As a *spokesperson*, the manager shares information with individuals outside the organization and provides visibility for the organization. Attending community meetings, offering continuing education, and participating in professional organizations are examples of ways in which the manager serves as a spokesperson.

Decisional Roles Mintzberg describes four decisional roles. The *entrepreneur* constantly seeks ways to solve problems and make improvements in the organization. Reorganization of supplies, staff redesign, and creation of new roles are all examples of entrepreneurship. The *disturbance handler* responds to unforeseen circumstances, such as replacement of staff for sick call, nosocomial outbreaks, or missing equipment. As *resource allocators*, managers schedule their own time, determine division and coordination of work, and authorize the timing and implementation of major decisions. Finally, the *negotiator* deals with outside forces mediating resources and decisions, such as resolving labor disputes or making business acquisitions.

A Contemporary Model of Managerial Work

Mintzberg (1994) proposed a new model to describe managerial functions depicted in Figure 4-8. In this model, managerial work is envisioned as occurring on three levels represented by concentric circles: *information, people,* and *action*. The manager, in the center, brings to the position a set of values, experiences, knowledge, and competencies. The manager conceives the frame, which includes the purpose of the job, the work needed, and how it should be done. This is the basic core of managing as shown in the center of Figure 4-8. Managerial work occurs through three levels represented by the three concentric circles shown: *information, people,* and *action*. Managing involves the following five roles, *communicating* and *controlling* at the information level, *leading* and *linking* at the people level, and *doing* at the action level.

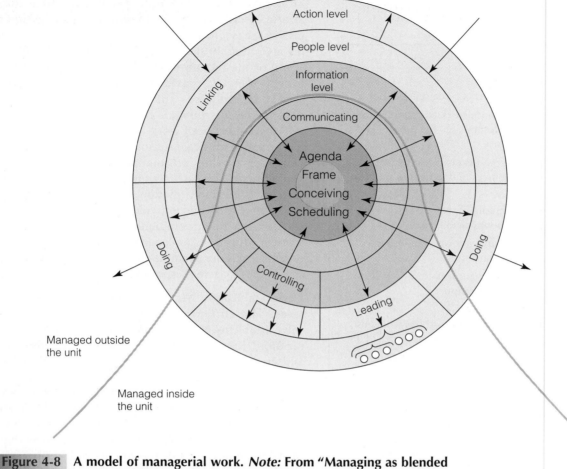

Figure 4-8   **A model of managerial work.** *Note:* From "Managing as blended care" by H. Mintzberg, 1994, *Journal of Nursing Administration, 24,* p. 30.

The first level of work, informational processing, is the most abstract and includes communicating and controlling. *Communicating* involves receiving and sharing information with others, whereas *controlling* is using information to manage the work of others.

The second level of managerial work involves leading and linking people in order to encourage people to take action. *Leading* is the encouraging and enabling of others—individually, as a team, or as an entire organization—to take effective action. *Linking* is the manager's establishment of networks outside the unit in order to relay needs and exchange influence.

At the third and most concrete level, the focus is on managing action by *doing.* Doing includes taking supervisory actions—directing change, handling disturbances, and negotiating external agreements.

Using this framework for an analysis of nursing management, Mintzberg (1994) found that the roles previously described are blended into an intricate

caring management style. Although still being tested, this model expands the role of human relations in management.

Roles and Functions of Nursing Managers

The American Organization of Nurse Executives (AONE) is an organization for the top nursing administrators in hospitals. AONE describes six roles and functions of the nurse manager (1992):

1. *The nurse manager is accountable for excellence in the clinical practice of nursing and the delivery of patient care on a selected unit or area within the health care institution.*

   This function is the primary focus of the nurse manager. To meet this responsibility, the nurse manager has the authority to plan and implement strategies and programs consistent with the organization's policies, goals, and objectives, as well as with professional standards and governmental rules and regulations. The manager is responsible for maintaining a safe and caring environment that promotes health teaching and maintenance. The manager is responsible for assessing patient and family response to nursing care as well as evaluating the effectiveness and quality of the care and services and their consistency with identified regimens. Supporting research and ensuring that research findings are incorporated into practice are also the responsibility of the manager.

2. *The nurse manager is accountable for managing human, fiscal, and other resources needed to manage clinical nursing practice and patient care.*

   With heightened awareness of the cost of health care, managers face a difficult task. Because nurses are the primary providers of patient care, nursing accounts for use of most of the resources. Therefore, nurse managers are accountable for efficient use of personnel, equipment, and supplies. Skill mix is important in meeting patient needs. Consequently, managers must prepare, monitor, and maintain budgets consistent with health care policy and economics. The nurse manager also must ensure that the staff are proficient in providing care and in using available equipment and resources wisely. It is the manager's responsibility to communicate to the staff constraints regarding resources and to coach and mentor the staff appropriately.

3. *The nurse manager is accountable for facilitating development of licensed and unlicensed nursing and health care personnel.*

   In order to maintain excellence in nursing practice and patient care, the staff must be competent to perform delegated roles and responsibilities. The manager is responsible for seeing that competency levels are maintained and that staff acquire new skills as needed. The nurse manager also plays an important role in providing a supportive environment for nursing and other health profession students.

4. *The nurse manager is accountable for ensuring institutional compliance with professional, regulatory, and government standards of care.*

   The provision of excellent nursing practice and patient care also involves compliance with standards of care. The nurse manager must be informed and be able to translate pertinent standards of care for staff and to implement required programs.

5. *The nurse manager is accountable for strategic planning as it relates to the unit(s) or area(s), department, and organization as a whole.*

   The manager is responsible for communicating input from the staff to the clinical director and chief nurse executive. The nurse manager also is responsible for developing and implementing a strategic plan for the unit that supports the department's and organization's plan. Finally, the manager is responsible for facilitating staff support for the strategic plan and modifying the plan as needed in response to changes in the environment.

6. *The nurse manager is accountable for facilitating cooperative and collaborative relationships among disciplines/departments to ensure effective quality patient care delivery.*

   Today, more than ever, cooperative and collaborative relationships are necessary to deliver efficient, cost-effective care. The nurse manager plays an important role in developing collegial relationships based on mutual respect and support. To do so, the manager must play an active role in interdisciplinary committees responsible for developing patient-focused programs.

Levels of Management

Whereas managers direct the work of a specified area, product line, or service, administrators (sometimes called executives) focus on establishing goals and on integrating work units to achieve the organization's mission. Generally, three levels of management are used in nursing: first (nurse manager), middle (director), and upper (executive) (Figure 4-9), although the tendency today is to continually push management decisions to lower and lower levels.

First-Level Management

The **first-level** manager, also known as a *first-line manager*, is responsible for supervising the work of nonmanagerial personnel and the day-to-day activities of a specific work unit or units. The manager is

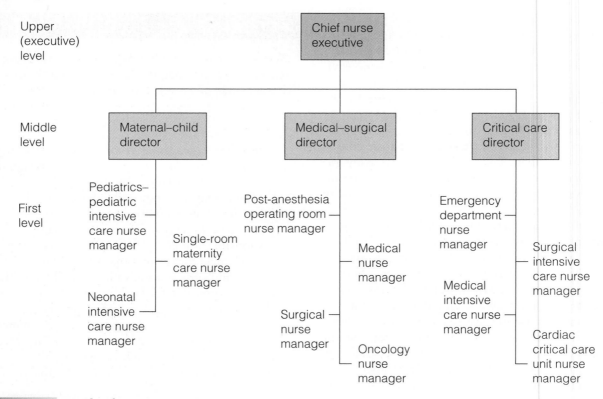

Figure 4-9   Levels of management.

responsible for clinical nursing practice; patient care delivery; use of human, fiscal, and other resources; personnel development; compliance with regulatory and professional standards; fostering interdisciplinary, collaborative relationships; and strategic planning (AONE, 1992). With primary responsibility for motivating the staff to achieve the organization's goals, the first-level manager represents staff to upper administration, and vice versa. Nurse managers have 24-hour accountability for the management of a unit(s) or area(s) within a health care organization. In the hospital setting, the first-level manager is usually the head nurse, nurse manager, or an assistant. In other settings, such as a home health care agency, a first-level manager may be referred to as a coordinator.

Bob is an example of a first-level manager. As the manager for a surgical intensive care unit (SICU), Bob is routinely responsible for supervising patient care, trouble-shooting, maintaining compliance with standards, and giving guidance and direction as needed. In addition, he has fiscal and committee responsibilities and is accountable to the organization for maintaining its philosophies and objectives. The following exemplifies a typical day.

As Bob came on duty, he learned that there had been a multiple car accident and that three of the victims were currently in surgery and destined for the unit. The assistant manager for nights had secured more staff for days: two part-time SICU nurses and a staff nurse from the surgical floor. However, she had not had time to arrange for two more patients to be moved out of the unit. From their assigned nurses, Bob obtained an update on the patients who were candidates for transfer and, in consultation with his assistant, made the appropriate arrangements for the transfers. Other staffing problems were at hand: In addition to the nurse who had been pulled from the floor, there were two orientees, and the staff needed to attend a safety inservice. As soon as the charge nurse came in, Bob apprised her of the situation. Together, they reviewed the operating room schedule and identified staffing arrangements. Fortunately, Bob had only one meeting today and would be available for backup staffing. In the meantime, he would work on evaluations.

After his discussions with the charge nurse, Bob met with each of the night nurses to get an update on the status of the other patients. Then he went to his office to review his messages and plan his day. Tamera, an RN, had just learned she was pregnant, but she stated that she planned to work until delivery. Bob learned that his budget hearing had been scheduled for the following Monday at 10 A.M. A pharmaceutical representative wanted to provide an inservice for the unit. Fortunately, there were no immediate crises. He called his supervisor to inform her of the status of affairs on the unit and learned that two other individuals in the accident had been transported to another hospital; one had since died. They discussed the ethical and legal ramifications. Bob would need to review the policies on relations with the press and law enforcement and to update his staff.

As the first patient returned from surgery, Bob went to help admit the patient and receive a report. Learning that the patient was stable, he informed the charge nurse that the patient they had just received was likely to be charged with manslaughter and reviewed media and legal policies with her. They also discussed how the staff were doing. There were some equipment problems in room 2110; the charge nurse had temporarily placed the patient on a transport monitor and was waiting for a biomedical technology staff member to check the monitor. Could Bob follow up? Bob agreed and commended the charge nurse for her problem solving. The charge nurse reminded Bob they would need backup for lunch and inservices.

As Bob returned to his office, he noted that the alarms were turned off on one of the patients. He pulled aside the nurse assigned to the patient and reminded her of the necessity to keep the alarms on at all times. Finally, back in his office he called biomedical technology to ascertain their plans to check the monitor and made notes regarding the charge nurse's problem-solving abilities and the staff nurse's negligence. He reviewed staffing for the next 24 hours and noted that an extra nurse was needed for both the evening and night shifts because of the increased workload. After finding staff, he was able to finish one evaluation before covering for the inservices and lunch and then attending the policy and procedure team meeting.

Middle-Level Management

The **middle-level manager** supervises a number of first-level managers, usually within related specialties or in a given geographic area. Middle-level managers are

responsible for the people and activities within the departments they supervise, and they too have 24-hour responsibility for their defined area. Typically, middle-level managers act as a liaison between upper management and first-level managers. A middle manager may be referred to as a supervisor, director, or assistant or associate director of nursing. Today, graduate education often is required for this position.

Alice is a middle-level manager. She is the director of maternal–child nursing at a large hospital. Within her division are the pediatric unit, pediatric intensive care unit (PICU), newborn intensive care unit (NICU), and the single-room maternity care (SRMC) area. Three nurse managers report to her. Alice routinely meets with her managers each day to identify patient or employee issues. She assists the managers in decision making and problem solving. She facilitates interdepartmental collaboration. In fact, much of her day is spent in meetings. A typical day might look like this.

Alice usually starts her day with personal organization, noting what meetings she has scheduled and planning when she will meet with her managers. From the bed census reports she notes that both the pediatric and PICUs are full; the newborn intensive care unit and single room maternity care area have low censuses. Today, the first thing on Alice's agenda is an interdisciplinary meeting with the obstetricians. As Alice enters the meeting, she thinks about the issues involved. Alice wants to know what plans her institution has for the residency program in light of another local hospital's closure of its obstetrical units. Will more residents be placed at her institution? What will be the impact on census and, subsequently, staffing? What, if any, fiscal effects will be noted? A great deal of discussion in the meeting revolves around the topic. Additional topics discussed are current quality improvement measures, departmental statistics, and recently released new care guidelines.

Following the interdisciplinary meeting, Alice meets with the SRMC nurse manager. They discuss the impact of an increase in residents. Alice suggests that the manager envision the direction the unit will take and present a plan for growth and development. They also discuss the status of the patients and staff. Since census is down in SRMC, the pediatric unit could use more staff. The manager informs Alice about a high-risk patient; her infant was admitted to NICU for a septic work-up. Alice next meets with the manager of NICU. She makes a point to get a report on the new infant. In addition, she learns two transport teams are out getting babies and that there is a potential for a third. The manager also identifies a need to set a meeting time to discuss the educational conference she proposed the hospital would offer that fall. The appointment is set, and Alice suggests the manager be prepared to identify a team to handle the arrangements. The meeting with the pediatric/PICU manager is brief because she is busy helping the staff. Alice learns the booming census is due to a number of respiratory illnesses. Because all patients are stable, she asks if some of the adolescents can be moved to adult units to make more room for smaller children. Alice agrees to make the arrangements and informs the manager that staffing assistance is available from SRMC.

Alice returns to her office, arranges for adolescent transfers to medical and surgical units, reads her mail, and returns phone calls. A distributor wants to talk about a new product, a nursing school faculty member wants to discuss new clinical opportunities, a graduate student wants to examine the potential for research, Dr. Smith wants to explore the possibility of implementing a new procedure, and the director of the laboratory wants to discuss a problem with maintaining hazard precautions with placentas.

After a quick lunch, Alice heads to the Continuous Quality Improvement meeting, which she chairs. The quarterly nurse council meeting is next. She returns the phone calls she received earlier before heading home for the day.

Many changes are occurring in first- and middle-level management in hospitals and other health care organizations today. In some, middle management positions are being consolidated and/or eliminated. Rather than holding the position of director of maternal–child nursing overseeing three managers and their subsequent units, the middle manager may hold the title of director of clinical services, with responsibility spanning all medical–surgical services. In addition, departments previously under separate management, such as laboratory and respiratory therapy, now may

be under the direction of nursing. These changes reflect attempts at cost containment, increased recognition of the professionalism of nursing, and the advanced preparation of nurse managers (Capozzoli, 1991). Movement toward a more participatory style of decentralized management also has encouraged such reorganization. Not only does the organization benefit, but so do the patients, staff, and the individual managers. Savings in management salaries can be used to meet cost-containment goals, purchase more equipment, or hire more caregivers. Decentralization empowers the manager and the staff, increasing job satisfaction and improving the quality of care.

Upper-Level Management

Upper-level management, or *executive-level management*, refers to top executives (administrators) such as the vice president for nursing or chief nurse executive, to whom middle managers report. This administrator is primarily responsible for establishing organizational goals and strategic plans for the entire division of nursing for integrating work units to achieve the organization's mission, and buffering the effects of the external environment on nurses within the organization. Some chief nurse executives have responsibilities for other departments, such as the respiratory therapy, housekeeping, or dietary departments. Nurses also are assuming systemwide administrative roles as directors of education, informatics, and quality (Krejci, 1999).

According to the American Organization of Nurse Executives (1990, p. 1), "A nurse executive is a registered nurse who is part of the executive management team and as such is responsible for the management of the nursing organization and the clinical practice of nursing throughout the organization." At this level, a graduate degree and a record of progressively increased management experience are necessary.

An example of a chief nurse executive (CNE) is Theresa, who is in charge of nursing at a 500-bed hospital. As such, she is intimately involved with the administration of the hospital. On any given day she may meet with other administrators or executives. She also may meet with community or professional leaders. Theresa spends much of her time gathering and sharing information.

Theresa has ultimate responsibility for the quality and cost effectiveness of the nursing care provided in the organization. As CNE, she is mutually responsible for establishing and maintaining a safe, caring environment for nursing practice and patient care. This involves an assessment of the internal and external environment. Internal factors include patient mix;

nursing staff mix, skills, and knowledge; research and education activities; available resources; and established health care outcomes. External factors include bioethical standards, legislation and regulations, public and health policy, community needs and expectations, economic climate, and technology.

Theresa also needs to be able to forecast trends, participate in strategic planning, and interpret the role of nursing to other disciplines in the strategic plan. She then develops and implements policies and programs based on available resources that support nursing practice and the mission of the organization. These policies and procedures address not only patient care issues but also the development of education and research programs. She also is responsible for evaluating nursing policies, programs, and services for effectiveness and consistency with the organization's mission, goals, and objectives. Another important role is the mentoring and career development of other nurse managers. Through role modeling, meetings, and education, Theresa provides examples of leadership and professionalism.

Charge Nurse

In health care, a number of roles that do not fit the traditional levels of management have evolved. The **charge nurse** is one of these. In some organizations, the position may be permanent and assigned and thus a part of the formal management team; in other organizations, the job may be rotated among experienced staff. In still other organizations, the assistant head nurse may perform the functions usually relegated to the charge nurse. In some organizations, a differential amount of compensation is paid to the person performing charge duties; in others, no differential is paid because the position is shared equally among staff or represents a higher rung of a career ladder (possibly the first rung of a management ladder).

Although the job description varies from organization to organization, the charge nurse position is an expanded staff nurse role with increased responsibility. The charge nurse functions as a liaison to the nurse manager, assisting in shift-by-shift coordination and promotion of quality patient care as well as efficient use of resources. The charge nurse often troubleshoots problems and assists other staff members in decision making. Role modeling, mentoring, and educating are additional roles that the charge nurse often assumes. Therefore, the charge nurse usually has extensive experience, skills, and knowledge in clinical practice and is familiar with the organization's standards and practices.

There are numerous ways in which the charge nurse's job differs from that of the first-level manager. First, the charge nurse's responsibilities are confined to a specific shift or task, whereas the first-level manager has 24-hour responsibility and accountability for all unit activities. Second, the charge nurse has limited authority; the charge nurse functions as an agent of the manager and is accountable to the manager for any actions taken or decisions made. Although often involved in planning and organizing the work to be done, the charge nurse has a limited scope of responsibility, usually restricted to the unit for a specific time period. In the past, the charge nurse had limited involvement in the formal evaluation of performance, but in today's climate of efficiency, the charge nurse may be involved in evaluations as well. With the trend toward participative management, charge nurses are assuming more of the roles and functions traditionally reserved for the first-level manager.

A charge nurse usually has considerable influence with the staff and may actually have more informal power than the manager. Therefore, the charge nurse is an important leader and can benefit by developing the skills considered necessary for a manager. Acting as charge nurse is often the first step toward a formal management position.

Staff Nurse

Although not formally a manager, the staff nurse working with other professionals and assistive personnel is also a manager who needs management and leadership skills. Management responsibilities involve supervising others to ensure safe, quality patient care. Therefore, communication, delegation, and motivation skills are indispensable.

In some organizations, shared governance has been implemented and traditional management responsibilities are allocated to the work team. In this case, staff nurses have considerable involvement in managing the unit. More information about shared governance and other innovative management methods is provided in Chapter 2.

Summary

- A leader employs specific behaviors and strategies to influence individuals and groups to attain goals.

- Managers are individuals who are responsible for efficiently accomplishing the goals of the organization.

- Exercise of power is an essential aspect of leadership. Power is positional or personal and is based on several different sources, including control over rewards, punishment, information, institutional authority, expertise, personal likability, or connections.

- Leadership approaches are not static; they can be adapted for different situations, tasks, individuals, and future expectations. In turn, leaders may change situations so as to maximize their leadership effectiveness.

- Trait theories attempt to identify the inborn characteristics of successful leaders whereas behavioral theorists focus on learned leadership abilities and behaviors.

- Four leadership styles are autocratic, democratic, laissez-faire, and bureaucratic.

- Likert's leadership model is based on employee involvement in decisions.

- A continuum of leadership styles based on production and people ranges from low concern for both production and people (impoverished) to high regard for production and people (team).

- Contingency theorists contend that leaders should adapt their style in relation to changing situations. Contingency theorists include Fiedler, Hersey and Blanchard, Vroom and Yetton, and House and Mitchell.

- Fayol first described management functions as planning, organizing, directing, and controlling.

- Mintzberg defines management functions in terms of human relations. He describes seven roles: conceiving the frame, scheduling the agenda, communicating, controlling, leading, linking, and doing.

- Levels of management common in nursing are first-level, middle-level, and upper-level. Charge nurses also carry management responsibilities and, increasingly, staff nurses manage other professionals and unlicensed personnel.

■ LEADERSHIP AND MANAGEMENT *in Action*

1. How does leadership differ from management?
2. What is power? How may the different bases of power be used during an interaction with a non-nursing department? A physician?
3. How do contemporary functions of management compare with the classical functions?

References

American Organization of Nurse Executives. (1990). The role and function of the hospital nurse executive. In *American Hospital Association Advisory*. Chicago: American Hospital Association.

American Organization of Nurse Executives. (1992). The role and functions of the hospital nurse manager. In *American Hospital Association Advisory*. Chicago: American Hospital Association.

Antrobus, S., & Kitson, A. (1999). Nursing leadership: Influencing and shaping health policy and nursing practice. *Journal of Advanced Nursing, 29*(3), 746–753.

Bass, B. (1985). *Leadership and performance beyond expectations*. New York: Free Press.

Bass, B. (1990). *Bass and Stogdill's handbook of leadership: Theory, research and managerial applications,* 3rd ed. New York: Free Press.

Blake, R. R., & McCanse, A. A. (1991). *Leadership dilemmas—grid solutions*. Houston: Gulf Publishing.

Block, P. (1991). *The empowered manager*. San Francisco: Jossey-Bass.

Bolman, L. G., & Deal, T. E. (1984). *Modern approaches to understanding and managing organizations*. San Francisco: Jossey-Bass.

Burns, J. M. (1978). *Leadership*. New York: Harper and Row.

Capozzoli, J. (1991). Consolidating middle management. *Pediatric Nursing, 17*(1), 65–66.

Charns, M. P., & Tewksbury, L. S. (1993). *Collaborative management in health care: Implementing the integrative organization*. San Francisco: Jossey-Bass.

Dienemann, J., & Shaffer, C. (1992). Manager responsibilities in community agencies and hospitals. *Journal of Nursing Administration, 22*(5), 40–45.

Fiedler, F. E. (1967). *A theory of leadership effectiveness*. New York: McGraw-Hill.

French, J. R. P., & Raven, B. (1959). The bases of social power. In C. Cartwright & A. Zander (Eds.), *Studies of social power.* Ann Arbor, MI: Institute for Social Research.

Gilbert, M. A. (1975). Personality profiles and leadership potential of medical-surgical and psychiatric nursing graduate students. *Nursing Research, 24,* 125–130.

Greenleaf, R. K. (1991). *The servant as leader.* Indianapolis: The Robert K. Greenleaf Center.

Hersey, P., & Blanchard, K. (1988). *Management of organizational behavior,* 5th ed. Englewood Cliffs, NJ: Prentice-Hall.

Hersey, P., Blanchard, K., & Natemeyer, W. E. (1979). Situational leadership perception and the impact of power. *Group and Organizational Studies, 4*(4), 418–428.

Homans, G. (1958). Social behavior as exchange. *American Journal of Sociology, 63*(6), 597–606.

House, R. J. (1971). A path–goal theory of leader effectiveness. *Administrative Science Quarterly, 16*(3), 321–338.

House, R. J., & Mitchell, T. R. (1974). Path–goal theory of leadership. *Journal of Contemporary Business, 3,* 81–98.

Jenkins, R. L., & Henderson, R. L. (1984). Motivating the staff: What nurses expect from their supervisors. *Nursing Management, 15*(2), 13–14.

Johnson, L. (1992). Strategic management in nursing administration. In P. J. Decker & E. J. Sullivan (Eds.), *Nursing management: A micro/macro approach for effective nurse executives.* Norwalk, CT: Appleton & Lange.

Kanter, R. M. (1982). The middle manager as innovator. *Harvard Business Review, 60*(4), 95–105.

Katz, D., & Kahn, R. L. (1952). Some recent findings in human relations research. In G. E. Swanson, E. M. Newcomb, & R. E. Hartley (Eds.), *Readings in social psychology.* New York: Holt, Rinehart & Winston.

Kerfoot, K. (1997). Leadership: Believing in followers. *Dermatology Nursing, 9*(3), 194–195.

Klakovich, M. D. (1994). Connective leadership for the 21st century: A historical perspective and future directions. *Advances in Nursing Science, 16*(4), 42–54.

Kouzes, J. M., & Posner, B. Z. (1987). *The leadership challenge: How to get extraordinary things done in organizations.* San Francisco: Jossey-Bass.

Krejci, J. W. (1999). Changing roles in nursing: Perceptions of nurse administrators. *Journal of Nursing Administration, 29*(3), 21–29.

Lewin, K., & Lippitt, R. (1938). An experimental approach to the study of autocracy and democracy: A preliminary note. *Sociometry, 1,* 292–300.

Lewin, K., Lippitt, R., & White, R. K. (1939). Patterns of aggressive behavior in experimentally created social climates. *Journal of Social Psychology, 10,* 271–301.

Likert, R. (1967). *The human organization: Its management and value.* New York: McGraw-Hill.

McCrea, M. (1998). Personal reflections on early learning in shared leadership. *Seminars for Nurse Managers, 6*(2), 83–88.

Miller, K. I., & Monge, P. R. (1986). Participation, satisfaction, and productivity: A meta-analytic view. *Academy of Management Journal, 29,* 727–753.

Mintzberg, H. (1973). *The nature of managerial work.* New York: Harper & Row.

Mintzberg, H. (1994). Managing as blended care. *Journal of Nursing Administration, 24,* 29–36.

Porter, L. W., & Lawler, E. E. (1968). *Managerial attitudes and performance.* Homewood, IL: Irwin-Dorsey.

Porter-O'Grady, T. (1999). Quantum leadership: New roles for a new age. *Journal of Nursing Administration, 29*(10), 37–42.

Porter-O'Grady, T. (1997). Quantum mechanics and the future of healthcare leadership. *Journal of Nursing Administration, 27*(1), 15–20.

Schermerhorn, J. R., Jr., Hunt, J. G., & Osborn, R. N. (1982). *Managing organizational behavior.* New York: Wiley.

Shortell, S. M., & Kaluzny, A. D. (1994). *Health care management: Organization design and behavior,* 3rd ed. Albany, NY: Delmar.

Stogdill, R. M. (1974). *Handbook of leadership: A survey of the literature.* New York: Free Press.

Stogdill, R. M., & Coons, A. E. (Eds.). (1957). *Leadership style: Its description and measurement.* Research Monograph O. 88. Columbus, OH: Bureau of Business Research, Ohio State University.

Tannenbaum R., & Schmidt, W. H. (1973). How to choose a leadership pattern. *Harvard Business Review, 51,* 164.

Thibaut, J. W., & Kelley, H. H. (1959). *The social psychology of groups.* New York: Wiley.

Vroom, V. H., & Yetton, P. W. (1973). *Leadership and decision making.* Pittsburgh: University of Pittsburgh Press.

Vroom, V. H. (1964). *Work and motivation.* New York: Wiley.

Yukl, G. A. (1989). *Leadership in organizations,* 2nd ed. Englewood Cliffs, NJ: Prentice-Hall.

Yukl, G. A., & Tabor, T. (1983, March/April). The effective use of managerial power. *Personnel, 60*(2), 37–44.

Zohar, D. (1990). *The quantum self.* New York: Quill/William Morrow.

Additional on-line resources for this chapter can be found on the World Wide Web at http://www.prenhall.com/sullivan_decker. Select Chapter 4 from the drop-down menu.

Legal and Ethical Issues

Looking Ahead

Chapter 5 outlines the legal and ethical issues facing nurses in management, beginning with a discussion of the theories and principles of ethical decision making and followed by an overview of the legal system and a more specific examination of legal issues in nursing.

Objectives

After reading this chapter, you will be able to:

- Compare and contrast the predominant ethical theories.
- Describe the three principles used in solving ethical dilemmas.
- Describe the sources and types of law.
- Define and delineate the types of liability.
- Discuss the legal issues facing nurses related to patient care, management, and employment.

Today's health care system presents many ethical and legal dilemmas for nurse managers. Advanced technology, escalating health care costs, a growing elderly population, and social and economic pressures are just a few of the factors posing ethical dilemmas. In addition, as the role of the professional nurse expands to include increased expertise, specialization, autonomy, and accountability, so does the number of legal issues involving nurses. This chapter provides an overview of ethical decision making and the legal system and describes common ethical and legal dilemmas in nursing.

Laws and Ethics

Laws are rules of conduct, established and enforced by authority, which prohibit extremes in behavior so that one can live without fear for oneself or one's property. **Ethics** is a science that deals with principles of right and wrong, good and bad; it governs our relationships with others. Ethics are based on personal beliefs and values that guide the decision-making process. Each ethical dilemma is subject to philosophical, moral, and individual interpretations by all the involved parties. Everyone has a system of right and wrong that guides decision making. Although the

KEY TERMS

Laws Rules of conduct, established and enforced by authority, which prohibit extremes in behavior so that one can live without fear for oneself or one's property.

Ethics The science that deals with the principles of right and wrong, good and bad, and governs our relationships with others and that is based on personal beliefs and values.

definitions of law and ethics may seem clear, there is a fine line between ethics and law, and in some health care encounters there is overlap between the two. In some cases, the overlap may be congruent; in others, conflictual. For example, what is ethical may not be legal, and what is legal may not be ethical. Making this distinction between ethics and law is important because the outcomes are very different. When you violate legal principles, you may be held liable for your actions. When you violate ethical principles, you may feel badly because of the results of your actions (Hall, 1990).

The American Nurses Association's Code of Ethics, found in Box 5-1, makes explicit the profession's values

Box 5-1   American Nurses Association Code of Ethics

1. The nurse provides services with respect for human dignity and the uniqueness of the client unrestricted by considerations of social or economic status, personal attributes, or the nature of health problems.
2. The nurse safeguards the client's right to privacy by judiciously protecting information of a confidential nature.
3. The nurse acts to safeguard the client and the public when health care and safety are affected by the incompetent, unethical, or illegal practice of any person.
4. The nurse assumes responsibility and accountability for individual nursing judgments and actions.
5. The nurse maintains competence in nursing.
6. The nurse exercises informed judgment and uses individual competence and qualifications as criteria in seeking consultation, accepting responsibilities, and delegating nursing activities to others.
7. The nurse participates in activities that contribute to the ongoing development of the profession's body of knowledge.
8. The nurse participates in the profession's efforts to implement and improve standards of nursing.
9. The nurse participates in the profession's efforts to establish and maintain conditions of employment conducive to high quality nursing care.
10. The nurse participates in the profession's efforts to protect the public from misinformation and misrepresentation and to maintain the integrity of nursing.
11. The nurse collaborates with members of the health professions and other citizens in promoting community and national efforts to meet the health needs of the public.

Note: From *Code for Nurses with Interpretive Statements*, by the American Nurses Association, 1985. Kansas City, MO: Author.

and standards of conduct. This document was adopted originally in 1950 and is revised periodically to reflect changes in the profession and society. It serves to inform the nurse and the public of the profession's expectations in ethical matters. It also provides a decision-making framework for solving ethical problems. Although the code of ethics is not legally enforceable, violation of these standards often results in violation of laws that have been enacted to ensure protection of the public; for example, violation of guidelines in the code regarding issues of confidentiality and incompetent practice also constitutes violation of law. A revision of the code is currently under consideration (ANA, 2000).

Ethical Decision Making

Ethical Theories

Ethical theories guide our actions and provide an overall framework for ethical decision making. Two major ethical theories dominate ethical decision making in the health care professions: utilitarianism and deontology.

Utilitarianism   Utilitarianism promotes making decisions based on what will provide the greatest good for the greatest number. The intent is to maximize happiness and minimize suffering for the greatest number of people. A utilitarian thinker judges the goodness or badness of an act according to the consequences of the act, even if the act itself is in violation of a moral rule or principle. If the consequences of the act produce happiness for the greatest number of people, then the act is considered good.

Deontology   Deontology emphasizes that an act is good only if it springs from good will. The act is judged to be good if the fundamental principles of the act are deemed to be good, regardless of the consequences of the act. This theory holds that because unforeseen circumstances cannot always be controlled, people should not be held responsible for the consequences of their actions, because the act was performed with good intentions and the outcome was not due to negligence.

A deontological thinker who believes that truth telling is good might tell the truth regardless of the consequences, whereas a utilitarian thinker might not tell the truth if he or she believed that the truth would create more harm than good. Persons holding different ethical values might well come to different conclusions about what ought to be done in a given situation.

KEY TERMS

Utilitarianism   An ethical theory that promotes making decisions based on what will provide the greatest good for the greatest number.

Deontology   An ethical theory that emphasizes that an act is good if the fundamental principles of the act are deemed to be good regardless of the consequences of the act.

Autonomy   The right of individuals to take action for themselves.

Beneficence/nonmaleficence   The duty to help others by doing what is best for them without inflicting evil or harm.

Distributive justice   Giving a person that which is deserved.

Allocation   The decision of a society about how much of its resources will be devoted to a particular effort.

Rationing   The process by which decisions are made about who will get the resources and who will not.

Ethical Principles

In addition to ethical theories, there are several key principles that play a role in solving ethical dilemmas. The principles most directly related to nursing management are the principles of autonomy, beneficence, and distributive justice.

Autonomy   Autonomy is the right of individuals to take action for themselves. It includes respect for individuals and the right of individuals to make decisions for and about themselves, even if those decisions are not congruent with others' goals. To respect autonomy is to respect others. It requires recognizing the uniqueness of others and listening to and understanding another person in a way that allows you to put yourself in that other person's position.

People engaged in autonomous and self-determining actions must have the capability of self-governance, operate from a stable and internalized set of principles, and view themselves as capable of implementing autonomous decisions. Inherent in this principle is the understanding that a person acts with intention and with knowledge and without external control or influence. Like most rights, autonomy is not an absolute right: Under certain circumstances, the individual's rights do not prevail over the rights of others. Individual autonomy does not prevail, for example, when it interferes with the rights, health, or well-being of another. For example, a nurse has the right to refuse to render care to a patient because of religious beliefs; however, if the safety of the patient is jeopardized because of that lack of care, the nurse may suffer legal consequences if care is not provided.

Beneficence and Nonmaleficence **Beneficence** is the duty to help others by doing what is best for them. This belief also implies the principle of **nonmaleficence,** or to "do no harm." Not only does one have the duty to do good, but one also has the duty not to inflict evil or harm or to risk harm to others. A beneficent nurse manager acts with empathy for the patients and staff and without resentment or malice. A manager who acts in bad faith or out of ill will or who makes false accusations concerning a patient or employee violates the principle of beneficence.

In many instances, the demands of beneficence and the functions required in a health care setting come into conflict. Sometimes, for example, treatment decisions are viewed as harmful from the patient's perspective. When an individual does not desire what others determine to be in that person's best interest—such as when a patient refuses treatment—the principles of beneficence and autonomy conflict. Generally speaking, in conflict situations involving patient care decisions, the principle of autonomy overrides the principle of beneficence, and this has been affirmed by the courts (Furrow, Johnson, Jost, & Schwartz, 1991).

Distributive Justice **Distributive justice** is giving a person that which he or she deserves. It implies that benefits and burdens ought to be distributed equally and fairly, regardless of race, gender, religion, or socioeconomic status so that no one person bears a disproportionate share of benefits or burdens. As health care technology increases and health care costs soar, nurse managers find themselves entrenched in conflicts between cost containment and the equal distribution of finite health care resources regardless of the patient's ability to pay.

Allocation (macroallocation) and rationing (microallocation) of scarce resources are the most important ethical issues facing nurse managers today. **Allocation** is a decision society makes regarding how many of its resources will be devoted to a particular effort, for example, organ transplants. **Rationing** is a decision regarding who gets the transplant and who does not. Allocation and rationing decisions require that some

societal values take precedence over some individual values.

The goal-driven or patient-centered model of care, which was traditionally taught to nurses in the past, does not suffice in the current health care delivery system, in which resources are finite. The traditional model stressed nurses' commitment to the patient regardless of the person's ability to pay or the cost of the person's care to society. Resource allocation was viewed as an absolute individual right that allowed individuals to make unlimited claims on societal resources. Ideally, nurses were taught to identify goals and then find the resources to meet those goals. Frequently, nurses did a good job with limited resources, but they did not feel right about the care they provided because it was less than ideal. In the current resource-driven model, nurses must learn to use finite resources efficiently and to be satisfied that resources were used wisely (Camunas, 1994). Allocation of scarce resources is not an issue that can be addressed by individual nurses or even by the nursing profession alone. It requires cooperative efforts and interdisciplinary understanding among a variety of participants, including policy makers and economists, as well as a new perspective on nursing ethics. There is no way to discuss issues of resource allocation without looking at the process by which resources are made available, the constraints on decision makers who must allocate those resources, and the comparative values of health care and other goods of society. Box 5-2 lists some common ethical dilemmas cited by nurse managers in a nationwide study conducted by Camunas (1994).

The Legal System

Law comes from a variety of sources. Understanding the sources of law and the various types of laws helps determine their impact on nursing practice. Nurses must understand the changing legal climate and their responsibilities as viewed by the public and the legal system (Luquire, 1989).

Sources of Law

Three branches of government contribute to the creation of law. They, in conjunction with the Constitution, form the basis of the judicial system of this country. The Constitution is the supreme law of the land. It defines the structure, power, and limits of the government and guarantees people certain fundamental rights as individuals. Influences of the legislative, judicial, and executive branches of government are

Box 5-2   Common Ethical Dilemmas for Nurse Managers

Allocation of Resources

Making staffing mix decisions
Meeting regulations requirements
Providing care to individuals who are medically indigent and have long-term care needs
Providing needed patient care programs

Access to Care

Providing or limiting access for certain groups of patients (e.g., obstetric patients, psychiatric patients, substance abuse patients, patients who are homeless)

Setting and Maintaining Standards of Care

Problems with controlled substances

• Substance abuse by patients and health care workers
• Diversion of narcotics
• Drug screening without consent

Poor judgment and incompetence of nurses, physicians, others
Lying, cheating, and stealing by patients, staff, physicians

Note: From "Ethical Dilemmas of Nurse Executives" by C. Camunas, 1994. *Journal of Nursing Administration, 24*(9), 19–23.

reflected in statutory law, common law, and administrative law.

Statutory Law   **Statutory laws** are enacted by the legislative branch of government. They are designed to declare, command, or prohibit something. Licensing laws for health care providers, including nurses, are examples of statutory laws, which are designed to protect the public from incompetent practitioners. Other statutory laws affecting nursing practice are guardianship codes, statutes of limitation, informed consent, living will legislation, and protective and reporting laws.

Common Law   **Common law** is judge-made law. This type of law is derived from earlier decisions made by courts. Common law establishes a custom or tradition by which other similar cases are judged; this custom is referred to as legal precedent. Common law

is not absolute; earlier decisions can be and frequently are overruled. As time and circumstances change, court decisions become obsolete and may require a different opinion. Each state has its own body of common law related to the delivery of health care within that state. These laws should be reviewed by health professionals as a basis for accountability, quality, and risk management within their professional practice. As the number of malpractice suits involving nurses increases, the body of common law regulating nursing practice also increases. Awareness of this law assists nurses to function within the boundaries of their role and to advocate for nursing practice when necessary.

Administrative Law   **Administrative laws** are made by administrative agencies. According to certain statutes, administrative agencies are granted authority to enact rules and regulations that will carry out specific intentions of the statute. This allows the legislature to delegate to an administrative agency of experts in the field the authority to create rules and regulations governing a specific area of practice. For example, state boards of nursing are authorized by nurse practice acts (statutory law) to write rules and regulations governing the practice of nursing. These rules and regulations are incorporated into the nurse practice act and are as binding as the statutory law itself. Another example of administrative law is the attorney general's opinion regarding the interpretation of a law, which also is binding.

Types of Law

Law also can be categorized according to specific types. The two basic types of law are public law and

KEY TERMS

Statutory laws   Laws enacted by the legislature that are designed to declare, command, or prohibit something.

Common law   A law derived from earlier decisions made by courts that establish a custom or tradition by which other cases are judged.

Administrative laws   Laws made by administrative agencies that have been given authority to create rules and regulations governing a specific area of practice.

private law (civil law). **Public law** consists of constitutional law, administrative law, and criminal law. **Private law** is further classified into tort law, contract law, and protecting and reporting law; however, the latter sometimes falls under the category of criminal law. All these have an impact on nursing practice; however, the most common law affecting nursing practice is that of torts.

Tort Law

Tort law is divided into two categories—*unintentional* and *intentional*. Negligence and malpractice (professional negligence) fall under the category of unintentional torts.

Unintentional Torts   **Negligence** is defined as the failure of an individual not to perform an act (omission) or to perform an act (commission) that a reasonable, prudent person would or would not perform in a similar set of circumstances. **Malpractice** is professional negligence; it evolves from negligence law and the premise that all individuals are responsible for the consequences of their actions or inactions. It refers to any misconduct or lack of skill in carrying out professional responsibilities. In order for malpractice to exist, four elements must be present: *duty, breach of duty, causation,* and *injury*. If any one of these elements cannot be proved beyond a reasonable doubt, then the malpractice claim may be dismissed.

Intentional Torts   In **intentional torts**, the intent to harm is present. Assault, battery, false imprisonment, invasion of privacy, libel, slander, and defamation of character are examples of actions considered to be intentional torts.

Liability

To understand malpractice, one must understand the various types of liability. As individuals, nurses are responsible and accountable for their own actions or inactions. This is referred to as **personal liability**. In addition, the law ascribes negligence to certain parties who may not be negligent themselves but whose negligence is assumed because of association with the negligent person. This is called **vicarious liability**. It is based on the legal principle of **respondeat superior,** which means "let the master speak." This doctrine allows the courts to hold the employer responsible for the actions of the employee when the employee is performing services for the organization.

KEY TERMS

Public law   The domains of constitutional law, administrative law, and criminal law.

Private law   The domains of tort law, contract law, and protecting and reporting law.

Tort law   A law that addresses wrongful acts, whether unintentional or intentional, against a person or property.

Negligence   The unintentional failure of an individual to perform or not perform an act that a reasonable person would or would not perform in a similar set of circumstances.

Malpractice   Professional negligence that refers to any misconduct or lack of skill in carrying out professional responsibilities.

Intentional torts   Action in which the intent to harm was present.

Personal liability   The responsibility and accountability of individuals for their own actions or inactions.

Vicarious liability   The assignment of negligence to certain parties, whose negligence is assumed due to their association with a negligent person.

Respondeat superior   The legal principle that allows the court to hold an employer responsible for the actions of an employee when performing services for the organization.

All too frequently, nurses have a false sense of security concerning the doctrines of respondeat superior and vicarious liability. Employees sometimes believe that the organization's responsibility protects them from being sued as individuals; this is not the case. Patients have the right to sue both the employee and the organization when they have suffered an injury as a result of substandard care. Also, the organization has the right to sue the employee for damages incurred as a result of the nurse's substandard care. This is why it is important for nurses to carry their own personal liability insurance. Nurse managers are not responsible for the actions of others but are responsible for their own acts of delegation and supervision of others. Failure to delegate and supervise properly can result in liability for the nurse manager. This is not a result of vicarious liability, but an issue of personal liability.

Corporate liability holds that the organization is responsible for its own wrongful conduct. The health care organization has the responsibility of maintaining an environment conducive to quality health care for its consumers. Corporate liability includes (a) the duty to hire, supervise, and maintain qualified, competent, and adequate staff; (b) the duty to provide, inspect, repair, and maintain reasonably adequate equipment; and (c) the duty to maintain safety in the physical environment. Responsibility to achieve these goals is delegated to managers even though the organization is ultimately responsible. For example, the organization has a responsibility to have a mechanism in place for reporting incompetent, unethical, and illegal practice; however, if the nurse manager is aware of such practice but does not report it, the nurse manager also is liable. Many states have statutory laws regarding mandatory reporting of legal and ethical problems.

Legal Issues in Nursing

Nursing Licensure

Licensure is a type of credential provided for by state statutes that authorizes qualified individuals to perform designated skills and services (Guido, 1997). In nursing, these statutes are referred to as **Nurse Prac-**

tice Acts. Nurse Practice Acts establish *boards of nursing*, whose members are granted the authority to set and enforce rules and regulations pertaining to the practice of nursing. Currently, each state's board of nursing establishes requirements for licensure in that state. Licensure protects the use of the titles, registered or practical nurse, and establishes educational, examination, and behavioral standards intended to protect the health, safety and welfare of the public.

Changes in licensure are on the horizon. These changes are designed to allow nurses mobility while protecting the public.

Uniform Licensure Requirements   One remedy proposed by the National Council of State Boards of Nursing (NCSBN) is to develop uniform licensure requirements among the states that would facilitate nurse mobility, but also assure public access to qualified practitioners (Box 5-3). The framework for these requirements is competence—competence in development, assessment, and conduct (NCSBN, 1999).

Multistate Licensure   Another initiative by the NCSBN is multistate licensure. **Multistate licensure** is a process similar to obtaining a driver's license. Each state that agrees to the interstate compact would mutually recognize the nurse's license, allowing practice in more than one state. As of July 2000, seven states had entered an interstate compact to allow multistate licensure privilege: Arkansas, Iowa, Maryland, North Carolina, Texas, Utah, and Wisconsin. Legislation is pending or goes into effect at a later date in several

---

Box 5-3   Uniform Core Licensure Requirements

I. Competence Development: Nursing education—registered nurses (RN)
- Graduation from or verification of completion and eligibility for graduation from state-approved registered nursing program.

II. Competence Assessment: Assessment of U.S. candidates—RN
- Nursing Knowledge, Skills and Abilities
- NCLEX-RN® examination, unlimited attempts

III. Competence Conduct:
Criminal convictions—RN and LPN/VN
- Self-report regarding all felony convictions.

- Conviction of lesser-included offenses arising from felony arrests.
- Local/state and federal background checks using current technology (i.e., fingerprinting) to validate self-reports.

Chemical dependency—RN and LPN/VN
- Self report regarding any drug-related behavior that affects the candidate's ability to provide safe and effective nursing care.

Functional abilities—RN and LPN/VN
- Self-report regarding any functional ability deficit that would require accommodation to perform essential nursing functions.

Note: National Council State Boards of Nursing (1999). Uniform core licensure requirements for initial licensure of RNs and LPN/VNs. *Issues,* 20(3), 1–2.

KEY TERMS

Corporate liability   The responsibility of an organization for its own wrongful conduct.

Licensure   A credential provided for by state statute that authorizes qualified individuals to perform designated skills and services.

Nurse Practice Acts   State statutes that authorize individuals to perform designated skills and services.

Multistate licensure   A licensure process whereby more than one state mutually recognizes licensure.

Invasion of privacy   The right to be left alone without being subjected to unwarranted or uninvited publicity and to make personal choices without interference.

Confidentiality   The right to privacy of records.

other states (NCSBN, 2000). The state of residence is considered the home state. All other states in the contract are remote states. The nurse is still responsible for meeting the standards set forth by the nurse practice acts where practice occurs. Disciplinary actions may be taken by both the home and remote state (NCSBN, 1998).

Patient Care Issues

Patient's Rights   When individuals enter the health care system, they retain their basic fundamental rights ascribed to individuals by the Constitution and courts of law. These rights are spelled out in the Patient's Bill of Rights (American Hospital Association [AHA], 1992), a document frequently given to individuals when they enter the health care system. Although not always legally binding, this document frequently is used as a standard for judging the nursing care rendered. Some argue that a bill of rights for patients is not necessary because it simply reiterates the basic rights already recognized; however, this document is designed to protect the rights of the individual at a time when he or she is most vulnerable to abuse (Guido, 1988). The Patient's Bill of Rights is designed to protect such basic rights as privacy, confidentiality, informed consent, and refusal of treatment.

Invasion of Privacy   The tort **invasion of privacy** is the violation of a person's right to be left alone without being subjected to unwarranted or uninvited publicity and to make personal choices without interference. Information disclosed by patients is confidential and as such is available to authorized personnel only. Patients can sue for invasion of privacy when confidential information is revealed to any unauthorized person. Similarly, a patient can sue for invasion of privacy when unauthorized personnel, directly or indirectly, observe the patient without permission. Authorized personnel are those involved in the diagnosis, treatment, and related care of the patient. Generally speaking, these are members of the health care team.

Nurses, as well as others, cannot use photographs, videotapes, or research data without the explicit permission of the involved patient. Also, the nurse should be discreet about the release of information over the telephone regarding the patient's status because it is difficult, if not impossible, to identify the caller accurately over the telephone. The nurse must even obtain the patient's permission to release information to family members and close friends.

Other cases regarding invasion of privacy involve the freedom to make choices without interference. Patients have the right to make informed choices, such as contraception use, abortion, and the right to refuse treatment, and they should be assured that these decisions will be respected and upheld even if they are not the same decisions or choices the health professional may make. Nurses often serve as advocates to safeguard these rights.

The same guiding principles regarding release of information about patients also apply to release of information about employees. Information regarding employees is considered confidential and must not be released outside the organization without the explicit consent of the employee except to verify employment or to comply with legal investigation. The Privacy Act of 1974 outlines stringent requirements for handling personnel matters related to privacy issues. The nurse manager needs to be familiar with this law, especially as it relates to giving references and recommendations.

Confidentiality is the right to privacy of records. Individuals have the right to believe that information disclosed to health professionals is to be used strictly for the purpose of diagnosis and treatment and will not be released to others without permission of the individual. This is considered protected information by the privilege doctrine. According to this doctrine, people who have protected relationships cannot be forced to reveal communication between them unless

KEY TERMS

Informed consent   The consent for treatment given by a patient after three requirements are met: the individual has the capacity to consent, consent is voluntary, and the individual receives information regarding treatment in a manner that is understandable to him or her.

Capacity   An individual's ability to consent as determined by age and competence.

Patient Self-Determination Act   A federal law requiring every health care facility receiving Medicare or Medicaid to provide written information to adult patients concerning their right to make health care decisions.

Advance directive   A document that allows the competent patient to make choices regarding health care prior to its need.

Living will   An advance directive that indicates what an individual wants done regarding treatment or lifesaving measures in the future.

Durable power of attorney for health care   A document that permits an individual to give a surrogate or proxy the authority to make decisions for that person in the event that she or he becomes incompetent.

the person who would benefit from the relationship agrees to it. Physician–patient relationships are considered privileged relationships. Some states extend this doctrine to nurse–patient relationships by law; even without such statutory requirements, courts by analogy have applied this premise to nurse–patient relationships (Northrop & Kelly, 1987). Also, the ANA Code of Ethics (Box 5-1) states that it is the nurse's duty to protect information of a confidential nature (ANA, 1985). Under certain circumstances, the nurse can lawfully disclose confidential information about the patient, such as when the welfare of a person or a group is at stake or when a personal injury or worker's compensation claim is being filed.

Informed Consent   To provide treatment without the patient's consent, except in an emergency situation, could result in liability for unauthorized touching, or battery. There are three basic requirements necessary

for **informed consent**: capacity, voluntariness, and information.

Individual **capacity** to consent is determined by age and competence. Generally, one must be an adult in the technical and legal sense in order to consent to treatment. The legal age for adult status is established by state statute and varies from state to state. Based on state statute, minors may consent to certain types of treatment, such as abortion and substance abuse treatment. Adults are considered competent when they can make choices and understand the consequences of their choices.

Individuals act *voluntarily* when they exercise freedom of choice without force, fraud, deceit, duress, or any other form of coercion. Consent that is compelled by threats or provoked by fraud is legally considered to be no consent at all. Because patients are exceptionally vulnerable when they need medical care, they may believe, or be led to believe, that they must comply with the recommendations of health care professionals. Often patients believe if they don't comply they may get less than adequate care or no care at all. All too frequently, nurses and other health professionals take it for granted that because a patient is under their care, the patient will agree to whatever care is deemed necessary. Nurses have an obligation to create an atmosphere that avoids any indication of coercion or manipulation.

The third element of informed consent is *information*. Information must be supplied to patients in a manner that is understandable to them. Lay terminology is preferred to professional terminology. The information must include the following:

1. An explanation of the treatment to be performed and the expected results
2. A description of the anticipated risks and discomforts
3. A list of potential benefits
4. A disclosure of possible alternatives
5. An offer to answer the patient's questions
6. A statement that the patient may withdraw his or her consent at any time

The legal responsibility to provide the necessary information for informed consent rests with the individual who will perform the treatment. When a nurse asks a patient to sign a consent form, the nurse is merely attesting to the fact that there is reason to believe that the patient is informed regarding the impending treatment and is witnessing the signature. If the nurse asks the patient to sign a consent form knowing that the patient has had no prior explanation of the treatment, the consent is invalid.

Right to Refuse Treatment   Just as competent adults have the right to consent to treatment, they also have the *right to refuse treatment*. In addition, guardians of incompetent adults have the right to refuse treatment for them. The right of competent adults to refuse treatment is guaranteed by the Constitution and has been tested in court with several landmark cases (Quinlan v. New Jersey, 1976; Cruzan v. Director, Missouri Department of Health, 1990). In recent years, most states have adopted statutory laws to protect these rights and to protect the health care provider who agrees to not treat even when treatment could be considered medically indicated. These laws are referred to as living wills, durable power of attorney, and advance directives.

In 1990, Congress enacted the **Patient Self-Determination Act**. This is a federal law that requires every health care facility that receives Medicare or Medicaid funds to provide written information to adult patients concerning their right under state law to make health care decisions. These decisions include the right to accept or refuse treatment and the right to formulate advance directives (Omnibus Budget Reconciliation Act [OBRA], 1990). An **advance directive** is a document that allows the competent patient to make choices prior to the need for medical treatment. Examples include decisions such as refusing treatment, being placed on life support, and stopping treatment. The two most common advance directives are the **living will** and the **durable power of attorney for health care** (Figure 5-1). With the living will, the competent adult signs a form indicating what health care the person wants done in the future. These decisions will be upheld should that adult's decision-making capacity be lost. The durable power of attorney permits a competent adult to appoint a surrogate or proxy to make decisions for that person in the event that he or she becomes incompetent. The health care provider must follow the expressed wishes as stated in these documents. Difficulties arise when the patient is incompetent and does not have an advance directive or the directive is vague. In these cases, the health provider often relies on family members to make these decisions. In most states, however, family members do not have the legal authority to make such decisions unless they are the legally appointed guardians or parents (Aiken, 1994).

Freedom from Restraint   Another potential area of liability is the use of *restraints*. The Omnibus Budget

Reconciliation Act (OBRA) of 1987 provides patients the right to be free from any physical or chemical restraint imposed for the purpose of discipline or convenience and not required to treat medical symptoms (OBRA, 1987). These regulations apply to nursing homes, state and federal agencies, and other health care organizations that receive Medicare and Medicaid funds. According to these rules, health professionals are required to assess the need for restraints and consider the use of alternative measures. When restraints are deemed necessary, a physician's order specifying duration and circumstances is required. No orders for as-needed (PRN) restraints are permitted. When restraints are used, the patient must be monitored closely and reassessed periodically to evaluate the continued need for restraints. In addition to federal regulations, most states have laws governing the use of restrictive devices.

Federal mandates also call for the judicious use of psychotropic drugs, which are frequently used as chemical restraints. Psychotropic drugs no longer may be used for the purpose of controlling behavior; they may be prescribed only for diagnosis-related conditions. The intention is to prevent indiscriminate use of psychotropic drugs that frequently cause patients to become deeply sedated, agitated, or combative.

In July 1992, the Food and Drug Administration (FDA) issued a warning to health care providers concerning the potential hazards associated with the use of physical restraint devices. Nurses frequently believe restraints protect the patient from injury to self or others, yet there is no proof that restraints actually prevent injury. On the contrary, there is more evidence that restraints cause injury: The FDA (1992) estimates at least 100 deaths or injuries per year are associated with the use of restraints.

The use of restraints should be based on the principles of informed consent. If patients are unable to consent, then reliable proxy consent should be obtained with full disclosure of risks and benefits (Moss & LaPuma, 1991). Restraining patients without consent or sufficient justification may be interpreted as false imprisonment. In addition to legal rights, the use of restraints clearly involves ethical issues such as autonomy and beneficence.

Management Issues

Delegation and Supervision   With the redesign of health care delivery systems and the use of more unlicensed workers, the professional nurse's responsibility

This is a Durable Power of Attorney for Health Care Decisions, and the authority of my agent shall not terminate if I become incapacitated. I grant my agent full authority to make decisions for me regarding my health care. In exercising this authority, my agent shall follow my desires as stated in my Health Care Treatment Directive or otherwise known to my agent. My agent's authority to interpret my desires is intended to be as broad as possible and any expenses incurred should be paid by my resources. My agent may not delegate the authority to make decisions. My agent is authorized as follows to:

> If there is a statement in paragraphs 1 through 6 below with which you do not agree, draw a line through it and add your initials.

1. Consent, refuse or withdraw consent to any care, treatment, service or procedure, (including artificiality supplied nutrition and/or hydration/tube feeding) used to maintain, diagnose or treat a physical or mental condition;
2. Make decisions regarding organ donation, autopsy and the disposition of my body;
3. Make all necessary arrangements for any hospital, psychiatric hospital or psychiatric treatment facility, hospice, nursing home or similar institution; to employ or discharge health care personnel (any person who is licensed, certified or otherwise authorized or permitted by the laws of the state to administer health care) as the agent shall deem necessary for my physical, mental and emotional well being;
4. Request, receive and review any information, verbal or written, regarding my personal affairs or physical or mental health including medical and hospital records and to execute any releases of other documents that may be required in order to obtain such information;
5. Move me into or out of any state for the purpose of complying with my Health Care Treatment Directive or the decisions of my agent;
6. Take any legal action reasonably necessary to do what I have directed.

I appoint the following person to be my agent to make health care decisions for me WHEN AND ONLY WHEN I lack the capacity to make or communicate a choice regarding a particular health care decision and my Health Care Treatment Directive does not adequately cover circumstances. I request that the person serving as my agent be my guardian if one is needed.

> If you do not wish to name an agent, write "None" in the space provided below.

Agent's Name: _____ Telephone: _____

Address: _____

_____

If my agent is not available or not willing to make health care decisions for me or, if my agent is my spouse and is legally separated or divorced from me, I appoint the person or persons named below (in the order named if more than one listed) as my agent: (It is not necessary to name an alternate agent.)

First Alternate Agent   Second Alternate Agent

Name: _____   Name: _____

Address: _____   Address: _____

Telephone: _____   Telephone: _____

Protection of Persons Who Rely on My Agent: I and my estate hold my agent and my caregivers harmless and protect them against any claim for following this durable power of attorney.
Severability: If any part of this document is held to be unenforceable under law, I direct that all of the other provisions of the document shall remain in force and effect.

Date: _____ X Signature _____

Witness _____ Date _____ Witness _____ Date _____

Figure 5-1 **Sample durable power of attorney for health care decisions.** *Note:* **Used with the permission of the Midwest Bioethics Center, Kansas City, MO.**

Health Care Treatment Directive

I _____ make this Health Care Treatment Directive to exercise my
Print Name

my right to determine the course of my health care and to provide clear and convincing proof of my treatment decisions when I lack the capacity to make or communicate my decisions and there is no realistic hope that I will regain such capacity.

If my physician believes that a certain life prolonging procedure or other health care treatment may provide me with comfort, relieve pain or lead to a significant recovery, I direct my physician to try the treatment for a reasonable period of time. However, if such treatment proves to be ineffective, I direct treatment be withdrawn even if so doing may shorten my life.

I direct I be given health care treatment to relieve pain or to provide comfort even if such treatment might shorten my life, suppress my appetite or my breathing, or be habit-forming.

I direct all life prolonging procedures be withheld or withdrawn when there is no hope of significant recovery, and I have:
- a terminal condition; or
- a condition, disease or injury without reasonable expectation that I will regain an acceptable quality of life; or
- substantial brain damage or brain disease which cannot be significantly reversed.

1. When any of the above conditions exist, I DO NOT WANT the life prolonging procedures which I have initialed below. (You should assume any treatments not initialed may be administered to you.)
   - surgery . . . . _____ initials
   - heart-lung resuscitation (CPR) . . . . _____ initials
   - antibiotics . . . . _____ initials
   - dialysis . . . . _____ initials
   - mechanical ventilator (respirator) . . . . _____ initials
   - tube feedings (food and water delivered through a tube in the vein,
     nose, or stomach) . . . . _____ initials
   - other _____ _____ initials
2. I make other instructions as follows: (You may describe what a minimally acceptable quality of life is for you.)

   _____

   _____

   _____

   _____

If you do not wish to name an agent as referred to on the reverse side, initial here _____ ,
write "None" in the space provided for agent's name, sign and have witnessed and/or notarized.

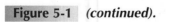 **Figure 5-1**   *(continued).*

Notarization

> Notarization of the Durable Power of Attorney is required in some states (e.g., Missouri but not Kansas). If this document is both witnessed and notarized, it is more likely to be honored in other states.

On this _____ day of _____ , _____ , before me personally appeared the aforesaid declarant, to me known to be the person described in and who executed the foregoing instrument and acknowledged that he/she executed the same as his/her free act and deed. IN WITNESS WHEREOF, I

have hereunto set my hand and affixed my official seal in the County of _____ ,

State of _____ , the day and year first above written.

_____   _____
Notary Public   My Commission Expires

Acceptance: (Optional) I have discussed this document with the person making this durable power of attorney and I accept the responsibility designated to me as stated above.

Date _____   Agent _____

Figure 5-1   **Sample durable power of attorney for health care decisions** *(continued).*

has increased. Now, more than ever, nurses must understand the legal responsibilities they assume when delegating and supervising unlicensed assistive personnel (Barter & Furmidge, 1994).

Nursing management encompasses supervision of nursing care and the personnel who provide that care. The nurse is personally liable for the reasonable exercise of their delegation and supervision activities. The nurse must be aware of the staff's knowledge, skills, and competencies when delegating tasks and should supervise appropriately. Nurses have a legal duty to ensure that staff members under their supervision are performing in a manner consistent with the desired standard of practice. If a nurse makes an assignment to an individual whom the nurse knows is not competent to perform that assignment, the nurse will be liable if the patient is injured. (See Chapter 14.)

Staffing   According to established standards, the organization must provide adequate staffing with qualified personnel (Joint Commission on the Accreditation of Healthcare Organizations [JCAHO], 1995). The organization that fails to retain the level of nursing personnel required to provide safe quality care may be held liable under the doctrines of respondeat superior and corporate liability if an injury occurs related to short staffing (Fiesta, 1990). The responsibility of the organization to maintain an adequate staffing level is the nurse manager's. What constitutes adequate personnel is not specified in JCAHO guidelines

because what is satisfactory under one set of circumstances may not be satisfactory under another.

Although retaining appropriate nursing personnel is the responsibility of the organization, if it can be shown that the staff nurse acted unreasonably under the circumstances, the individual nurse also can be held liable for acts of omission or commission. In other words, inadequate staff is no excuse for negligent acts; however, if the nurse acts reasonably under the circumstances, the individual may not be found culpable for malpractice. And if the hospital can demonstrate that it has taken appropriate actions to alleviate the staffing crisis, then they may not be held liable (Fiesta, 1990).

Staffing an organization is not as clear-cut as it may seem. Although the organization has some guidelines to follow, such as those mandated by JCAHO and federal and state regulatory bodies, these guidelines are broad and require a certain amount of judgment. Other factors involved in providing adequate staff are somewhat subjective and the responsibility of the organization. Patient classification systems help provide an objective measure of the number of staff needed; however, they do not take into consideration whether the staff are experienced or inexperienced. They also do not take into consideration whether adequate equipment is accessible, appropriate policies exist, and sufficient supervision is available, all of which are helpful adjuncts during a staffing crunch (Fiesta, 1990).

Job Reassignment The hospital has a legal duty to ensure that all areas of the hospital are adequately staffed. With fluctuating patient census, this often places the hospital in a position in which reassigning nurses' duties is the only way to balance the needs of the unit and the safety of patients. **Job reassignment** (floating) is the process of pulling nurses from one area of the hospital to another. This practice is commonplace in today's health care organization, but concerns are raised by both staff and administration. Floating nurses to unfamiliar areas, especially specialty areas, increases the chance of error and may increase the nurse's anxiety, which in turn may affect job satisfaction and morale.

Reassigning hospital personnel is a necessary evil that in many instances cannot be avoided. Nurses have no legal ground to refuse to float unless it has been previously specified in their contract, or unless the organization has policies and procedures to the contrary. The nurse who refuses to float may face the possibility of discharge on the grounds of insubordination. Nurses must realize they have a professional responsibility to serve in the best interest of the patient. Open communication regarding limitations and concerns, creative problem solving, and cross-training are some solutions to the problem of reassignment.

Policies and Procedures When the nurse is responsible for performing procedures that require judgments beyond the usual scope of nursing practice, a standardized procedure, or protocol, is necessary. These procedures must be written and authorized by the organization. Routinely, the standardized protocol must specify (a) the functions the nurse may perform under specific circumstances; (b) any requirements that must be followed in performing the function; (c) education, experience, and training requisites of the nurse performing the procedures; and (d) the method for evaluating the competence of the nurse performing the practice (Walker, 1980).

Policies and procedures are required for all health care organizations. These documents serve to standardize care, set standards, and guide practices. They should be well delineated, clearly stated, and based on current and actual practice.

Incompetent Practice The "due care" standard requires nurse managers to confront unsafe practice. It is important for the nurse manager to be familiar with both the organization's procedures for addressing safety and professional conduct and state boards of nursing guidelines. Many states have instituted mandatory reporting of unsafe practices to safeguard public

health. Mandatory reporting is a complex process involving both legal and ethical parameters. The vast majority of the complaints and disciplinary actions are for impairment or drug diversion (Luckenbill-Brett & Stuhler-Schlag, 1987). Chapter 21 provides more information about impaired nursing practice.

Employment Issues

Increasingly, nurse managers are responsible and liable for employment decisions within health care organizations. For this reason, the nurse manager needs to be familiar with the growing body of antidiscrimination laws. These statutes have a profound effect on hiring, advancement, and termination practices of the employer. Matters of employee rights have been pronounced since the passage of the Civil Rights Act of 1964. Today, we continue to see increased activity related to discrimination of various kinds, and many states have enacted laws governing civil rights and antidiscrimination (McConnell, 1990).

Civil Rights Act of 1964 Title VII of the 1964 Civil Rights Act (CRA) bars discrimination on the basis of race, color, sex, or national origin. It governs all public and private agencies with 15 or more employees and addresses all aspects of employment (e.g., hiring, promotion, discipline, supervision, performance appraisal, dismissal). The Equal Employment Opportunity Commission (EEOC) is the federal agency that administers and enforces Title VII. In 1978, the CRA was extended to include discriminatory treatment of pregnant women; as a result, employers who require mandatory maternity leave without regard to the employee's ability to work are in violation of Title VII. Two exceptions are the *bona fide occupational qualifications (BFOQ)* and *bona fide seniority* or *merit system*. The BFOQ states that it is lawful to make employment decisions on the basis of national origin, religion, and sex (but not race or color) if this is necessary for the job. Proof of necessity may be difficult to verify. The bona fide seniority or merit system contends that it is permissible to make decisions about promotions and layoffs based on seniority.

Sexual Harassment In 1980, the EEOC established guidelines stating that sexual harassment in the workplace violates Title VII. Under these guidelines, the employer can be held liable for acts of sexual harassment committed by employees whether or not the employer had any prior knowledge of the reported acts. For these reasons, employers frequently establish proactive policies to sensitize employees to the problem and to help prevent instances of sexual harassment in the workplace. The guidelines define sexual harassment to include conduct in which (a) submission to sexual advances is explicitly or implicitly a term or condition of an individual's employment, (b) submission to or rejection of sexual advances is used as a basis for employment decisions, and (c) the nature of the sexual advances has the purpose or effect of interfering with work performance or creating an intimidating, hostile, or offensive work environment.

Age Discrimination in Employment Act (ADEA) Passage of the Age Discrimination in Employment Act (ADEA) in 1967 made it unlawful for employers to discriminate against older men and women in decisions regarding all phases of employment. In 1986, this act was extended to prohibit discrimination against individuals over the age of 40, and mandatory retirement for persons at any age is prohibited. The ADEA applies to public and private organizations with 20 or more employees. Again, as with Title VII, an employer may exercise bona fide occupational qualifications (BFOQ) and the bona fide seniority system as exemptions.

Americans with Disabilities Act (ADA) Title I of the Americans with Disabilities Act (ADA) (1990), which became effective July 1992, is designed to eliminate discrimination against disabled persons in employment by enforcing equal access to jobs and accommodations.

In general, no employer, public or private, with 15 or more employees may discriminate against a qualified individual with a disability because of the disability (Cross, 1992). The ADA broadly defines disability as (a) a physical or mental impairment that substantially limits one or more of the major life activities of such individuals, (b) a record of such impairment, and (c) being regarded as having such impairment. Some disabilities that qualify under ADA are listed in Box 5-4.

These guidelines apply to all phases of the employment process, including hiring, advancement, compensation, training, discharge, or other conditions of employment. Furthermore, the ADA not only prohibits discrimination but also requires employers to provide reasonable accommodations for disabled employees, which includes employees who have been identified as recovering from alcohol or drug addiction. (See Chapter 21 for more on employees with substance abuse problems.)

Reasonable accommodations might include providing leaves of absence with or without pay, job reassignment, and job restructuring. The exact recommendations for providing these accommodations are not yet clear. Other suggestions from the courts include keeping disabled employees informed of other, more suitable, job openings within the agency, allowing the employee to work at home, and assigning another employee to work with the disabled employee as part of a team. Until such time when there are enough consistent data from the test cases, the nurse manager should be open-minded, flexible, and creative when it comes to making reasonable accommodations for disabled employees.

Just as what constitutes making accommodations is vague, so are the definition itself and the EEOC's implementation regulations. Therefore, many alleged

---

Box 5-4 Classifications of Disability

Mental retardation	HIV infection/AIDS
Organic brain syndrome	Cancer, diabetes, heart disease
Emotional or mental illness	Orthopedic impairments
Alcoholism/drug abuse (individual participating in supervised rehabilitation program)	Hearing, vision, and speech impairment
	Communication disorders
Cerebral palsy, epilepsy	Learning disabilities
Muscular dystrophy, multiple sclerosis	

Note: Developed from "Cost Containment Strategies for Worker's Compensation" by J. Frieden, 1989, *Business Health*, 7(10), 48–54; "Federal Disabilities Act Increases Litigation Risks for Providers" by P. O'Hare and W. Schmidt, 1991, *Health Progress 4*, 43–46; "The Top Ten Issues under the ADA" by L. M. Schumaker, 1994, *Journal of the Missouri Bar 5*, 283–289; "Employers and the Disability Act" by R. S. Wray and N. M. O'Connor, 1990, *Business Health*, 8(10), 66.

violations are being decided by the courts on a case-by-case basis. As these court decisions are handed down, the working definition of "disability" as well as key issues and answers surrounding this act are becoming clearer. Nurse managers are urged to keep abreast of these latest court decisions.

The Family and Medical Leave Act (FMLA) of 1993 provides eligible employees with a leave of up to 12 weeks during any 12-month period for the employee's own serious illness, the birth or adoption of a child, the placement of a foster child into the household, or the care of a seriously ill child, spouse, or parent. Knowledge of this act, which is described in more detail in Chapter 21, provides guidance for leave issues.

Occupational Safety and Health Act The **Occupational Safety and Health Act (OSHA)** of 1970 was established to ensure a safe and healthful work environment for employees and to preserve human resources. OSHA standards are sets of rules designed to minimize specific on-the-job risks to employees. These risks include exposure to toxic chemicals, infectious agents, hazardous waste, and hazardous equipment. When OSHA deems agencies to be in violation of these standards, severe penalties are assessed. This act created three administrative bodies to carry out its mission:

1. The Occupational Safety and Health Administration (OSHA) is primarily responsible for creating and enforcing standards and procedures to enhance employee safety and health.
2. The National Institute of Occupational Safety and Health (NIOSH) engages in safety research and makes recommendations to OSHA.
3. The Occupational Safety and Health Review Committee (OSHRC) reviews contested actions made by employers following citations for noncompliance.

With the increased awareness of AIDS and the dangers of hepatitis infections, OSHA published regulations in 1991 designed to reduce occupational risks of infection from blood-borne pathogens. This standard is the most pervasive regulation imposed by OSHA on health care organizations. It applies to all occupational exposure to blood and other body fluids. Although most health care organizations comply with the Center for Disease Control and Prevention's universal precautions, OSHA regulations mandate several additional guidelines (White, 1992):

1. Develop an exposure control plan to eliminate or minimize exposure.

KEY TERMS

Occupational Safety and Health Act A law established to ensure a safe and healthful work environment for employees and to preserve human resources.

2. Make hepatitis B vaccine available to all employees at risk for exposure.
3. After an exposure, ensure that the employee is tested and provided with follow-up treatment and counseling.
4. Implement certain engineering and work practice controls to eliminate or minimize on-the-job risks.
5. Store or maintain sharps or contaminated materials in accordance with regulations.
6. Communicate to employees and the public the nature of contaminated waste by affixing appropriate labels bearing biohazard symbols.
7. Provide training programs for all employees at the time of initial employment and annually thereafter.
8. Maintain accurate and confidential records related to personnel training, vaccination, and management of exposures.

Although the number of guidelines regarding patient care, management, and employment may seem overwhelming, it is important to realize the improvements these guidelines have contributed to the work environment. They have helped to improve the quality of care and minimize risks. In addition, they have helped make efforts to eliminate discrimination successful.

Summary

- Both ethical and legal principles guide the practice of nurses and nurse managers.
- Ethics is a science that deals with principles of right and wrong, good and bad. Ethics are based on personal beliefs and values and govern our relationships with others.
- Actions that are based on achieving the greatest good for the greatest number correspond to the theory of utilitarianism. Deontology emphasizes the intent to do good without regard to the outcome of an action.
- Three principles guide ethical decision making. Autonomy is the principle that individuals have the right to make their own decisions. Beneficence is a duty to help others by doing what is best for them. The principle of distributive justice involves ensuring

that a person fairly receives the benefits or burdens due him or her.

- The American Nurses Association Code of Ethics explicitly defines the profession's values and standards of conduct.

- Laws are rules of conduct, established and enforced by authority, that prohibit extremes in behavior so that one can live without fear for self or property. The Constitution, statutes, common laws, and administrative rules and regulations make up the body of legislation that governs nursing practice.

- The area of law that most commonly affects nursing is tort law, specifically, negligence. Negligence is the failure of an individual to perform or not perform an act that a reasonably prudent person under the same circumstances would or would not perform. Malpractice is professional negligence. In order for malpractice to exist, the elements of duty, breach of duty, causation, and injury must be proved beyond a reasonable doubt.

- Liability may be personal, vicarious (as in the principle of respondeat superior), or corporate.

- Patients' rights are spelled out in the AHA Patient's Bill of Rights and include privacy, confidentiality, informed consent, right to refuse treatment, and limitations on the use of restraints.

- Liability issues that directly concern management are delegation and supervision, staffing, floating, policies and procedures, confronting unsafe practice, and employment regulations.

- Nurse managers must be knowledgeable about OSHA standards and the laws regarding antidiscrimination and sexual harassment.

■ LEADERSHIP AND MANAGEMENT
in Action

1. List and describe the three principles that guide ethical decision making.
2. What is malpractice? List the four elements that must be proved for malpractice to exist.
3. Describe several liability issues that directly concern management.

References

Aiken, T. D. (1994). *Legal, ethical, and political issues in nursing.* Philadelphia: F. A. Davis.

American Hospital Association (AHA). (1992). *A patient's bill of rights.* Chicago: Author.

American Nurses Association (ANA). (1985). *Code for nurses with interpretive statements.* Kansas City, MO: Author.

American Nurses Association (ANA). (2000). A new code of ethics for nurses. *American Journal of Nursing, 100*(7), 69–71.

Americans with Disabilities Act. (1990). 42 U.S.C. Subsection 12101 P.L. 101–336.

Barter, M., & Furmidge, M. (1994). Unlicensed assistive personnel. Issues relating to delegation and supervision. *Journal of Nursing Administration, 24*(4), 36–40.

Camunas, C. (1994). Ethical dilemmas of nurse executives. *Journal of Nursing Administration, 24*(9), 19–23.

Cross, L. (1992). Americans with Disabilities Act: Meeting requirements. *AAOHN Journal, 40*(6), 284–286.

Cruzan v. Director, Missouri Department of Health (1990), 110 S. Ct. 2841.

Fiesta, J. (1990). The nursing shortage: Whose liability problem? Part I. *Nursing Management, 21*(1), 24.

Food and Drug Administration. (1992). *FDA safety alert: Potential hazards with restraint devices.* Rockville, MD: Department of Health and Human Services.

Frieden, J. (1989). Cost containment strategies for worker's compensation. *Business Health, 7*(10), 48–54.

Furrow, B., Johnson, S., Jost, T., & Schwartz, R. (1991). *Bioethics: Health care law and ethics.* St. Paul, MN: West.

Guido, G. W. (1988). *Legal issues in nursing: A source book for practice.* Norwalk, CT: Appleton & Lange.

Guido, G. (1997). *Legal issues in nursing,* 2nd ed. Stamford, CT: Appleton & Lange.

Hall, J. (1990). Understanding the fine line between law and ethics. *Nursing, 20*(10), 34–39.

Joint Commission for the Accreditation of Healthcare Organizations (JCAHO). (1995). *Accreditation manual for hospitals.* Chicago: Author.

Luckenbill-Brett, J. L., & Stuhler-Schlag, M. K. (1987). Mandatory reporting. *Journal of Nursing Administration, 17*(12), 32–38.

Luquire, R. (1989). Nursing risk management. *Nursing Management, 20*(10), 56–58.

McConnell, C. R. (1990). The changing force of people management: Effects of the first-line supervisor. *The Health Care Supervisor, 9*(1), 65–74.

Moss, R. J., & LaPuma, J. (1991). The ethics of mechanical restraints. *Hastings Center Report, 1*, 22–25.

National Council of State Boards of Nursing [NCSBN] (1998). Mutual recognition model for nursing regulation: Frequently asked questions. *Issues, 19*(1), 1–4.

NCSBN (1999). Uniform core licensure requirements for initial licensure of RNs and LPN/VNs. *Issues, 20*(3), 1–2.

NCSBN (2000). State compact bill status. http://www.ncsbn.org/files/mutual/billstatus.asp Accessed June 22, 2000.

Northrop, C. E., & Kelly, M. E. (1987). *Legal issues in nursing.* St. Louis: Mosby.

Occupational Safety and Health Act of 1970, P.L. 91-596, 29 U.S.C. 651–678.

O'Hare, P., & Schmidt, W. (1991). Federal Disabilities Act increases litigation risks for providers. *Health Progress, 4*, 43–46.

Omnibus Budget Reconciliation Act (OBRA). (1987). P.L. 100–203 Sec. 420(a), 421(a).

Omnibus Budget Reconciliation Act (OBRA). (1990). P.L 101–508 Sec. 4206, 4751.

Quinlan v. New Jersey (NJ 1976). 355 A. zd 647.

Rehabilitation Act Amendments of 1986, P.L. 99–506 100 Stat 1808.

Schumaker, L. M. (1994). The top ten issues under the ADA. *Journal of the Missouri Bar, 5*, 283–289.

Walker, L. J. (1980). New responsibilities, new liabilities. *Trial, 16*(12), 42.

White, C. L. (1992). Protecting workers from pathogens. *Health Progress, 4*, 38–43.

Wray, R. S., & O'Connor, N. M. (1990). Employers and the disability act. *Business Health, 8*(10), 66.

Additional on-line resources for this chapter can be found on the World Wide Web at http://www.prenhall.com/sullivan_decker. Select Chapter 5 from the drop-down menu.

Power and Politics

Looking Ahead

What do politics mean to our everyday existence? How can political action influence the environment in which we live and work? How can power help reshape and improve nursing? In this turbulent time in health care, these are important questions for nurses to consider. Chapter 6 defines the role of politics in nursing and management, providing a framework of political action. In addition, the chapter addresses the relationship of power to leadership and image and provides an in-depth look at how political action in combination with power can have an impact on the future of health care.

Objectives

After reading this chapter, you will be able to:

- Define politics, power, and policy.
- Discuss the different sources of power.
- List reasons why nurses should know political strategies.
- Describe ways to use power for professional purposes.

As a nurse, do you want power? Do you need power? Do you have power? Are you politically savvy? Should you be more involved in the politics of nursing and health care? These are essential questions for nurses to consider. Although many nurses believe their work should be apolitical, failure to recognize the politics of patient care and nursing management can result in poor quality of care for the patient and frustration for the nurse (Mason, 1985).

It has become apparent that restructuring health care has enormous implications for professional nursing. Although agreement on the approaches and solutions to resolve the health care crisis has yet to be reached, we are confronted with a new pulse for change. Nurses must be ready to use their knowledge, expertise, and influence to make the system work (Costello-Nickitas, 1993). It is also incumbent on nurses to take leadership roles in transforming the health care system in order to ensure access to quality health care. This can be done only if nurses develop their power base and political skills.

This chapter presents a framework for political action, identifies sources and uses of power, discusses strategies for effective political action, discusses the principles of power and politics, and applies these principles to the practice of the staff nurse, the role of the nurse manager, and the role of nurse leaders in the community.

Politics: The Art of Influencing

Politics is the art of influencing the allocation of scarce resources (Mason & Talbott, 1985). These resources include money, time, personnel, and materials. Politics is a means to an end, a means for influencing events and the decisions of others (Stevens, 1980). Nurses who renounce politics are essentially saying they do not want to influence events in their everyday work.

Politics is an interpersonal endeavor. It involves skills of communication and persuasion. Their communication skills make nurses particularly effective in political activities. Nurses understand the importance of rapport and how to create meaningful connections with people. They understand the importance of time in developing these connections. They also understand the need to appeal to the other person's needs and interests if the goal is going to be reached. At a "Nurses Night" telephone bank to solicit support for a congressional candidate, the candidate's manager told the nurse organizer of the event, "You nurses are won-

> ### KEY TERMS
>
> ***Politics***   A means of influencing the allocation of scarce resources, events, and the decisions of others; a complex of relationships within an organization, including norms, values, and culture.

derful at this! I was listening to one nurse talking on the phone with a man who I thought must be her uncle or someone she knew well—it was a stranger, but they were talking as if they were old friends!"

Politics is a collective endeavor. It often requires the support and action of many people to bring effective politics to bear on a situation or issue. Furthermore, working with others for political action can be invigorating, more creative, and simply more effective because there are more people to do the work and provide the emotional support that may be needed to sustain long-term political action. The politically astute nurse develops and carefully uses a support base that crosses the hierarchical lines of each sphere. In the workplace, this means developing connections to other nurses, the maintenance people, top administrators, the social work department, physicians, and other workers at all levels of the organization. Certainly, this takes time, but it can and should be a part of the nurse's everyday work. For example, greet and speak to the person who is cleaning the floor every morning, sit with different people at lunch, and invite the new chief of the medical staff for a cup of coffee. It involves going to professional nursing meetings and exchanging business cards with those you meet. It involves providing support for others' agendas, knowing that they may be able to support you on an issue in the future. And it involves being able to organize and mobilize groups of nurses and coalitions of diverse groups. It is helpful to have a target list of people with whom you would like to connect to build your support base, remembering that the secretary to the chief officer in the organization may be one of the most powerful persons in the organization by virtue of his or her ability to control access to the top administrator.

Politics is also about analysis and planning. Just as the nursing process requires a thorough assessment, good politics arises from a careful and insightful political analysis of the situation, issue, or problem. A political analysis includes assessing the structure and functioning of the sphere in which you are operating. What is the organizational structure? What are the formal and informal lines of communication? Who holds legitimate power? Who holds informal power? What are the stated and unstated missions and agendas of the organization? What individuals are involved in the issue or situation? From a systems perspective, one change on the system can have far-reaching effects on the rest of the system. What are the values, interests, beliefs, priorities, and agendas of these players? What connections and power bases do they have? What is the current context of the situation or issue? What is the climate for change? What outside forces might be influencing the situation or potential solutions or changes? What recent events might influence how others view the situation and their openness to change?

A good political analysis also includes a thorough assessment of the issue or problem itself. Why does the issue exist? What are the contributing factors? Who is affected by the issue? Do efforts need to be devoted to creating an audience interested in the issue? What beliefs and feelings do people hold about the issue? Are more data needed?

Effective political action involves planning. Based on the analysis just described, a group trying to influence an issue or situation would brainstorm about alternative solutions and evaluate their risks and benefits. But the group also would develop a plan for introducing its alternative and persuading others to support its position. Political analysis tells you who can be counted on to play what role in this process. For example, who should introduce the alternative to the person with the formal authority to make the decision to adopt it? Sometimes, the most politically astute approach is not to have the originator of the alternative introduce it, but rather the individual who is most likely to be accepted by the decision maker(s). Is collective action needed? What coalitions need to be formed? The political analysis also will suggest strategies related to timing. Should the alternative be proposed now or in 2 months? Should it be proposed as a pilot project or demonstration project? Should it be gradually phased in or implemented fully at one time? Should group pressure be brought to bear now or later? Timing is often crucial to the effectiveness of political action. People usually are more willing to accept something as a trial or test. Pilot projects also enable those affected to adjust to the change gradually.

Politics is also about images. Do people think you can make the change? Do people think the change will be harmful to them? Do people trust you? Do people identify positively with the coalition involved? Your future ability to be politically effective may hinge on the image that others have of you or the group. For example, it is well known that when a workers' contract is settled in a collective-bargaining dispute, both the union and management sides try to come out of the negotiations with the appearance of having won the most. Even losses can be seen as victories, particularly if the effort resulted in the mobilization and empowerment of nurses so that the whole group's power and likelihood of future success are enhanced. Defining the message you want others to receive and effectively marketing that message can create the image needed to further your political agenda.

Some of these guidelines for effective political action stem from long-standing political tenets based on how people (men, in particular) have operated in politics. Machiavelli's *The Prince* is the classic work advocating the use of cutthroat strategies for getting what one wants. Some nursing literature has addressed how to "swim with the sharks," and certainly nurses need to be aware of how the game of politics traditionally is played. However, work by feminist scholars is suggesting that many women may be uncomfortable with cutthroat, Machiavellian politics. It is important for nurses to think about the ethics of their politics. According to Mason (1999) a new ethic is evolving in nursing based on women's ways of knowing and working together. This is particularly relevant to understanding what power is, how to get it, and how it can be used and abused.

A Framework for Political Action

Although most people associate the word *politics* with government, it pertains to every aspect of life that involves competition for allocating scarce resources or influencing decision making. As such, it is relevant to what nurses do in their daily practice, whether as a nurse in a home health agency, a nurse practitioner in a clinic, or a nurse manager in a hospital. What nurses do in their everyday practice is influenced by, and in turn influences, what governments do, what professional organizations do, and what communities do. What nurses do or do not do in one of these areas can have an effect on other areas and on their overall political power.

Politics in the Workplace

Politics in the workplace is often regarded with disdain, as reflected in the remark, "She plays politics." This statement is used to imply that the individual got what he or she wanted because of personal connections rather than on merit. And yet, would that same person want a chief nurse administrator who did not understand or use politics in advocating for nursing within the organization? Ehrat (1983) pointed out that politics is inherent in health care delivery because health care involves multiple special interest groups all competing for their piece of a limited pool of resources. A group's failure to recognize this fact ensures that the group's ability to influence decision making within the organization will be limited.

Politics in Government

Politics in government can influence who gets what kind of health care, where, and why. In spite of many efforts to limit health care costs, health care costs continued to rise much faster than inflation throughout the 1980s and early 1990s, acounting for an increase in consumption of 8.9 percent of the gross domestic product (GDP) to that of 13.4 percent. However, since 1992, health care expenditure has slowed, and health care's share of the GDP has remained the same at about 13.6 percent or $1 trillion. While Medicare savings have not been as dramatic, Medicare spending also has been more stable. A major factor in controlling these costs was the Balanced Budget Act of 1997 (Medicare Payment Advisory Commission, 1998).

Interestingly, little change has occurred in the number of uninsured Americans. The rate remains around 45 million (Monheit & Vistnes, 1997). However, the trend in insurance coverage has been away from indemnity insurance plans and toward managed care plans (Medicare Payment Advisory Commission, 1998).

Following a national election, Towers (1995) suggests that nurses take responsibility for educating and communicating with new legislators. Nurses must be attuned to the priorities of the administration and the majority party. Nurses must use their authoritative voices and political muscle to shift resources to expand community-based services that promote greater access to and availability of health care. Warner (1991) recommends that to be effective in forming public policy, nurses must establish standards of care and advocate changes in financing and health care organizations for persons who lack access to adequate care.

Politics in Financing

Which individuals qualify to be cared for by a nurse in an organization is, to a certain extent, determined by the politics of health care financing in the United States. Financing also influences where patients receive their care. In metropolitan regions, one can find at least two tiers of health care—one for the poor (the public hospital, the well-child clinic) and one for the middle and upper classes (the private institution and private physician). Although public health care institutions and agencies can often provide excellent care, they frequently are underfinanced and have limited resources (staff, equipment, medications).

To manage with shrinking health care dollars, market forces have caused a shift from fee-for-service reimbursements to managed care contractual arrangements and, more recently, to new integrated delivery systems and managed competition (Weis, 1995). In this competitive environment, health insurers have attempted to create cost-control pressures and slow the rate of reimbursement of high and rapidly escalating health care costs. These various arrangements are designed to create a capitated payment system, whereby health care providers (or health maintenance organizations) are paid a set sum per patient per year (known as "covered lives") rather than fees for specific services rendered to individuals at the time of service.

Managed care environments offer increasing opportunities for nurses to gain influence and prominence in health care delivery. As managed care plans seek to reduce costs, nursing's ability to provide cost-effective, high-quality care should be viewed as a political asset. In health maintenance organizations (HMOs), productivity is increased by using more nurse practitioners and by reducing the number of physicians (Hicks, Stallmeyer & Coleman, 1993).

The outcome of these redesign efforts is to emphasize primary, preventive care and avoid using high-cost services, including acute care hospitalization (Porter-O'Grady, 1994). The driving force behind the health care equation is economics. The politics of financing will depend on future market forces and responsiveness to patients' needs.

Politics in the Organization

Once a patient gets into a hospital bed, the kind and quality of nursing care he or she receives also can be influenced by politics. For example, the nurse may not find the time to sit with the elderly patient who needs to be fed but will unquestioningly take the time to give the tube feeding that the physician has now ordered (and which will be reimbursed) for a patient who is not eating. The politics of this situation involves what values and policies the organization and third-party payers have embraced. In this case, nursing care requiring a physician's order—and particularly care that involves a technical procedure—is valued, expected, and reimbursed before humanistic, low-technology, personal care.

Are nurses involved in defining the mission and philosophy of the organization or third-party payers? They should be. Are nurses participating as equals in committees that set organizational policy? They should be. This is political action.

Something as mundane as which health care providers have reserved parking spaces, a reserved dining room, or the largest offices (or any office!) becomes an important symbol of the power and influence of particular groups. The resources available for nurses to provide safe, effective patient care also reflect the power of nursing within the organization. For example, staff nurses in a medical clinic may waste precious time trying to locate one of the clinic's two tympanic thermometers. Why does the clinic have only two tympanic thermometers available? Most organizations do not purchase the thermometers—the manufacturers often provide them free because the company makes its profit from the sheaths made specifically for the company's thermometer, which must be replaced with each use. Why will the organization spend money on expensive diagnostic equipment such as a nuclear magnetic imager but not on relatively inexpensive equipment that would facilitate cost-effective use of the nurses' time? In organizations where nurses have a high degree of power and influence, the nurse manager controls a budget and is able to negotiate for necessary time-saving equipment.

Policy can be defined as "the principles that govern action directed toward given ends. This concept denotes action about means as well as ends and therefore implies change: changing situations, systems practices, and behavior" (Titmus, 1974, p. 23). Whether in government or the workplace, nurses need to bring their valuable expertise and perspectives to the places where policies are made. While individual nurses can and should participate in developing organizational and health care policy, professional nursing organizations provide a mechanism for nurses to influence policy collectively. Most nursing organizations, such

as the American Nurses Association (ANA), its constituent state nurses associations, the National League for Nursing, the American Association of Colleges of Nursing, and a variety of specialty nursing organizations, monitor and influence governmental legislation and regulations.

The primary focus for many of these organizations is furthering nurses' practice in a variety of ways. For example, nursing organizations on local, state, and national levels collaborated to prevent implementation of the American Medical Association's proposal for a Registered Care Technician (RCT) in the late 1980s. The AMA proposed that the RCT could provide bedside patient care that nursing organizations believed required the preparation and skill of a registered nurse. Organized nursing's successful effort to protect its practice and ensure that quality care continued to be delivered to the public was preceded by years of work by state nurses associations to update state laws that defined the scope of nursing practice—that is, nurse practice acts. Nursing organizations also monitor governmental regulations and patterns of organizational policies that can jeopardize nursing practice and have worked to secure adequate reimbursement for nursing services.

Increasingly, these associations also are playing a major role in developing and influencing broader health and social policies that affect the quality of health care and the health of communities, such as developing a national policy on long-term care, securing the rights of employees to take an unpaid leave of absence from work to care for a sick family member or new child, and working with state legislatures to reform Medicaid services.

For many of these nursing organizations, the increasing attention that they are giving to broader health care issues came about as a result of the political action of many of their members, who believed that nurses' voices should be heard on these larger issues. Nurse members developed resolutions that addressed these issues and lobbied for their passage at the business meetings of their organizations. Just as politics decides policies of government, they also determine the shape and focus of nursing organizations. These organizations are an important forum for nurses to learn, develop, and apply their political skills.

Politics in the Community

The workplace, government, and organizations all interact with the community, whether local, regional, national, or international. One nurse found that her leadership in a community effort to eliminate improper garbage dumping in her town enabled her to develop important connections to government officials on both the state and local levels. It also brought her to the attention of her hospital administrator in a positive and powerful way. The administrator knew that she had developed a positive reputation in the community and made significant connections to other persons of influence as a result of her actions. For many nurses who have children, an important forum for developing their political skills and power is the school's PTA or school board. An identity as a nurse in these groups can and should be made known. The connections developed can be used to further other purposes in the future.

This framework suggests that nurses need to understand the connections between what they do in their everyday work and what takes place in the rest of the community, nation, and world. Such a macroscopic view is particularly needed for the nurse manager. Although the nurse manager is rightfully concerned about how the work group is functioning, she or he must recognize that it does not function in a vacuum. Understanding and considering the broader context in which the unit is functioning makes the difference in whether the nurse manager is seen as visionary, whether the unit is on the cutting edge of nursing practice, and whether the unit sets the standard for excellence in the organization.

Power and Leadership

Real **power**—principle-centered power—is based on honor, respect, loyalty, and commitment. Principle-centered power is not forced; it is invited (Covey, 1990). It is defined by the capacity to act and to make choices and decisions. How you choose and what you choose is based on deeply held values. If you choose to live up to your own values and potential, you have an infinite amount of power available. By recognizing your power and the capacity to use it, you can influence and lead others in promoting and creating changes in health care and in your community.

Leadership power then becomes the capacity to create order from conflict, contradictions, and chaos. Leadership power comes from the ability to sustain proactive influence, which is sustained because followers trust and respect the leader to do the right thing for the right reason. As leaders in health care, nurses must understand and select behaviors that activate principle-centered leadership:

KEY TERMS

Power The capacity to act and make choices and decisions; the capacity to create order and sustain influence.

- *Getting to know people.* Understanding what other people want is not always simple.
- *Being open.* Keep others informed. Trust, honor, and respect spread just as equally as fear, suspicion, and deceit.
- *Knowing your values and visions.* The power to define your goals is the power to choose.
- *Sharpening your interpersonal competence.* Actively listen to others, and learn to express your ideas well.
- *Using your power to enable others.* Be attentive to the dynamics of power, and give attention to ground rules, such as encouraging dissenting voices and respecting disagreement.
- *Enlarging the sphere of influence and connectedness.* Power sometimes grows out of someone else's need.

Image as Power

A major source of power for individual nurses and for the profession is an image of power. Even if one does not have actual power from other sources, the perception by others that one is powerful bestows a degree of power. The same is true for the profession as a whole. If the public or legislators see the profession of nursing as powerful, the profession's ability to achieve its goals and agendas is enhanced.

Kotler (1984, p. 57) states that "an image is the sum of beliefs, ideas, and impressions that a person has of an object." Images emerge from interactions and communications with others. If nurses present themselves as caring and compassionate experts in health care through their interactions and communications with the public, then a strong, favorable image develops for both the individual nurse and the profession. Nurses, as the ambassadors of care, must understand the importance and benefit of positive therapeutic communications and image. Developing a positive image of power is important for both the individual and the profession.

Individual nurses can promote an image of power by a variety of means.

1. Appropriately introducing yourself by saying your name, using eye contact, and shaking hands can immediately establish you as a powerful person. If nurses introduce themselves by first name to the physician, Dr. Smith, they have immediately set forth an unequal power relationship unless the physician also uses his or her first name. Although women are not socialized to initiate handshakes, it is a power strategy in male-dominated circles, including health care organizations. In Western cultures, eye contact conveys a sense of confidence and connection to the individual to whom one is speaking. These seemingly minor behaviors can have a major impact on whether the nurse is perceived as competent and powerful.

2. Appropriate attire can symbolize power and success. Although nurses may believe that they are limited in choice of attire by uniform codes, it is in fact the presentation of the uniform that can hold the key to power. For example, a nurse manager needs a powerful image both with unit staff and with administrators and other professionals who are setting organizational policy. An astute nurse manager might wear a suit rather than a uniform to work on the day of a high-level interdisciplinary committee meeting. Certainly, attention to details of grooming and uniform selection can enhance the power of the staff nurse as well.

3. Conveying a positive and energetic attitude sends the message that you are a "doer" and someone to be sought out for involvement in important issues. Chronic complaining conveys a sense of powerlessness, whereas the problem solver and optimist promotes a "can do" attitude that suggests power and instills confidence in others.

4. Pay attention to how you speak and how you act when you speak. Nonverbal signs and signals say more about you than words. Make sure your words are reflected in your body language. In other words, keep your facial expression consistent with your message. Stand erect and move energetically. Speak with an even pace and enunciate words clearly. Use only body movements and gestures necessary to make your point.

5. Use facts and figures when you need to demonstrate your point. Policy changes usually evolve from data presented in a compelling story. To position yourself as a powerful player requires the ability to collect and analyze data. Data can be obtained to describe nursing care issues, activities, or concerns. These include patient acuity, daily census, length of stay, overtime budgets, or any data that reflect nursing's overall contribution. Remember that power is a matter of perception; therefore, you must use whatever data are available to support your judgment.

6. Knowing when to be at the right place at the right time is crucial to gain access to key personnel in the organization. This means being invited to events, meetings, and parties not necessarily intended for nurses. It means demanding to sit at the policy table when decisions affecting staffing and patient care are made. Influence is more effective when it is based on personal relationships and when people see others in person: "If I don't see you, I can't ask you for needed information, analysis, and alternative recommendations." Become visible. Be available. Offer assistance. You can be invaluable in providing policy makers with information, interpreting data, and teaching them about the nursing side of health care.

7. In dealing with people outside of nursing, it is important to develop powerful partnerships. Be very careful to use "we" instead of "they." Learn how to share both credit and blame. When working on collaborative projects, be clear about what is needed. If something isn't working well, say so. Never accept another's opinion as fact. Facts can be easily manipulated to fit one's personal agenda. Learn how to probe and obtain additional information. Don't assume you have all the information. Beware of unsolicited commentary. Don't be fearful of giving strong criticism, but always put criticisms in context. Before giving any criticism, give a compliment, if appropriate. Also, make sure your partners are ready to hear all sides of the issue. It's never superfluous to ask, "Do you want to talk about such and such right now?" Once an issue is decided—really decided—don't raise it again.

8. Make it a point to get to know the people who matter in your sphere of influence. Become a part of the power network so that when people are discussing issues or seeking people for important appointments of leadership, your name comes to mind. Be sure to deal with senior people. The more contact you have with the "power brokers," the more support you can generate in the future should the need arise. The more power you use, the more you get.

9. Know who holds the power. Identify the key power brokers. Develop a strategy for gaining access to power brokers through joining alliances and coalitions. Learn how to question others and

how to become part of the organizational infra-structure. There is an art to determining when, what, and how much information is exchanged and communicated at any one time and to determining who does so. Powerful people have a keen sense of timing. Be sure to position yourself to be at the right place at the right time. Any strategy will involve a good deal of energy and effort. Direct influence and efforts toward issues of highest priority or when greatest benefits are likely to result.

10. Use power appropriately to promote consensus in organizational goals, develop common means to achieve these goals, and enhance a common culture to bind organizational members together.

The concern with images of power has extended to the profession as a whole. A recent survey demonstrated that the American public has more confidence, trust, and favorable regard for nurses than for physicians and organization administrators (Mason, Costello-Nickitas, Scanlan & Magnuson, 1991). As the health care providers closest to the patient, nurses best understand patients' needs and wants. In the hospital, nurses are present on the first patient contact and thereafter for 24 hours a day, 7 days a week. In the clinic, the nurse may be the person the patient sees first and most frequently. By capitalizing on the special relationship that they have with patients, nurses can use marketing principles to enhance their position and image as professional caregivers.

Nursing as a profession must market its professional expertise and ability to achieve the objectives of health care organizations. Kotler and Clarke (1987, p. 5) describe marketing as "the analysis, planning, implementation, and control of carefully formulated programs designed to bring about voluntary exchanges of values with target markets for the purpose of achieving organizational objectives." From a marketing perspective, nursing's goal is to ensure that identified markets (e.g., patients, physicians, other health professionals, community members) have a clear understanding of what nursing is, what it does, and what it is going to do. In doing so, nursing is seen as a profession that gives expert care with a scientific knowledge base. Nursing care often is seen as an indicator of an organization's overall quality. Regardless of the setting, quality nursing care is something that is desired and valued. Through understanding patients' needs and preferences for programs that promote wellness and maintain and restore health, nurses become the organization's competitive edge to enhancing

revenues. Marketing an image of expertise linked with quality and cost can position nursing powerfully and competitively in the health care marketplace.

Using Power to Increase Your Professional Influence

To manage patient care successfully and to be more effective, nurses must understand the concept and importance of power. Then they must be willing to acquire power.

Why Power?

Power emerges in every human encounter, whether you choose to acknowledge it or not. Often, the content, meaning, and purpose of power use or abuse are misunderstood or ignored. Power needs to be your ally, and you must seek to understand its dynamic qualities. It is also important to understand why power is used. The most common reasons are to gain a competitive advantage, acquire information, motivate, communicate, improve performance, and improve processes. By developing a power base, you gain the potential for maximum influence. The willingness to use power increases a nurse's ability to acquire the resources needed to improve patient care (Carter, 1988).

Regardless of when, why, and where care takes place, power centers around an individual's ability to influence others or the behavior of others. Power also is defined as the potential to achieve goals. Bennis and Nannus (1985) suggest that power is the basic energy needed to initiate and sustain action, translating intention into reality. To acquire power, maintain it effectively, and use it skillfully, nurses must be aware of the sources and types of power that they will use to influence and transform patient care.

Power can be acquired through a variety of sources. Reward, coercive, referent, legitimate, charismatic, and expert power are defined and discussed in Chapter 4. In addition, there are two other bases of power related to political action.

- *Connection or network power* is developed through relationships with other people. Both the quantity and the quality of these relationships can determine how much power is derived from this source. Ferguson (1985) suggests that nursing as a profession has a right to and a need for collective or collaborative power. Developing connections and networks can further this collective power.

• *Informational power* is the possession and judicious sharing of valued information that another individual desires. Informational power is related to connection power, because what information one has may depend on one's networks and access to information. If a person has a reputation as a reliable confidant, he or she is more likely to have access to valued information. Conversely, someone who is known to be a gossip will be given only the information that others want made public.

Despite an increase in pride and self-esteem that comes with using power and influence, some nurses still consider power unattractive. The association of power with aggression and coercion remains strong. In a profession that prides itself on care and compassion, power is viewed as alien. How, then, can nurses bridge the disparity between power as good versus power as bad?

Several authors have noted that women and nurses are not as comfortable with power grabbing, which has been the traditionally accepted means of relating to power for one's own self-interests and use (Mason et al., 1991; Wheeler & Chinn, 1989). Rather, women and nurses tend to be more comfortable with power sharing and empowerment: power "with" rather than power "over" others. Although nurses need power to ensure that patients have access to cost-effective quality nursing care, nurses can help transform health care organizations by bringing a vision of power acquisition and usage that embraces equality and caring. Still, nurses must beware of power plays, in which others attempt to diminish or demolish their opponents. Table 6-1 describes several common power plays and their consequences. It is essential that nurses not accept these statements at face value. Often, restating one's initial point in a firm manner is a useful strategy. It is not necessary to respond directly to statements such as those shown in Table 6-1.

In a health care environment driven by competition and cost, nurses can make an important contribution, using their knowledge and expertise to influence health care legislation and reimbursement policies. To transform the notion that power is good and can be used to gain, maintain, and expand resources, nurses need to combine the various sources of power presented here and in Chapter 4 and apply them to the advancement of excellence in nursing practice. Promoting the positive effects of power can sustain nursing's power base in the health care arena and foster quality patient care. To use power to change and improve patient care is to recognize that power is natural and desirable.

Nursing must perceive power for what it really is—the ability to mobilize and focus energy and resources. What better position can nurses be in but to assume power to face new problems and responsibilities in reshaping nursing practice to adapt to environmental changes? Power is the means, not the end, to seek new ways for doing things in this uncertain and unsettling time in health care.

Power plus Vision

The key to understanding and gaining power is to identify what you and other people really desire. Once you have decided what you want, look at the total situation or encounter. Take into account, for example, the whole organization, not just your workplace or unit. Rank your wants or needs in order of importance. Determine who controls what you want and who or what stands in your way of achieving it. Identify the resources you control and the individuals who might desire those resources. Power resides not in aggressiveness or assertiveness but in the ability to make a conscious choice. Focus on the choice, not the action.

Table 6-1   Power Plays

Power Play	Recipient's Response
"Let's be fair."	Feelings of insecurity; insecure about choices because the power game is played by someone else's rule.
"Can you prove that?"	Embarrassed by inability to defend self.
"Be specific."	Feelings of incompetence if facts and figures cannot be generated to support position.
"It's either this or that. Which is it? Take your pick."	Angered at being forced to pick between limited options.
"But you said . . . and now you say . . ."	Confused about what was meant; believe position is illogical.

By making choices about what you want, you develop a strong sense of self-confidence and are aware of and feel good about your true capabilities. Your self-respect depends not on maintaining your role or position of power, but rather on your sense of purpose and direction. A clear vision pulls it all together by building consensus and support; identifying present capabilities; determining success factors; and identifying resources of people, time, and money.

Once you understand how power influences what choices are made and how these choices affect behaviors and feelings, you can appreciate its usefulness. In a constantly dynamic universe, power is a fundamental ingredient. You must ask yourself: Are you willing to use your power to know yourself, set goals, ignite the imagination, direct nursing care, build teams, and reach beyond the unknown into what could be? Survival in this turbulent health care environment calls for nursing's knowledge and expertise to initiate and sustain influence at all levels of care: the workplace, government, financing, organizations, and community.

Applying Power and Politics to Managing Nursing Care

The delivery of nursing services occurs at many levels in health care organizations. The effectiveness of care delivery is linked to the application of power, politics, and marketing. For the staff nurse, the politics of bedside care involves influencing the allocation of scarce resources (e.g., equipment, supplies, time, or personnel) for the delivery of nursing care. To maintain access to the resources needed for patient care, nurses must connect to the whole organization and beyond, not just their own nursing unit. Staff nurses need to understand that they belong to a complex organization that is continually confronted with limited resources and is in competition for those resources. With this understanding in mind, staff nurses can use their power when the limitations interfere with and place restrictions on patient care. Whether the restrictions come in the form of limited supplies, money, or time, nurses can use their power and the political skills of artful negotiation, collaboration, and networking to obtain the necessary resources to provide care. Speaking on behalf of patient care, access, and quality are what drives the politics of nursing care.

The politics of nursing care calls for an action plan, not just a care plan. It is time to force those who seek to establish policy without nursing's input to listen to what nurses have to say. Using power often means moving from being a passive observer to an active player. It means responding in politically astute ways by influencing and drafting policies rather than solely abiding by them. Mason (1999) suggests that there are two ways to lose power: by allowing others to take away your power and to become fragmented and self destruct. Unfortunately, both have occurred in nursing.

To respond effectively to the limits placed on clinical nursing practice, nurses must be visible and speak out about the "things nurses do": physical assessment, patient education, primary care, home and hospice care, and other health-related activities. How can nursing become a powerful force in the workplace and the community? How can nurses change the way power, politics, and policy are developed and used? One strategy is to write letters to the editor of your local newspaper or to contact television or radio talk shows explaining what nurses do and how their work improves care and individual lives.

In addition to becoming directly involved with policy makers, nurses can hold grass-roots organizational meetings to prepare new policy initiatives or changes. Other strategies include identifying a group of nurses to write letters to the hospital paper explaining the impact the new policy will have on nursing and educating doctors about the public good that can be gained by working together.

What happens in the workplace both depends on and influences what is happening in the larger community, professional organizations, and government. The effective nurse manager understands the connections among these groups and uses them to the advantage of nursing, patients, and the health care organization. Developing influence in each of these three groups takes time and a long-range plan of action. Although the nurse's first priority should be to establish influence in the workplace, the nurse can gradually increase connections and influence with other groups and, later on, make these other groups a priority.

How Nursing's Voice Can Become Powerful

The first step in improving nursing's power is to seek out opportunities for change. When you are ready to influence policy, start in your own workplace, where individuals and families know and understand the difference nurses make in the health and healing process. Don't stop at the bedside. Be sure to move beyond the workplace to the larger community and professional organizations. Identify where decisions are made and ask to be invited (e.g., nursing council, policy and procedure committee, the quality improvement committee). Focus your power on political and policy issues that evolve from personal and professional values and visions. Do your homework; knowledge is power.

The professional organization provides an opportunity for developing political skills that its members can use both in the association and in other areas. Obviously, the first step is to join a local and state nurses' association and/or a specialty organization. Attending meetings provides an opportunity to network with other influential nurses and to become known within the organization. Professional organizations depend on volunteer effort to accomplish their mission. Volunteering for one of the many committees that these organizations usually have gives you the opportunity to learn more about how the organization operates and to influence its actions and decisions. Seeking a leadership position with the committee provides additional influence and visibility. Such visibility often is needed if you are interested in serving on the major policy-making body of the organization, such as the board of directors.

Serving in various capacities provides you with the opportunity to develop some political skills, influence, and connections. However, most organizations also provide opportunities for the general membership to influence the organization's direction and decisions. This is usually done through making and passing motions at a regular meeting and/or through resolutions brought forth for action at the annual business meeting, which often is held in conjunction with the annual convention of the association.

Whether in committee, at a board meeting, or at a membership meeting, securing passage of motions and resolutions requires an understanding of formal and informal political processes. Support must be garnered for the motion or resolution. Just getting the item on the agenda may require a formal motion or some behind-the-scenes pressure on the individual who controls the agenda. Once an item is on the agenda, it is important to make sure people are prepared to speak in favor of the motion or resolution or in opposition, if that is preferred. On the one hand, because the image of power can be as important as actual power, some people will not bring a motion or resolution forward unless there is a certainty of passage. This may mean contacting people before the meeting and garnering their support for the motion, much like Congress does. On the other hand, raising

the issue may be an important first step in a long-range plan to eventually secure support. It is not uncommon for someone to float an issue or motion at one meeting to get a sense of the nature and strength of opposing arguments so preparations can be made to reduce the opposition in the future. In addition, the issue may be so important to some individuals that their convictions dictate that concerns about power images be put aside. Regardless, the politically astute nurse will reflect on these options.

By knowing your bottom line before you enter into any situation, you will be more open and flexible to the ideas of others. Develop a systems perspective; focus on the whole system rather than parts. To interact harmoniously, know how the system works. Power and influence are successful in securing scarce resources only when you understand what the system is and what it has to offer. Start with exploring relationships, structures, roles, and connections. These are resources that can be used to exchange power and influence.

Your vision and values allow you to connect to, relate to, and understand those you seek to influence. Find the common ground between your visions and values and those of others. Identify common threads, and speak your mind. Remember to keep communication open. Listen to understand; speak to be understood. Start the dialogue from the point of agreement, and move slowly into areas of disagreement. Assume good faith. Seek to resolve differences in perception. Help others to see your point of view. Establish relationships built on honor and trust, and you will earn legitimate power. Power created and sustained on integrity and goodwill is everlasting. Coercion and control lead to deceit, dishonesty, and suspicion, and are short-lived.

There is no quick fix or perfect strategy to using power and politics to manage nursing care. It requires skill, tact, and relationship building. Integrity—saying what you mean, and meaning what you say—is essential. If you try to use manipulative strategies and tactics to get others to do what you want, you will fail.

In difficult times, in pressing moments, remember to ask yourself, "How can I best respond to this situation?" Covey (1990) suggests the following power rules:

1. Never make a promise you cannot keep.
2. Make meaningful promises only to do better and better.
3. Consider promises as a measure of your integrity and faith.
4. Personal integrity is a basis for success with others.

The Impact of Power and Politics on Nursing's Future

How can nursing apply the principles of power and politics in the health care environment? Health care is in a state of constant change. Acute care hospitals are downsizing and reorganizing while, at the same time, community sites to deliver nursing care are expanding.

Nurses know the problems and have many of the solutions. Making a case for nursing input into health care policy is no longer an option for nurses. Nurses must be prepared to demand a seat at the policy table, whether that seat is in the board room; at federal, state, or local levels of government; or in any other setting where nurses remain a strong, vital component in health care delivery.

Nurses can have a tremendous impact on health care policy. The best impact is often made with a bit of luck and timing, but never without knowledge of the whole system. This includes knowledge of the policy agenda, the policy makers, and the politics that are involved. Once you gain this knowledge, you are ready to move forward with a political base to promote nursing.

To convert your policy ideas into political realities, consider the following power points:

- Use persuasion over coercion. Persuasion is the ability to share reasons and rationale when making a strong case for your position while maintaining a genuine respect for another's perspective.
- Use patience over impatience. Despite the inconveniences and failings caused by health care restructuring, impatience in the nursing community can be detrimental. Patience, along with a long-term perspective on the health care system, is needed.
- Be open-minded rather than closed-minded. Acquiring accurate information is essential if you want to influence others effectively.
- Use compassion over confrontation. In times of change, errors and mistakes are easy to pinpoint. It takes genuine care and concern to make course corrections.
- Use integrity over dishonesty. Honest discourse must be matched with kind thoughts and actions. Control, manipulations, and malice must be pushed aside for change to occur.

To manage nursing care in the future, nurses must come to realize that nursing expertise and clinical judgment are the best combination to effectively influence nursing practice and policy changes. By applying power and politics to the workplace, nurses increase their professional influence. Using influence, knowledge, and expertise can make the health care delivery system work.

Summary

- Politics is the ability to influence the allocation of scarce resources and events in our everyday world.
- Power is the means, not the end, to seek new ways of doing things in this uncertain and unsettling time in health care.
- Nursing must perceive power for what it really is— the ability to mobilize and focus energy and resources. What better position can nurses be in but to assume responsibilities for reshaping nursing practice to adapt to environmental changes?
- To use power and politics to change and improve patient care helps achieve nursing's goals of autonomy, economic independence, and professional status.
- Survival in this turbulent health care environment calls for nursing's knowledge and expertise to initiate and sustain influence at all levels of care: the workplace, government, financing, organization, and community.

■ LEADERSHIP AND MANAGEMENT
in Action

1. What is politics? How can nurses use politics in the organizational setting?
2. How does power differ from politics? How are they related?
3. Identify five ways nurses can promote an image of power.

References

Bennis, W., & Nannus, B. (1985). *Leaders.* New York: Harper & Row.

Carter, M. A. (1988). One step forward, one step back. *Journal of Professional Nursing, 4*(6), 96.

Cobrin, D. (1993). *Believe it or not: Incredible facts about America's health care crisis.* (Special Report No. SR15-Health) Washington, DC: Democratic Policy Committee.

Costello-Nickitas, D. (1993). Making a case for nursing: Earning a seat at the policy table. *Revolution: Journal of Nurse Empowerment, 3*(4), 58–60, 94.

Covey, S. (1990). *Principle-centered leadership.* New York: Simon & Schuster.

Ehrat, K. S. (1983). A model for politically astute planning and decision making. *Journal of Nursing Administration, 13*(9), 29–35.

Ferguson, V. D. (1985). Two perspectives on power. In D. Mason & S. Talbott (Eds.), *Political action handbook for nurses: Changing the workplace, government, organization and community* (pp. 88–93). Menlo Park, CA: Addison-Wesley Nursing.

Hicks, L., Stallmeyer, J., & Coleman, J. (1993). *Role of the nurse in managed care.* Kansas City, MO: American Nurses Association.

Institute of Medicine. (1988). *Prenatal care: Reaching mothers, reaching infants.* Washington, DC: National Academy Press.

Kotler, P. (1984). *Marketing management: Analysis, planning, and control,* 5th ed. Englewood Cliffs, NJ: Prentice-Hall.

Kotler, P., & Clarke, R. N. (1987). *Marketing for health care organizations.* Englewood Cliffs, NJ: Prentice-Hall.

Mason, D. (1985). The politics of patient care. In D. Mason & S. Talbott (Eds.), *Political action handbook for nurses: Changing the workplace, government, organization and community* (pp. 38–52). Menlo Park, CA: Addison-Wesley Nursing.

Mason, D., & Talbott, S. (Eds.). (1985). *Political action handbook for nurses: Changing the workplace, government, organization and community.* Menlo Park, CA: Addison-Wesley Nursing.

Mason, D., Costello-Nickitas, D., Scanlan, J., & Magnuson, B. (1991). Empowering nurses for politically astute change in the workplace. *Journal of Continuing Education in Nursing, 1*(22), 5–10.

Mason, D. J. (1999). Nurses dancing with wolves. *American Journal of Nursing, 99*(8), 7.

Medicare Payment Advisory Commission (1998). *Health care spending and the Medicare program: A databook.* Washington, DC: Author.

Monheit, A. C., & Vistnes, J. P. (1997). *Health insurance status of workers and their families.* 1996. Rockville, MD: Agency for Healthcare Policy and Research, Pub. No. 97-0065.

Porter-O'Grady, T. (1994). Working with consultants on redesign. *American Journal of Nursing, 94*(10), 32–37.

Stevens, B. J. (1980). Power and politics for the nurse executive. *Nursing and Health Care, 1*(4), 208–210.

Titmus, R. M. (1974). *Social policy.* New York: Pantheon Books.

Towers, J. (1995). A call to action: The GNE-GME-NEA debate. *Nursing Policy Forum, 1*(1), 40–45.

Warner, D. (1991). Nursing and public policy: What is the high ground? *Journal of Nursing Administration, 21*(5), 52–57.

Weis, D. (1995). Challenging our values: Directing health care reform. *Nursing Policy Forum, 1*(1), 22–26.

Wheeler, C. E., & Chinn, P. L. (1989). *Peace and power: A handbook for feminist process,* 2nd ed. New York: National League for Nursing.

PART 2

Key Skills in Nursing Management

CHAPTER 7

Budgeting and Resource Allocation

The Budgeting Process

Approaches to Budgeting

>Incremental Budget
>Zero-Based Budget
>Fixed or Variable Budgets

The Operating Budget

>The Revenue Budget
>The Expense Budget

Determining the Salary (Personnel) Budget

>Benefits
>Shift Differentials
>Overtime
>On-Call Hours
>Bonuses and Premiums
>Salary Increases
>Final Considerations

Managing the Supply and Nonsalary Expense Budget

Developing the Capital Budget

Timetable for the Budgeting Process

Monitoring Budgetary Performance during the Year

>Variance Analysis
>Position Control
>Staff Impact on Budgetary Performance

Future Trends

Looking Ahead

Chapters in Part I outlined management theory, structure, environment, and political issues. Building on that base, Part II outlines essential components to becoming an effective manager. This chapter examines one of the most important factors contributing to changes in health care and the role of the nurse manager: the economic climate. It is crucial that nurses be able to allocate resources effectively, plan and develop different types of budgets, and monitor expenditures. The challenge is to be able to juggle these responsibilities competently in an increasingly cost-conscious climate.

Objectives

After reading the chapter, you will be able to:

- Describe the budgeting process.
- Compare and contrast different types of budgets.
- Discuss guidelines for developing different types of budgets.
- Explain how to monitor and control budgetary performance.
- Determine budget variance.
- Describe the impact of staff on budgetary performance.

With the economic climate of health care in turmoil, greater attention is being given to cost containment and operational efficiency. The move toward capitated systems, increased competition, and the scarcity of financial resources are key forces behind the current focus on financial accountability. Because the nursing budget can account for as much as half of an organization's total expenses, nurse managers at all levels are facing significant pressure to become proficient in the budgeting process, to allocate resources, and to control and monitor expenditures (Villemaire & Lane-McGraw, 1986). This level of fiscal accountability is new to many managers and comes at a time when nursing must compete with other departments within the organization for limited resources. To compete, new and innovative methods are being tried, such as evidence-based budgeting (Massel, 1999) and the use of a professional salary model for staff nurses (Borromeo, Windle & Eagen, 1996). This chapter explains the budgeting process, defines budget terms, and presents guidelines for developing a budget, including how to determine salary expenses as well as operating and capital equipment budgets. The chapter also explains how to monitor and control budgetary performance and how to project costs based on current and anticipated needs.

A **budget** is a quantitative statement, usually in monetary terms, of the plans and expectations of a defined area over a specified period of time. Budgets provide a foundation for managing and evaluating financial performance. Budgets detail how resources (money, time, people) will be acquired and used to support planned services within the defined time period. The budget's purpose is to allow management to project action plans and their economic impact on the future so that objectives of the organization are coordinated and met. The budget process also helps ensure that resources necessary to achieve these objectives are available at the appropriate time and that operations are carried out within the resources available. The budgeting process increases the awareness of costs and also helps employees understand the relationships among goals, expenses, and revenues. As a result, employees are committed to the goals and objectives of the organization, and various departments are able to coordinate activities and collaborate to achieve the organization's objectives.

Budgets also help management control the resources expended through an organizational awareness of costs (Smeltzer & Hyland, 1989). Finally, budget

KEY TERMS

Budget A quantitative statement, usually in monetary terms, of the expectations of a defined area of the organization over a specified period of time in order to manage financial performance.

Budgeting The process of planning and controlling future operations by comparing actual results with planned expectations.

performance provides management with feedback about resources management and the impact on the budget.

The Budgeting Process

Budgeting is a process of planning and controlling future operations by comparing actual results with planned expectations. Planning first involves reviewing established *goals* and *objectives* of both nursing and the organization. Goals and objectives help identify the organization's priorities and direct the organization's efforts. In order to plan, the organization must anticipate the future by gathering information about the following:

- Demographics of the population served, community influences, and competitors.
- Sources of revenue, especially managed care contracts, as well as public payers such as Medicare, Medicaid, and commercial insurance companies, because payment arrangements and mechanisms determine the projected revenues of the organization.
- Statistical data, including the number of admissions or patient visits, patient days, average length of stay, and projected occupancy or visits.
- Projected salary increases and price increases, including inflation rate, for supplies and other costs.
- Information about regulatory changes (e.g., Medicare regulations) for the budgetary period.

The organization may use sophisticated and complex forecasting methods, including statistical techniques, to assist in making projections related to the budgetary period. Management normally uses the past as the common starting point for projecting the future, but in today's volatile payment environment, the past may be a poor predictor of the future. This is one of the major drawbacks of the budgeting process. In a rapidly changing industry, basing budgets on historical data often requires readjustment during the actual budget period.

Controlling is the process of comparing actual results with the results projected in the budget. Two techniques for controlling budgetary performance are *variance analysis* and *position control*. By measuring the differences between the projected and the actual results, management is better able to make modifications and corrections. Therefore, controlling depends on planning.

Approaches to Budgeting

The organization may choose one of two approaches, or a combination of both, for requesting departmental managers to prepare their budget requests. These approaches are incremental (line-by-line) budgeting and zero-based budgeting.

Incremental Budget

With an **incremental**, or **line-by-line budget**, the finance department distributes a budget worksheet listing each expense item or category on a separate expense line (Figure 7-1). The expense line is usually divided into salary and nonsalary items. A budget worksheet is commonly used for mathematical calculations to be submitted for the next year. It may include several columns for the amount budgeted for the current year, the amount actually spent year-to-date, the projected total for the year based on the actual amount spent, increases and decreases in the expense amount for the new budget, and the request for the next year with an explanation attached.

The base or starting point for calculating next year's budget request may be either the previous year's actual results or projected expenditures for the current year. For salary expenses, the adjustment might be the average salary increase projected for next year. For nonsalary expenses, the finance department may provide an estimate of the average increase for supplies or opt to use a standard measure of cost increases, perhaps the consumer or medical price index projected for the next year.

KEY TERMS

Incremental (line-by-line) budget   A budget worksheet listing expense items on separate lines that is usually divided into salary and nonsalary expenses.

Zero-based budget   A budgetary approach that assumes the base for projecting next year's budget is zero; managers are required to justify all activities and every proposed expenditure.

Fixed budget   A budget in which budgeted amounts are set regardless of changes that occur during the year.

Variable budget   A budget developed with the understanding that adjustments to the budget may be made during the year.

Operating budget   The organization's statement of expected revenues and expenses for the upcoming year.

Fiscal year   A specified 12-month time period during which operational and financial performance is measured.

For nurse managers to complete budget worksheets accurately, they must be familiar with expense account categories. The manager should understand what type of expenses, such as instruments and minor equipment, are included under each line item. In addition, the manager has to keep abreast of different factors that have affected the expenditure level for each expense line during the current year. The projected impact of next year's activities will be translated into increases or decreases in expense levels of the nursing unit's expenditures for the coming year.

The advantage of the line-by-line budget method is its simplicity of preparation. The disadvantage of this method is that it discourages cost efficiency. In order to avoid budget cuts for the next year, an astute manager learns to spend the entire budget amount established for the current year, because this amount becomes the base for the next year.

Zero-Based Budget

The **zero-based budget** approach assumes the base for projecting next year's budget is zero. Managers are

2002 Budget Preparation

Nonsalary Worksheet

Nursing Unit: 12 Tower

Nonsalary	2001 Budget	6/01 YTD Actual	Total 2002 Department Projection	Additions or Deletions	2002 Budget Request	Comments
Dressings	$1,013	$953	_____	_____	_____	_____
Syringes and needles	$1,009	$1,130	_____	_____	_____	_____
Instruments and minor equipment	$279	$1,150	_____	_____	_____	_____
Other medical/ surgical supplies	$1,494	$1,989	_____	_____	_____	_____
Lab supplies	$850	$409	_____	_____	_____	_____
IV solutions	$2,671	$2,698	_____	_____	_____	_____
Stationery and office supplies	$505	$1,090	_____	_____	_____	_____
Data processing supplies	$258	$125	_____	_____	_____	_____
Disposable linen	$1,487	$987	_____	_____	_____	_____
Housekeeping supplies	$484	$218	_____	_____	_____	_____
Total nonsalary	$10,050	$10,749	_____	_____	_____	_____

Figure 7-1   Budget preparation worksheet.

required to justify all activities and programs as if they were being initiated for the first time. Regardless of the level of expenditure in previous years, every proposed expenditure for the new year must be justified under the current environment and its fit with the organization's objectives. Because zero-based budgeting is time-consuming, organizations may not use this process every year. An adaptation of the zero-based budget is to start the budget with a lower base, for example, 80% of the current expenses. Managers then have to justify any budgetary expenses requested above the 80% base.

Fixed or Variable Budgets

Budgets also can be categorized as fixed or variable. Budgets are considered **fixed budgets** when the bud-

geted amounts are set without regard to changes that may occur during the year, such as patient volume or program activities, that have an impact on the cost assumptions originally used for the coming year. In contrast, **variable budgets** are developed with the understanding that adjustments to the budget may be made during the year based on changes in revenues, patient census, utilization of supplies, and other expenses.

The Operating Budget

The **operating budget,** also known as the annual budget, is the organization's statement of expected revenues and expenses for the coming year. It coincides with the **fiscal year** of the organization, a specified

12-month period during which the operational and financial performance of the organization is measured. The fiscal year may correspond with the calendar year—January to December—or another time frame. Many organizations use July 1 to June 30; the federal government begins its fiscal year on October 1. The operating budget may be further broken down into smaller periods of 6 months or 4 quarters; each quarter may be further separated into three 1-month periods. The revenues and expenses are organized separately, with a bottom-line net profit or loss calculated.

The Revenue Budget

The **revenue budget** represents the patient care income expected for the budget period. As a result of the acceleration of competition among health care organizations for patient revenues, the number of payers that pay customary or listed charges continues to decline. More commonly, health care payers pay a predetermined rate based on *discounts* or allowances. In many cases, actual payment generated by a given service or procedure will not equal the charges that appear on the patient bill. Instead, the health care provider will be reimbursed based on a variety of methods. These include reimbursement of a predetermined amount, such as fixed costs per case (Medicare recipients); negotiated rates, such as *per diems* (a specified reimbursement amount per patient, per day); negotiated discounts; or capitation (one rate per member, per month, regardless of the service provided).

Revenue projections for the next year are based on the volume and mix of patients, rates, and discounts that will prevail during the budget period. Projections are developed from historical volume data, impact of new or modified clinical programs, shifts from inpatient to outpatient procedures, and other influences. The impact of the payers' mix and the percentage that each of them contributes to projected revenues of the organization also is taken into consideration, such as the percentage of revenues derived from Medicare, Medicaid, commercial insurance companies, HMOs, and other third-party payers.

Medicare payments for inpatient services are made at a predetermined specific rate for each Medicare recipient based on the patient's diagnosis. Under the Medicare Prospective Payment System (PPS), adopted by the federal government in 1983, care is classified into diagnosis-related groups (DRGs). Payments are made based on the assumption that patients with the same DRG use similar resources.

DRGs are based on primary and secondary diagnoses, age, and treatment received. Within each DRG is the assumption that a certain number of resources are required for a specific patient treatment. It also is assumed that the use of resources varies according to the patient's age, sex, primary and secondary diagnosis, and discharge status. Currently the government uses 494 Medicare DRGs. The health care organization has a financial incentive to provide care at a cost below the fixed DRG price because it can keep the difference between the cost of treating the patient and the amount the organization is paid. Because of this incentive, organizations have used different methods to minimize the costs of caring for that patient, including reducing the patient's length of stay.

The Expense Budget

The **expense budget** consists of salary and nonsalary items. Expenses should reflect patient care objectives and activity parameters established for the nursing unit. The expense budget should be comprehensive and thorough; it should also take into consideration all available information regarding the next year's expectations. Described below are several concepts and definitions related to the budgetary process in a health care setting.

Cost Centers In hospitals, nursing units are typically considered cost centers. A **cost center** is described as the smallest area of activity within an organization for which costs are accumulated. Cost centers may be revenue producing, such as laboratory and radiology, or non–revenue producing, such as environmental services and administration. Nursing managers are commonly given the responsibility for costs incurred by their department, but they have no revenue responsibilities. In contrast, if managers are responsible for controlling both costs and revenues and if their financial performance is measured in terms of **profit** (the difference between revenues and expenses), then the manager is responsible for a profit center. Customarily, nursing is not directly reimbursed for its services. Nursing-related costs usually are included in the room charge. In addition, nursing lacks a method to categorize its activities, although work has been done in developing a taxonomy and minimum data set for nursing. (See Chapter 8 for more information about a taxonomy for nursing.)

Classification of Costs   Costs are commonly classified as fixed, variable, and semivariable or mixed. **Fixed costs** are costs that will remain the same for the budget period regardless of the activity level of the organization, such as rental payments and insurance premiums. **Variable costs** depend on and change in direct proportion to patient volume and patient acuity, such as patient care supply expenses. If more patients are admitted to a nursing unit, more supplies are used, causing higher supply expenses. Some costs contain both fixed and variable elements. These costs, called **mixed,** or **semivariable costs,** may vary with volume, but not directly. An example of this type of cost is utility bills. Utility bills are regular costs that vary with increases or decreases in census.

Expenditures also may be direct or indirect. **Direct costs** are expenses that directly affect patient care. For example, salaries for nursing personnel who provide hands-on patient care are considered direct costs. **Indirect costs** are expenditures that are necessary but don't affect patient care directly. Salaries for dietary or housekeeping personnel, for example, are classified as indirect costs.

Determining the Salary (Personnel) Budget

The **salary budget,** also known as the **personnel budget,** projects the salary costs that will be paid

and charged to the cost center in the budget period (Villemaire & Lane-McGraw, 1986). If available, labor reports (Table 7-1) are useful tools for projecting salary expenses for the upcoming period. Labor reports list employees' names, hours, and salary dollars charged to the unit. The information may be summarized by job classification (RNs, LPNs, nursing assistants, technicians) and by pay period for both year-to-date and total for the fiscal year. Labor reports are generally prepared every pay period in conjunction with paychecks, using payroll information derived from time cards or other time-keeping mechanisms. In addition to determining annual salaries based on number of employees in each job classification, other cost factors, such as premiums and operational components, must be considered for the budget request.

Benefits

After the number of required full-time equivalents (FTEs) is determined (see Chapter 18), it is also necessary to determine how many FTEs are necessary to

Table 7-1 Labor Report

Date 8/10/00
Period Ending 8/6/00   POSITION—AHN

Employee Name	Reg Day	Reg Evening	Reg Night	O/T Day	O/T Evening	O/T Night	Holiday	Benefit	Bonus	Total
Pietro, A.	80.00	0.00	0.00	2.50	0.00	0.00	0.00	0.00	0.00	82.50
	$1,440.00	$0.00	$0.00	$67.50	$0.00	$0.00	$0.00	$0.00	$0.00	$1,507.50
AHN HOUR	80.00	0.00	0.00	2.50	0.00	0.00	0.00	0.00	0.00	82.50
AHN DOLL	$1,440.00	$0.00	$0.00	$67.50	$0.00	$0.00	$0.00	$0.00	$0.00	$1,507.50

POSITION—RN

Employee Name	Reg Day	Reg Evening	Reg Night	O/T Day	O/T Evening	O/T Night	Holiday	Benefit	Bonus	Total
Seldridge, H.	0.00	0.00	40.00	0.00	0.00	0.00	0.00	40.00	0.00	80.00
	$0.00	$0.00	$678.50	$0.00	$0.00	$0.00	$0.00	$678.50	$0.00	$1,357.00
Werner, L.	16.00	24.00	0.00	0.00	0.00	0.00	0.00	0.00	0.00	40.00
	$236.00	$396.48	0.00	0.00	0.00	0.00	0.00	0.00	0.00	$632.48
Jabari, K.	0.00	0.00	80.00	0.00	0.00	0.00	0.00	0.00	0.00	80.00
	$0.00	$0.00	$1,357.00	$0.00	$0.00	$0.00	$0.00	$0.00	$0.00	$1,357.00
RN HOUR	16.00	24.00	120.00	0.00	0.00	0.00	0.00	40.00	0.00	200.00
RN DOLL	$236.00	$396.48	$2,035.50	$0.00	$0.00	$0.00	$0.00	$678.50	$0.00	$3,346.48

POSITION—UAP

Employee Name	Reg Day	Reg Evening	Reg Night	O/T Day	O/T Evening	O/T Night	Holiday	Benefit	Bonus	Total
Townsend, D.	40.00	0.00	40.00	0.00	0.00	0.00	0.00	0.00	0.00	80.00
	$260.00	$0.00	$299.00	$0.00	$0.00	$0.00	$0.00	$0.00	$0.00	$559.00

replace personnel for **benefit time** (vacations, holidays, personal days, and so on). This factor can be calculated by determining the average number of vacation days, paid holidays, personal days, bereavement days, or other days off with pay that the organization provides and the average number of sick days per employee as experienced by the cost center. By definition, replacement time is not calculated for indirect staff.

To determine FTEs required for replacement

1. Determine hours of replacement time per individual.

Benefit time	Hours/shift	Replacement hours
15 vacation days	× 8 hours	= 120
8 holidays	× 8 hours	= 64
4 personal days	× 8 hours	= 32
5 sick days	× 8 hours	= 40
	Total	256

2. Then determine FTE requirement

Divide replacement time by annual FTE base $\frac{256}{2080} = 0.12$

From the FTE calculations an FTE budget is calculated (see Table 7-2). This budget provides the base for the salary budget (Jones, 1989). However, shift differentials, overtime, and bonuses or premiums also may affect budget performance and need to be considered.

Shift Differentials

A fixed premium dollar amount may be set for all personnel working the evening or night shifts. The budget for these differentials can be calculated by multiplying the projected total number of hours that employees will work those shifts during the year. For example, on the night shift, RNs receive a premium set at $1.75 per hour. The total additional salary cost per RN position for the year on the night shift is added to the salary budget request.

Benefit time   Paid time, such as vacation, holidays, and sick days for which there is no work output.

To determine shift differentials

1. Multiply shift differential per hour by hours/shift

$$
\begin{array}{rr}
\$ & 1.75 \\
\times & 8 \\
\hline
\$ & 14.00
\end{array}
$$

2. Multiply differential/ by days/year

$$
\begin{array}{rr}
\$ & 14.00 \\
\times & 356 \\
\hline
\$ & 5096.00
\end{array}
$$

Overtime

Fluctuations in workload, patient volume, variability in admission patterns, and temporary replacement of staff due to illness or time off all create overtime in the nursing unit. A projection of overtime for the next year can be calculated by determining by staff classification (RN, LPN, nursing assistant, and other employee classifications) the historical or typical number of hours of overtime worked and multiplying that number by 1.5 times the hourly rate. For example, if the average number of overtime hours paid in a unit for RNs is 35 hours per 2-week pay period and the average hourly rate is $16.75, the projected overtime cost for the year would be $22,864 for the RN category.

To determine overtime costs

1. Multiply average salary for classification by factor to obtain overtime rate

$$
\begin{array}{rr}
\$ & 16.75 \\
\times & 1.50 \\
\hline
\$ & 25.125
\end{array}
$$

2. Multiply average overtime hours by overtime rate to obtain expenditure per pay period

$$
\begin{array}{rr}
 & 35 \\
\times & 25.125 \\
\hline
\$ & 879.375
\end{array}
$$

3. Multiply number of pay periods by overtime expenditure to obtain annual overtime costs

$$
\begin{array}{rr}
 & 26 \\
\times & \$879.375 \\
\hline
 & \$22,863.75
\end{array}
$$

Clearly, overtime can rapidly deplete finite budget dollars allocated to a nursing unit. The nurse manager should explore options to overtime such as using part-time or per diem workers in order to keep the cost per hour more in line with the regular hourly rates. A competent manager certainly would also evaluate unit productivity to decrease overtime. (See Chapter 8.)

On-Call Hours

If the nursing unit uses a paid on-call system, the approximate number of hours that employees are put on call for the year should be estimated and that cost added to the budget. Typically under the on-call system, staff are requested to be available to be called back to work if patient need arises, and the number of hours on call are paid at a flat rate per hour.

Bonuses and Premiums

The approximate number of lump sum bonuses, such as night bonuses, also should be added to the budget request. Some organizations also offer premiums for certifications or clinical ladder steps. In this situation, a fixed dollar amount may be added to the base hourly rate of eligible personnel; for example, an additional $0.50 per hour paid for professional certifications. This would result in the hourly rate of the employee being adjusted from a base of $16.75 to $17.25. In this case, if the employee is full time and works 2080 hours a year (40 hours a week multiplied by 52 weeks a year), the annual new salary would be $35,880, or $17.25 multiplied by 2080.

Salary Increases

Merit increases or cost-of-living raises also need to be factored into budget projections. These increases are usually calculated on base pay. For example, if a 3% cost-of-living raise is projected and the base salary for an RN is $35,000, then the new base becomes $36,050.

Final Considerations

Other important factors to consider when developing the salary budget are changes in technology, clinical supports, delivery systems, clinical programs or procedures, and regulatory requirements. Changes in patient care technology or introduction of new equipment may influence the number, skill, or time that unit personnel may spend in becoming oriented to the new equipment and, later, operating and maintaining it. If significant, the projected number of additional labor hours for the new budgetary period should be incorporated into the request.

The Joint Commission on Accreditation for Healthcare Organizations (JCAHO) and government regulations often establish the number and level of nursing personnel for specific clinical units to maintain safety requirements. For example, in critical care units and some other specialty units, a minimum of two staff members are required at all times, regardless of patient number or acuity. This may mean that even during times when no patients are in the unit, two employees must be paid to stay there.

Departments such as environmental services, dietary, escort, or laboratory may provide the nursing unit with support in performing certain tasks, such as transporting patients or specimens. Any change in the level of support they provide should be reviewed, and the effect of such change on the unit's staffing levels should be quantified for the next year's budget request. Changes in the method of delivering care (primary, team, differentiated practice, or functional nursing) or staff mix (RNs, LPNs, unlicensed assistive personnel) also will affect staffing patterns for the next year. Any changes in staffing can place new demands on the unit. Therefore, orientation and additional workload needs also should be considered.

Managing the Supply and Nonsalary Expense Budget

The supply and nonsalary expense budget identifies patient-related supplies needed to operate the nursing unit. In addition to supplies, other operating expenses, such as office supplies, rental fees, maintenance costs, and equipment service contracts, also may be paid out of the nursing unit's nonsalary budget.

An analysis of the current expense pattern and a determination of its applicability for the next budget period should be performed first. Any projected changes in patient volume, acuity, and patient mix also should be considered because they will affect next year's supply use and other nonsalary expenses. As an example, if patient days for a particular type of patient are projected to multiply and cause a 5% increase in the use of intravenous solutions, this increase should be addressed in the budget request by requesting an additional 5% for intravenous solution supplies for the next year.

Increases due to an inflation rate index, or at a rate estimated by the finance or purchasing department, are included as part of the budget request. A simple way of calculating the effect of a price increase is to take the estimated total ending expense for the year and multiply it by the inflationary factor.

To determine projected price increases

Multiply current total line item expense by inflation factor plus 1.0	$12,758
	$\times$ 1.05
	$13,396

Increases in expenses, such as maintenance agreements and rental fees, should also be incorporated as part of the budget request. The introduction of new technology and changes in programs and regulatory requirements may require additional resources for supplies as well as increased salaries.

Developing the Capital Budget

The **capital budget** is an important component of the plan to meet the organization's long-term goals. This budget identifies physical renovations, new construction, and new or replacement equipment planned within the budget period. Organizations define capital items based on certain conditions or criteria. Usually, capital items must have an expected performance of 1 year or more and exceed a certain dollar value, such as $500 or $1,000. Capital budgets also may be designed with a time horizon longer than 1 year, such as 3, 5, 10, or more years.

Nurse managers usually provide input into the capital budget by indicating needs. Request forms such as the sample provided in Figure 7-2 are used. As part of the request, additional related costs, such as installation, delivery charges, and service contracts must be estimated.

Priority Listing # _____

1. Department _____Nursing_____

   Location _____

2. Cost center title _____

3. Cost center number _____6062_____

4. 5 physiologic monitor (ECG and Respiratory)

   _____
   Request title and quantity

5. _____788338_____

   Model no., type, catalog no., size, etc.

6. _____Hewlett-Packard_____

   Potential vendor, tel. no. or vendor location

   (alternate vendor, if available)

Justification

Current monitors are constantly down for repair.
This model is outdated and has been phased out.
With the type of patients that are admitted to this
unit, we need a more sophisticated and reliable
system to monitor continuously the cardiac and
respiratory status of sick infants. This is phase II of
the planning for replacement in a systematic
approach. We have 12 more monitors to be
replaced over the next 3 years.

If more space is needed, please turn over.

Purchasing's Comment	Electronic/eng's Comment

Budget use only

Budget request   # _____

Equipment cost $ _____

Total cost $ _____

7. Equipment Cost $5,705.70 ea x 5 = $28,528.50

8. Cost _____

9. Tax _____$1,854.35_____

10. Freight _____

11. UL Approval _____

12. Other _____

13. Total Costs _____$30,682.35 + freight_____

14. Related New Operating Costs:

    a. Salaries (No. of FTE's) _____

    b. Nonwage supplies _____

    Repair and

    maintenance _____

15. Reason for Request:

    [x] Patient care

    [ ] Nonpatient

    [x] Replacement of equipment specify ID
        #F-13-576, F13-577, F13-575,
        F13-584, F-13-580

    [ ] Enhancement of existing equip

    [ ] Compliance with statutory mandate

    [ ] Expanding or new program

    [ ] Will increase revenue or cut expenses

    [ ] Other

16. Funding source, if any, other than
    hospital funds:

    Grant/account   # _____

    Contract/account   # _____

    Special Fund   # _____

    Other/account   # _____

17. Projected month of purchase _____

18. Person to contact _____
                        (please print)

_____ _____ _____
Date   Exten.   Division Head

_____ _____ _____
Date   Exten.   Department Head

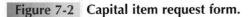

Figure 7-2   Capital item request form.

Because organizations typically set aside a fixed amount for total capital purchases, the nurse manager competes with other cost centers for limited resources. The expected benefits, including how the request fits into the organization's goals or programs, should be stated. To strengthen the capital budget request, the nurse manager should include information on features, price quotes, and a product comparison.

The impact of the new equipment on the unit's expenses, such as the number of staff needed to run the equipment, use of supplies, and maintenance costs, needs to be considered either as part of the capital budget request or the operating budget. For example, if monitoring equipment is being requested, the cost of electrocardiogram paper and electrodes should be determined, documented, and included in the supply budget. Likewise, the need for additional nursing and non-nursing personnel to operate the new equipment, additional workload, and training of personnel should be quantified for the next year's budget.

Timetable for the Budgeting Process

Depending on the size and complexity of the organization, the budgeting process takes 3 to 6 months. The process begins with the first-level manager. The individual at this level of management may or may not have formalized budget responsibilities, but he or she is key to identifying needed resources for the upcoming budget period. The manager seeks information from staff about areas of needed improvement or change and reviews unit productivity and the need for updated technology or supplies. The manager uses this information to prepare the first draft of the budget proposal. Depending on the levels of organizational management, this proposal ascends through the managerial hierarchy. Each subsequent manager evaluates the budget proposal, making adjustments as needed. By the time the budget is approved by executive management, significant changes to the original proposal usually have been made. The final step in the process is approval by a governing board, such as a board of directors or designated shareholders. Typically, the budget process timetable is structured so that the budget is approved a few months before the beginning of the new fiscal year.

Nurse managers must recognize the importance of clearly articulating their budgetary needs. Senior management must prioritize budget requests for the

---

entire organization and they base those decisions on strong supporting documentation. Nurse managers should not expect to receive all of their budget requests, but they need to be prepared to defend their priorities.

Monitoring Budgetary Performance during the Year

In many organizations, nurse managers receive a monthly report prepared by the accounting department summarizing the expenses for the department (Table 7-2). This report shows expense line items with the budgeted amount, actual expenditure, variance from budget, and the percentage from the budgeted amount that such variance represents. Commonly these monthly reports also show the comparison between actual year-to-date results and the year-to-date budget.

The difference between the amount that was budgeted for a specific revenue or cost and the actual revenue or cost that resulted during the course of activities is known as the **variance**. In the case of nursing units, variance might occur in the actual cost of delivering patient care for a certain expense line item in a specified period of time. Nurse managers are commonly asked to justify the reason for variances and present an action plan to reduce or eliminate these variances.

Variance Analysis

In the daily course of events in the unit, it is unlikely that projected budget items will be completely on target in all situations (Wilburn, 1992). When expenses occur that differ from the budgeted amounts, organizations usually have an established level at which a variance needs to be investigated and explained or justified by the manager of the department. This level may be a certain dollar amount, such as $500, or it

Table 7–2 | **Sample Salary Budget**

Monthly Budget to Actual Comparison Report
Fiscal Year through Period Ending 07/31/00

Month to Date					Year to Date		
Actual Balance	Budget Balance	Variance	Expense Line	Description	Actual Balance	Budget Balance	Variance
$7,875	$7,827	($48)	100	Assistant head nurse	$57,623	$54,789	($2,834)
$83,759	$85,450	$1,691	150	Registered nurses	$584,314	$598,150	$13,836
$11,655	$15,149	$3,494	250	Nursing assistants	$81,501	$106,043	$24,542
$4,462	$5,260	$798	700	Unit secretaries	$31,436	$38,820	$5,384
$107,751	$113,686	$5,935	XX	Subtotal—salary	$754,873	$795,802	$40,929
$6,815	$7,282	$467	302	Dressings and bandages	$47,505	$50,976	$3,471
$465	$672	$207	303	Syringes and needles	$3,775	$4,704	$929
$2,308	$2,410	$102	308	Instruments and minor equipment	$16,031	$16,869	$838
$16,105	$15,894	($211)	309	Other med/surg supplies	$120,985	$111,261	($9,724)
$33	$373	$340	320	Lab supplies	$1,121	$2,610	$1,489
$5,390	$3,881	($1,509)	350	IV Solutions	$37,988	$27,170	($10,818)
$398	$568	$170	401	Stationery and office supplies	$2,528	$3,974	$1,446
$31,514	$31,081	($433)	XX	Subtotal—nonsalary	$229,933	$217,564	($12,369)
$139,265	$144,767	$5,501	XXX	Total cost center	$964,806	$1,013,366	$28,560

may be a percentage, such as a 5% or 10% increase above the budget.

In determining causes for variance, the nurse manager must review the activity level of the unit for the same period (Wilburn, 1992). There may have been increases in census or patient acuity that generated additional expense in salary and supplies. While reviewing the causes for variance, the manager must remember that in many situations, variances might not be independent of one another. Variances may result from expenses that follow a seasonal pattern, occurring only at determined times in the year; renewal of a maintenance agreement is one example. Expenses may also follow a tendency or trend either to increase or to decrease during the year (Tzirides, Waterstraat, & Chamberlin, 1991). Even if the situation is outside the manager's usual responsibility or control, the manager

needs to understand and be able to identify the cause or reason for the variance (Francisco, 1989).

To determine when a variance is favorable or unfavorable, it is important to relate the variance to its impact on the organization in terms of revenues and expenses. If more earnings came in than expected, the variance is favorable; if less, the variance is negative. Likewise, if less was spent than expected, the variance is favorable; if more was spent, the variance is negative.

For instance, the nurse manager might receive the following expense report:

Medical/surgical supplies

Budgeted Expenditures	Actual Expenditures	Variance (in $)	Percent
34,560	36,958	(2398)	−6.9

This expense variance is considered unfavorable because the actual expense was greater than the budget. In this example, more money was spent on medical/surgical supplies than was projected in the budget.

If the variance of the actual budget amount is not presented in the reports, it can be calculated as follows:

To determine variance percentage

Divide the dollar variance by the budget amount then multiply by 100:

$$\frac{\$\,2398}{\$34,560} = 0.069$$

$$0.069 \times 100 = 6.9\% \text{ over budget}$$

Salary Variances With salary expenditures, variances may occur in volume, efficiency, or rate. Typically these factors are related and have an impact on each other. **Volume variances** result when there is a difference in the budgeted and actual workload requirements as would occur with increases in patient days. An increase in the actual number of patient days will increase the salary expense, resulting in an unfavorable volume variance. Although the variance is unfavorable, concomitant increases in revenues for the organization should be apparent. Thus, the impact to the organization should be welcomed, even though it generated higher salary costs at the nursing unit level.

Efficiency variance, also called quantity or use variance, reflects the difference between budgeted and actual nursing care hours provided. Patient acuity, nursing skill, unit management, technology, and productivity all affect the number of patient care hours actually provided versus the original number planned or required. At the same time, if the census had been higher than expected, it would be understandable if more hours of nursing care were provided and paid. A favorable efficiency, or fewer nursing care hours paid, could suggest that patient acuity was lower than projected, that staff was more efficient, or that higher-skilled employees were used. An unfavorable efficiency may be due to greater patient acuity than allowed for in the budget, overstaffing of the unit, or the use of less experienced or less efficient employees. Chapter 8 explains efficiency and productivity in greater detail.

Rate variances, also known as price or spending variance, reflect the difference in budgeted and actual hourly rates paid. A favorable rate variance may reflect the use of new employees who were paid lower salaries. Unfavorable rate variance may reflect unantic-

KEY TERMS

Volume variances Differences in the budget as a result of increases or decreases in patient volume.

Efficiency variance The difference between budgeted and actual nursing care hours provided.

Rate variance The difference between budgeted and actual hourly rates paid.

Nonsalary expenditure variance Deviation from the budget as a result of changes in patient volume, supply quantities, or prices paid.

Position control A monitoring tool used to compare actual numbers of employees to the number of budgeted FTEs for the nursing unit.

ipated salary increases or increased use of personnel paid at higher wages, such as agency personnel.

Nonsalary Expenditure Variances Nonsalary expenditure variances may be due to changes in patient volume, patient mix, supply quantities, or prices paid. New, additional, or more expensive supplies used at the nursing unit because of technology changes or new regulations also could influence expenditure totals.

Position Control

Another monitoring tool used by nurse managers is the position control. The **position control** is used to compare actual numbers of employees to the number of budgeted FTEs for the nursing unit. The position control is a list of approved, budgeted FTE positions for the nursing cost center. The positions are displayed by category or job classification, such as nurse manager, RNs, LPNs, and so on. The nurse manager updates the position control with employee names and FTE factors for each individual with respect to personnel changes, new hires, and resignations that take place during the year.

Staff Impact on Budgetary Performance

Staff can acutely affect the organization's finances. Misuse of sick time, excessive overtime, and wasteful use of resources can result in negative variance. Organizations have implemented a number of different programs and incentives for increasing employee awareness and minimizing costs. Techniques to decrease absenteeism may be instituted (see Chapter 21). Displaying equipment costs on supply stickers or requisitions and indicating medication costs on medication sheets increase staff awareness of costs. Participation in quality improvement and action teams also serves to inform staff of cost factors. Bonuses based on net gains have been shared with employees, in addition to cost-of-living raises.

Future Trends

A major trend in financial management of health care organizations is the shift from a revenue-based to a cost-based accounting system. Formerly, hospitals emphasized generating revenues to cover the costs of health care. With the impending shift to managed care, however, the focus is on decreasing costs to maintain adequate profit margins in an area of diminishing compensation. In the managed care environment, payment is prospectively determined in a competitive arrangement between provider and payer. In an effort to be a low-cost provider of health care, agencies are strongly motivated to be cost effective. This trend has serious implications for nursing. Nursing has always been considered a cost, not a source of revenue. It is nursing's challenge to be consistently cost-conscious and to measure, manage, and document nursing's cost-effectiveness in this new financial environment (Diers, & Bozzo, 1997).

Summary

- A budget is a quantitative statement, usually written in monetary terms, of plans and expectations over a specified period of time.
- The operating or annual budget is the organization's statement of expected revenues and expenses for the coming year.
- The revenue budget represents the patient care revenues expected for the budget period based on volume and mix of patients, rates, and discounts that will prevail during the same period of time.
- Nursing units are typically considered cost centers. A cost center is described as the smallest area of

activity within an organization for which costs are accumulated.

- A full-time equivalent (FTE) is a full-time position that can be equated to 40 hours of work per week for 52 weeks, or 2080 hours per year.
- The position control is a list of approved, budgeted FTEs that compares the budgeted number of FTEs by classification (RN, LPN), shift, and status to the actual available employees of the unit.
- Variance is the difference between the amount that was budgeted for a specific revenue or cost and the actual revenue or cost that resulted during the course of activities.
- The capital budget identifies physical renovations, new construction, and the purchase of new or replacement equipment planned within a period of time, usually longer than 1 year.
- The shift from a revenue- to a cost-based accounting system requires nurses to remain cost-conscious and to demonstrate nursing's cost-effectiveness.

■ LEADERSHIP AND MANAGEMENT
in Action

1. Identify four different types of budgets. What are the advantages and disadvantages of each?
2. What factors influence the development of the personnel budget?
3. List five items that would be considered capital expenditures.

References

Borromeo, A. R., Windle, P. E., & Eagen, M. K. (1996). The professional salary model: Meeting the bottom lines. *Nursing Economics, 14*(4), 241–244.

Diers, D. & Bozzo, J. (1997). Nursing resource definition in DRGs. *Nursing Economics, 15*(3), 124–130, 137.

Francisco, P. D. (1989). Flexible budgeting and variance analysis. *Nursing Management, 20*(11), 40–43.

Jones, R. A. (1989). Taking the 'guesstimates' out of FTE budgeting. *Nursing Management, 20*(2), 65–73.

Massel, D. (1999). Evidence based budgeting is now necessary. *British Medical Journal, 319*(7206), 384.

Smeltzer, C. H., & Hyland, J. (1989). A working plan to

understand and control financial pressures. *Nursing Economics, 7*(4), 208–214.

Tzirides, E., Waterstraat, V., & Chamberlin, W. (1991). Managing the budget with a fluctuating census. *Nursing Management, 22*(3), 80B–80H.

Villemaire, M., & Lane-McGraw, C. (1986). Nursing personnel budgets: A step-by-step guide. *Nursing Management, 17*(11), 28–32.

Wilburn, D. (1992). Budget response to volume variability. *Nursing Management, 23*(2), 42–44.

CHAPTER 8

Effectiveness, Efficiency, and Productivity

Looking Ahead

As changes in the health care industry occur and as costs rise, nurses and nurse managers are being asked to identify and implement effective strategies and processes that will create a more efficient and productive workplace environment in hospitals, homes, and the community. This chapter looks at calculating input and output, measuring productivity, and identifying strategies to improve effectiveness.

Objectives

After reading this chapter, you will be able to:

- Define effectiveness, efficiency, and productivity.
- Describe ways to measure nursing productivity.
- Discuss methods by which productivity can be improved.

Despite efforts by the health care industry to contain costs, health care expenditures continue to increase at a rate greater than the overall rate of inflation. Concerned about the billions spent each year on health care, consumers and policy makers are now demanding that the escalating costs of health care decrease without diminishing the quality of care they have come to expect. These expectations have driven the movement by government and health care management to evaluate allocation of scarce resources carefully and to begin to identify what constitutes quality care; others suggest that evidence-based budgeting is necessary (Massel, 1999).

Congress responded to these concerns by creating the Agency for Health Care Policy and Research (AHCPR) in the U.S. Department of Health and Human Services in 1989. AHCPR has been charged with identifying effective clinical practices with an emphasis on cost-effectiveness. The primary activity of the AHCPR is to conduct research projects to evaluate existing technologies and practices. Multidisciplinary patient outcomes research teams (PORTS) have been created to study selected practice areas and identify effective diagnostic, curative, and caregiving strategies. Currently these PORTS are studying many important areas of health care to improve effectiveness.

At the same time, the health care industry has undertaken a massive effort to identify the professional care delivery systems, technologies, and processes that create a productive, effective, and efficient workplace. Nursing, which comprises the largest single group of health care providers, can account for 50% or more of the operating budgets of organizations such as hospitals, home care agencies, and long-term–care facilities, but because it does not directly generate revenue, it is perceived as an expense. Therefore, nursing is targeted as a logical choice when costs are scrutinized. Reductions in the nursing service budget appear to result in sizable savings. Although this is not necessarily correct, nursing currently lacks an adequate definition and measurement of nursing effectiveness, efficiency, and productivity to challenge this common belief.

What Are Effectiveness, Efficiency, and Productivity in Health Care?

Effectiveness, efficiency, and *productivity* are terms that relate to outcomes of care. **Effectiveness** is an outcome measure of the interventions that improve people's health under ordinary circumstances and in ordinary settings. This is in contrast to the word *efficacy*, used frequently in medical research, which identifies only whether an intervention can improve health in *ideal* circumstances (U.S. Congress, Office of Technology Assessment, 1994). Another author defines *effectiveness* as the safety, appropriateness, and excellence of care, which encompasses the issues of health status, patient outcomes, and patient satisfaction (American Management Sciences, Inc. [AMSI], 1980). If one considers effectiveness in terms of achievement of objectives, then **efficiency** can be described as the relationship between achieving objectives and consumption of resources (Smalley & Freeman, 1966). **Productivity** describes the relationship between the output (product) of an industry and the resources required to produce that output (output per input), but this single-factor output:input ratio usually fails to take into account the complexity of defining productivity in a service sector such as health care. Fundamental questions remain about what should be considered an input and how output should be measured.

Organizational Effectiveness in Health Care Today

From an open systems perspective, organizational effectiveness means sensing a change in the environment, inputting and digesting relevant information, using that information rather than past organizational history to make creative decisions, changing the throughput according to those decisions while managing undesired side effects, outputting new products or services in line with perceived environmental demands, and obtaining feedback on the change. Open systems have multiple functions that exist within uncertain environments and whose effectiveness is measured by their ability to survive, adapt, maintain themselves, and grow. Effectiveness is defined by how well an organization copes with its environment; nothing could be more meaningful for health care today.

Many factors today make it difficult for bureaucratically structured organizations such as health care organizations to be effective. A bureaucracy's strength is its capacity to manage routine and predictable activities in a stable environment with its well-defined chain of command and rules. But many health care organizations are not equipped to deal with today's rapid and continuous environmental change. In addition, growth of an organization introduces complexity in a bureaucratic pyramid. Increased administrative overhead, tighter controls, rigid rules, and greater impersonality can all result when an organization grows.

Increased diversity also results from growth. Today's environment demands diverse, highly specialized competence that is often incompatible with a bureaucracy's hierarchy and rigidity. Managerial philosophies must change to allow innovative, non–status quo thinking to be integrated into organizational decision making. Any organization designed to function in a stable environment will not be able to react effectively to rapid environmental change.

Health Care Inputs

Inputs include labor, materials, and equipment used in the production of services (Figure 8-1). Inputs usually can be measured in physical units, such as hours of labor; dollars spent on equipment, remodeling or building expense; and the number of supplies used. The measurement of some inputs is not as simple as it seems. Nursing personnel, for example, are not a homogeneous group; nurses vary in their level of education, experience, and skill. Even two nurses with equivalent education and years of experience can differ considerably in their ability to care for patients.

Health Care Outputs

In the past, hospital **output** (products) was most frequently defined in **patient days**, that is, the total number of days all patients were hospitalized in a facility over a period of time (Feldstein, 1971). Then it was

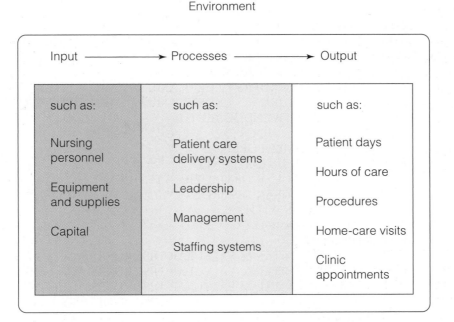

Figure 8-1 **Nursing productivity framework.** *Note:* **From** *A review and evaluation of nursing productivity* **by R. C. Jelinek and L. C. Dennis, 1976, DHEW Publication no. (HRA) 77-15, Bethesda, MD: Health Resources Administration.**

realized that some patient days required the use of many more resources than others. A day of care for a transplant patient is much more costly than a day of postpartum care, for example.

Newer concepts of hospital output are more specific than the patient days. **Case mix** is a method of clustering patients into groups that are homogeneous with respect to the use of resources. Factors used to cluster patients have included diagnosis, prognosis, resource utilization, organ system, hospital department, and patient demographic characteristics (Hornbrook, 1982). The best known of these case-mix measures is the diagnosis-related groups (DRGs) system introduced by the federal government in 1983 as a prospective payment system to reduce reimbursement costs for Medicare patients. Patients are assigned into 494 resource-use groups based on information about their diagnosis, age, and the use of certain procedures. Using the DRG case-mix measure, the hospital could potentially produce 494 distinct products that vary from one another in the cost of production. (See Box 8-1 for examples of DRGs.) Each DRG is weighted to represent the average cost of providing care to patients in that category. Although there are many

Box 8-1		**Sample List of Diagnosis-Related Groups (DRGs)**
106	05	SURG	CORONARY BYPASS W CARDIAC CATH
107	05	SURG	CORONARY BYPASS W/O CARDIAC CATH
108	05	SURG	OTHER CARDIOTHORACIC PROCEDURES
109			NO LONGER VALID
110	05	SURG	MAJOR CARDIOVASCULAR PROCEDURES WITH CC
111	05	SURG	MAJOR CARDIOVASCULAR PROCEDURES W/O CC
112	05	SURG	PERCUTANEOUS CARDIOVASCULAR PROCEDURES
113	05	SURG	AMPUTATION FOR CIRC SYSTEM DISORDERS EXCEPT UPPER LIMB & TOE
114	05	SURG	UPPER LIMB & TOE AMPUTATION FOR CIRC SYSTEM DISORDERS
115	05	SURG	PERM CARDIAC PACEMAKER IMPLANT W AMI. HEART FAILURE OR SHOCK
116	05	SURG	OTH PERM CARDIAC PACEMAKER IMPLANT OR AICD LEAD OR GEN PROC
117	05	SURG	CARDIAC PACEMAKER REVISION EXCEPT DEVICE REPLACEMENT
118	05	SURG	CARDIAC PACEMAKER DEVICE REPLACEMENT
119	05	SURG	VEIN LIGATION & STRIPPING
120	05	SURG	OTHER CIRCULATORY SYSTEM O.R. PROCEDURES
121	05	MED	CIRCULATORY DISORDERS W AMI. & C.V. COMP DISCH ALIVE
122	05	MED	CIRCULATORY DISORDERS W AMI. W/O C.V. COMP DISCH ALIVE
123	05	MED	CIRCULATORY DISORDERS W AMI. EXPIRED
124	05	MED	CIRCULATORY DISORDERS EXCEPT AMI. W CARD CATH & COMPLEX DIAG
125	05	MED	CIRCULATORY DISORDERS EXCEPT AMI. W CARD CATH W/O COMPLEX DIAG
126	05	MED	ACUTE & SUBACUTE ENDOCARDITIS
127	05	MED	HEART FAILURE & SHOCK
128	05	MED	DEEP VEIN THROMBOPHLEBITIS
129	05	MED	CARDIAC ARREST, UNEXPLAINED
130	05	MED	PERIPHERAL VASCULAR DISORDERS WITH CC
131	05	MED	PERIPHERAL VASCULAR DISORDERS W/O CC
132	05	MED	ATHEROSCLEROSIS WITH CC
133	05	MED	ATHEROSCLEROSIS W/O CC
134	05	MED	HYPERTENSION
135	05	MED	CARDIAC CONGENITAL & VALVULAR DISORDERS AGE > 17 WITH CC
136	05	MED	CARDIAC CONGENITAL & VALVULAR DISORDERS AGE > 17 W/O CC
137	05	MED	CARDIAC CONGENITAL & VALVULAR DISORDERS AGE 0–17
138	05	MED	CARDIAC ARRHYTHMIA & CONDUCTION DISORDERS WITH CC
139	05	MED	CARDIAC ARRHYTHMIA & CONDUCTION DISORDERS W/O CC
140	05	MED	ANGINA PECTORIS

Note: From *Federal Register*, September 1, 1992, *Rules and Regulations*, 57 (170).

KEY TERMS

Case mix A method of clustering patients into groups that are homogeneous with respect to the use of resources; the most well known of these are Diagnosis Related Groups (DRGs).

arguments about the validity of the DRG system, it or a case-mix method similar to it is likely to remain in use because it provides greater precision in the measurement of hospital output (Jones, 1989).

Home health care agencies frequently measure output in terms of number of visits made per interval of time. These visits are broken down by type of nursing care provided, by International Classification of Diseases (ICD-9) diagnosis coding, and by payer per ICD-9 diagnosis coding. Currently, home health care agencies are beginning to be reimbursed prospectively, although much research is needed to identify what critical variables affect the outputs of home health care nursing.

Output or Outcome?

Case-mix measures have refined how output quantity is measured, but they do not address the question of quality. Estimating the quality of health care services is a particularly vexing problem. In purchasing goods such as household appliances and automobiles, the consumer is usually able to judge the quality of a product by inspection or by referring to a consumer's guide for information on that product's durability and performance. If a manufacturer consistently creates inferior goods, consumers can express their quality preferences by not purchasing those products.

The purchase of health care services is fundamentally different. Because health care is a service, production and consumption of the service are simultaneous events. The consumer cannot return a defective product and often cannot reverse the effects of poor service. Furthermore, few consumers have access to a guide to health care services. Evaluation of quality is left to the consumer, who has neither the time nor the necessary knowledge on which to base this decision. Instead, the health care consumer must rely on the ethical obligation of the professional to exercise sound judgment about the type and quantity of health care required.

Effectiveness

Health care output is increasingly defined in terms of quality as well as quantity of services. (See Chapter 9 on Quality Management.) The goal is to describe output as a quality-adjusted output or as an outcome (Jones, 1993). Quality adjustments of outputs can be made in one of two ways: soundness of the care process or the quality of the output itself. The soundness of the care process is generally the most convenient to measure, but it is based on the assumption that there is a demonstrable link between the care given and the outcome achieved by the patient. Is there, for example, a cause-and-effect relationship between preoperative teaching and improved recovery following surgery? The best evidence of quality is a clear link between the process and the outcome. The effectiveness research being undertaken by the AHCPR is designed to test this premise. Measuring effectiveness is difficult because the ultimate outcome of many episodes of illness care or treatment encounters is not known for some time after the care ceases. It is expensive because of the large sample populations required and because follow-up may entail locating and evaluating the patient after care and treatment end. Although researchers have made considerable progress in demonstrating these links in nursing care, the work proceeds at a relatively slow pace (Holzemer, 1990; Townsend, 1991).

The alternative to measuring effectiveness is evaluation of the care process itself or quality of the output. *Total quality management* (TQM), sometimes called *continuous quality improvement* (CQI), is a management framework designed to improve quality through care processes (see Chapter 9 for more detail on TQM and CQI). Finding meaningful indicators of effective, quality care is likely to be a key task for years to come.

Efficiency

Finally, health care organizations are facing severe financial constraints in the future delivery of care. This emphasis on the financial aspects of care has led to an increased interest in the efficiency of providing care and care deliverers. Although sometimes difficult to separate from care effectiveness, *efficiency* refers to a state in which the inputs and methods used to produce a product or service result in the maximum feasible output/outcome (Pauly, 1970). The challenge is to identify what constitutes both efficient and effective care.

What Is Nursing Productivity?

There are two basic approaches to measuring productivity. The *economic/industrial concept* measures productivity as the ratio of work output to work input, that is, the units of output divided by units of input. The most common examples of this approach are nursing hours per patient day (NHPPD) or costs per unit of service, such as clinic visits or operative procedures.

This approach comes out of the scientific management tradition of the 1920s, which focused on the question, How can we design processes and procedures to produce the product most efficiently? An example of the use of scientific management principles in nursing is the development of patient classification systems for measuring nursing workload (see Chapter 18).

Although principles of scientific management have been applied to nursing productivity, a second, more comprehensive, model for evaluating productivity is currently being advocated in the health care and nursing literature. This model attempts to place productivity within a *systems framework* and incorporates the concept of effectiveness as well as efficiency (Jordan, 1994). R. C. Jelinek and L. C. Dennis (1976) were among the first to articulate the concept in nursing. They used an open systems model (see Figure 8-1) to show the relationship between inputs, processes, and outputs. This model also includes interactions with the environment.

Inputs include the number and type of nursing personnel, equipment, and supplies used, and the capital costs incurred in providing care. Processes include all of the activities and resources required to convert inputs into output, for example. Outputs, such as patient days or visits per day, represent the "product" resulting from the application of processes and inputs. The environment is everything external to the organization over which the nurse manager has little control, such as labor laws, health care financing policies, and personnel licensing laws.

In addition to developing a framework for understanding nursing productivity, Jelinek and Dennis (1976) proposed that in defining nursing productivity, we must be as concerned about the quality as the quantity of output. They suggest that the concept of productivity encompasses both the *effectiveness* of nursing care, which relates to its quality and appropriateness, and the *efficiency* of care, which is the production of nursing output with minimal resource waste.

KEY TERMS

Nursing hours per patient day   An indicator of productivity calculated by dividing total paid hours for nursing personnel for a specific time period by the total number of patient days in that same time period.

Nursing salary costs per patient day   An indicator of productivity calculated by dividing total payroll expenses of nursing personnel for a specific time period by the total number of patient days in that same time period.

This definition is consistent with standard economic definitions of productivity and also takes into account some of the special characteristics of nursing services, such as caring (Edwardson, 1986). There is an increasing tendency to incorporate both efficiency and effectiveness into the operational definition of the output of health care organizations (AMSI, 1980).

Measuring Nursing Productivity

Several performance measures are currently being used to evaluate the productivity of nursing services. Although some do not meet the strict definition of productivity as a ratio of output to input, they do provide important information about the efficiency of nursing care delivery. Table 8-1 compares the advantages and disadvantages of these measures.

Resources per Patient Day

Nursing Hours per Patient Day   **Nursing hours per patient day** is a commonly used indicator of labor productivity that is simple and easily understood. It is calculated by dividing

$$\frac{\text{Total paid hours for nursing personnel for time } X}{\text{Total number of patient days in time } X}$$

To reflect accurately the true cost of nursing care, the total paid hours should include the fringe benefit hours (e.g., vacation, holiday, and sick hours used) and the paid hours for nursing administrators, as well as the hours required for direct patient care, both professional and nonprofessional.

While nursing hours per patient day is one of the oldest and most frequently used performance measures, it considers only the number of hours of nursing care.

Table 8-1   Comparison of Nursing Productivity Measures

Measure	Advantages	Disadvantages
Nursing hours per patient day	• Simple and easy to use. • Provides indication of labor productivity.	• Reduces productivity to a single output. • Ignores changes in efficiency, effectiveness, skill level, intensity, or quality.
Nursing salary costs per patient day	• Provides information about skill mix. • Provides information about labor productivity.	• Does not provide information about quality or intensity of care.
Nursing hours or nursing salary standardized patient day	• Improves validity of comparisons between monitoring periods.	• None noted.
Degree of occupation	• Indication of adequacy of staff assignments.	• Informal. • Questionable validity.
Utilization rates	• Good day-to-day monitor.	• Poorly defines output.
Targeted hours of care	• Indicator of quantity and quality of care.	• When target hours exceed actual hours, productivity measure is uninterpretable.

It fails to consider any changes that may have been made in the process of care or in the supplies and equipment used—*changes that may have increased or decreased the efficiency or effectiveness of the care given.* It also fails to consider the skill level of staff, the type and intensity of patient days, or the quality of care.

Salary Costs per Patient Day   A second method is **nursing salary costs per patient day**. It is computed by dividing

$$\frac{\text{Total payroll expenses for nursing personnel in time } X}{\text{Total number of patient days in time } X}$$

It is a slightly more refined measure, however, in that the use of salary costs provides some information about the skill mix of the staff.

Standardizing Patient Days   Both nursing hours per patient day and salary costs per patient day are useful as measures of labor productivity (e.g., personnel costs per unit of output), but only if the nature of the patient day is held constant. If the patients' needs changed, it may be difficult to determine if productivity changed or not. For example, if a nursing unit provided the same number of hours of care in two time periods and the level of patient acuity remained the same, labor productivity would remain unchanged. But if the overall level of patient acuity increased in the second time period, productivity was higher; that

is, the nurses provided more care in the same amount of time.

One way to factor in patient dependency levels is to standardize patient days using information from the patient classification system designed to measure nursing workload. Patient days can be standardized by substituting the required hours of care as calculated by the patient classification system for patient days. Productivity ratios can then be calculated.

$$\frac{\text{Total paid hours for nursing personnel for time } X}{\text{Total required hours (or days) of care in time } X}$$

If desired, hours of care can be divided by 24 to produce required days of care. Standardizing patient days in this way allows nursing hours and nursing salary costs per patient day in two or more monitoring periods to be compared. Nursing salary costs are computed by

$$\frac{\text{Total payroll expenses for nursing personnel in time } X}{\text{Total required hours (or days) of care in time } X}$$

Utilization Rates

The ratio of required to actual staffing levels used by most nursing care delivery systems is based on patient classification. These classification systems are available as computer programs designed to determine skill mix requirements.

Table 8-2   Sample Productivity Report

	Actual Hours	Acuity Hours	Actual HPPD*	Acuity HPPD*	Acuity Variance	Variance Percentage
Totals						
Census	6.33	6.33				
RN	83.00	54.02	13.10	8.53	−28.97	65.09
LPN	0.00	0.00	0.00	0.00	0.00	***.**
NA	0.00	0.00	0.00	0.00	0.00	***.**
MT	16.25	24.00	2.56	3.78	7.75	147.69
DIR	0.00	4.00	0.00	0.63	4.00	***.**
CNS	9.75	8.00	1.53	1.26	−1.75	82.05
Grand Total	109.00	90.02	17.21	14.21	−18.98	82.59

*HPPD = Hours per patient day
Note: Used with permission from Lawrence Memorial Hospital, Lawrence, KS.

To calculate utilization rates, the patient classification system is used to predict the amount of care each patient will require in the near future (usually one or two shifts hence). The time required by all patients on a unit is added and then labeled "required hours of care." Additional time is factored in for indirect care activities (e.g., charting, making referrals), unit maintenance activities, and the nurses' break time. At the end of the shift for which the prediction was made, the actual hours of nursing time paid is calculated. The utilization rate is then calculated as

$$\frac{\text{Required hours of care}}{\text{Nursing hours paid}}$$

Table 8-2 shows an example of how utilization rates are frequently reported in nursing management information systems. The actual hours of care provided are subtracted from the required (or predicted) hours of care to give a variance. For example,

Predicted acuity hours = 90.02
Variance = 218.98 hr of care
Actual hours = 109

The percentage of productivity is then calculated by dividing the required hours of care by the actual hours provided and then multiplying the quotient by 100.

$$\frac{90.02}{109} = 82.59$$

A productivity rate of 100% indicates that the actual hours of care matched the required hours. A rate greater than 100% indicates that actual hours were fewer than required, whereas a rate less than 100% shows that more hours of care were provided than

were required. Most organizations set acceptable productivity ranges of 85% to 115%.

Although these rates are perhaps the single best day-to-day control monitor available to nursing managers, they are more appropriately called a **utilization rate** rather than a productivity indicator, unless certain assumptions are made about required hours of care. When compared to standard economic definitions of productivity, the ratio of required to actual hours of care has an input measurement (actual hours) but does not have a commonly used output measurement.

The ratio of required to actual hours of care is useful as a productivity measure only if the required number of nursing hours can provide the quantity and quality of care that the organization wishes to provide. In other words, the use of staff utilization ratios to judge productivity is based on one very important, but frequently unacknowledged, assumption: The standard hours of care used by the patient classification system to calculate required nurse hours are assumed to provide the desired level of service.

To be used as an output indicator, the required hours of care should be thought of as targeted hours of care (that is, the hours of care required to produce the desired level of quality of care). Either the nursing department must use the research findings of others to

KEY TERMS

Utilization rate   A calculated ratio of required versus actual staffing levels that monitors the productivity of an organization.

Box 8-2	Example of the Use of Targeted Hours of Care as an Output Indicator

Outcome Standard

Average length of stay: 2.9 days

Quality Indicators

Knowledge and skill	90% score above 90% on a post-teaching test of knowledge
	98% give satisfactory return baby bath demonstration
Satisfaction	90% satisfied or very satisfied on satisfaction questionnaire
Complications	2% postpartal and newborn infection rate
	50% of mothers continue to breast-feed at least 1 month

show that a certain amount of care produces the desired results, or it must do its own evaluation to demonstrate that care of a given level of quantity and quality can be produced by a given number of nursing-care hours.

An example from a maternity service illustrates this point. Assume that a maternity service has determined that 5 hours of professional and 2 hours of nonprofessional nursing care during the postpartum period meet the outcome standards set by the service (Box 8-2). Because the unit is able to meet the organization's standards of care, targeted hours of care could quite legitimately be substituted as an indicator of the appropriate quantity and quality of care, or output (Edwardson, 1986).

A second approach for calculating productivity uses utilization rates (Box 8-3). When the actual hours of care provided match the target, productivity is 100%. When actual hours exceed the target, productivity falls below 100%. A problem arises in calculating productivity when the actual hours provided are fewer than the target. Although most organizations might calculate productivity as more than 100%, it is questionable whether this is a legitimate calculation. When the actual use of staff is less than the targeted level, it suggests one of two things: (a) the standards used to establish the target are too high or (b) the organization is willing to compromise its standards with unknown consequences. For these reasons, some have suggested that productivity levels should never exceed 100% unless the clinical service can show that the care process has been made more efficient by using new methods or new equipment and that the quality of care has not suffered.

Improving Nursing Effectiveness, Efficiency, and Productivity

How can nursing productivity be improved and thus become more effective and efficient? As the productivity model in Figure 8-1 suggests, there are two possible points at which productivity gains may be made: (a) through changes in the use of inputs and (b) through changes in the care process itself. Changes to elements of the overall health care environment are

Box 8-3	Calculating Productivity

These standards can be met at 7 hours of care per patient day. Therefore, productivity can be calculated as follows, using hypothetical actual hours of care provided.

a. $\dfrac{\text{Target}}{\text{Actual}} = \dfrac{7}{7} = 100\%$

b. $\dfrac{\text{Target}}{\text{Actual}} = \dfrac{7}{7.9} = 89\%$

c. $\dfrac{\text{Target}}{\text{Actual}} = \dfrac{7}{6.5} = 108\%$

largely beyond the control of individual nurses and, often, the organization.

Changes in Use of Inputs

Inputs include the raw materials, personnel, supplies and equipment, and capital (money) used to provide a service or produce a product. Little attention has been given to the raw material of nursing services because it is uncommon to think of patients and clients as raw material. Nurses have traditionally had little control over the type of patients presented to them. Recent activities among health care organizations to identify areas of excellence and market those selected services to potential consumers may change that. Increasingly, nursing departments and individual nurse practitioners are marketing their services as well, thereby exerting some influence over the type of patients for whom they care.

Matching Supply with Demand The most costly input in the provision of nursing care is labor. Therefore, the greatest productivity gains can be achieved by careful selection and use of personnel. The key to efficient resource use is to match the required and available staff (Morrow, 1994). If more nurses are needed than are scheduled, other nurses will be needed from a float pool, on-call service, unscheduled employees, or a substitute nurse service. If more nurses are scheduled than are needed, some of the staff may be asked either to float to other units with greater need or not come to work that day.

Making Staff Substitutions Many would argue that to reduce personnel costs it is logical to employ more nonprofessional staff, who receive lower salaries. Increasing the number of LPNs and unlicensed assistive personnel (UAPs) in relation to the number of RNs, for example, would result in an increase in available hours of personnel time per patient day with no increase in cost. There are, however, theoretical arguments for and against staff substitution as a method for improving nursing productivity (Baer, 1994). Adherents of the scientific management tradition would predict that productivity would be greatest when the work of providing care to individual patients is divided into its component parts and the tasks assigned to staff members according to their ability to perform the task. Tasks would be assigned to the least costly personnel category capable of doing the task; the most qualified individuals would be assigned only those tasks requiring their special expertise. A key issue in such assignment of tasks is a clear understanding of

what constitutes professional nursing and which activities can be performed safely and appropriately by non-nurses. Cost reduction pressures of the early 1990s have led many acute care facilities to make such downward substitutions of functions once reserved for registered nurses (American Nurses Association [ANA], 1993; Kirby & Garfink, 1991).

In contrast to the scientific management approach, supporters of the human relations theoretical framework would argue that knowledge workers such as nurses will be most satisfied, and therefore most productive, when they are allowed to perform whole tasks, for example, to provide total patient care for a caseload of patients. They argue against dividing the work into component parts and assigning isolated tasks to individuals.

Continuing financial pressures on health care facilities have led health care organizations to search for new methods of extending the work of the professional nurse. These include differentiated practice, case management, and practice partnerships (see Chapter 3). In addition, some administrators advocate changing the hourly pay model to a professional salary model (Avigne, Guin, Pittman, & Surdez, 1998).

Controlling the Use of Supplies and Equipment Input costs also can be controlled by the wise use of supplies and equipment. One method is to compare the cost and features of roughly equivalent supplies and equipment, selecting products that have the desired qualities at the lowest cost. At times, the purchasing department may be able to obtain the lowest cost by using competitive bidding procedures for the organization's vendors.

Once supplies and equipment have been purchased, cost can be controlled by using them wisely by, for example, instituting systems that carefully monitor the use of supplies in order to reduce waste and prevent theft. One nurse manager was able to increase cost sensitivity and produce large savings by simply placing price tags on chargeable supplies. Nurses in the study hospital discovered that they could substitute less costly items and avoid using some items altogether with no adverse effects (McVay, 1983).

Nurse managers receive monthly reports that note variances between actual charges received from the unit and items charged to the unit's supply. Any discrepancies are investigated and corrected.

Changes in the Process of Care

Finding ways to improve productivity by making changes in the care process allows nurses and nurse managers to use their creativity to the fullest. Jelinek and Dennis (1976) called the care process the "technology of nursing." According to their definition, technology "comprises all methodologies employed in converting inputs into outputs" (p. 12). In this concept of productivity, technology includes the physical and managerial organization of nursing services, leadership and supervision, patient care delivery systems, staffing and scheduling practices, care planning and documentation procedures, and the performance of nursing activities themselves. Clearly, there are many opportunities to experiment with methods for improving the quantity and quality of nursing care given.

Changes in the direct care process may lead to improvements in the quantity and quality of care delivered. Experiments with new approaches to common clinical problems such as incontinence and situational confusion may be fruitful. Investigating alternative methods of nursing care delivery, such as primary nursing, case management (McIntosh, 1987), differentiated practice (Koerner & Karpiuk, 1994), or other restructuring methods may be needed (Brett & Tonges, 1990; Malloch, Milton, & Jobes, 1990).

Documenting Changes Regardless of the nature of the changes made in the process of care, it is essential that nurse managers measure and evaluate the changes and their consequences. Without careful documentation, it may be impossible to convince others that the innovations introduced are safe, effective, and efficient.

Consider the example of one nurse midwifery clinic. Several years ago, clinic staff decided that they could be more efficient if they replaced an individual approach to early prenatal teaching and orientation to the clinic with a group approach. After some time it became apparent that the clientele, who represented several ethnic groups and some of whom had a limited command of English and little formal education, were too diverse to make group teaching practical. Class members frequently were forced to wait while the instructor attended to language or other unique needs of individuals. According to the plan, the class was to be conducted in 1 hour. But as it turned out, the class required several hours, attendance dropped, and concerns grew about the women's ability to care for themselves in early pregnancy.

The staff decided that an evaluation of the patient teaching program was in order. By totaling the cost of staff time (including the time of staff who were largely unoccupied during the class) and the cost of the unused clinic rooms and comparing these costs with the attendance rate and knowledge outcomes, it became clear that the group approach for this set of patients

was inappropriate and at least as costly. The clinic reverted back to the one-on-one teaching strategy.

To evaluate the effects of changes, cost and outcome data should be collected as a part of all clinical studies. This is a less formidable task than it may appear on the surface. Cost-accounting methods are well understood and relatively easy to apply. Although outcome evaluation can be difficult, studies of outcome, when they are used for managerial purposes, need not meet all of the rigorous criteria applied to research studies.

Calculating Costs Costs can be calculated using one of two approaches. In some cases, it will be necessary to estimate only the direct costs of the change, for example, costs associated with changes in the brand of a product used or introduction of a new record-keeping system. In other cases, an episode of care (e.g., a home visit, clinic appointment, hospital admission) may be analyzed.

Table 8-3 shows how costs can be calculated. First, each patient is classified by hours of care. For this analysis, it is important that the data are recorded in a retrievable fashion, such as on the patient record or on a computer file. After discharge, the total hours of care are totaled and multiplied by the hourly nursing care salary cost (total salary costs/total number of paid hours). Then, all indirect nursing costs are added. (For a discussion of indirect costs, see Chapter 7.) To obtain an average cost for all patients being studied, the costs of each patient's care are totaled and divided by the number of patients in the sample. To identify cost savings, the average costs before introduction of the innovation can be compared to costs after its introduction.

Measuring Outcome Measuring the effects of a change in care processes can be complex. Increasingly, process outcomes have been evaluated in research studies reported in the literature. Clinical application of this research is a critical step in standardizing cost-effective and efficient care.

In other instances, however, the nursing staff will need to design its own outcome evaluation method (Sovie, 1994). The first question to be asked in developing an evaluation strategy is, What is the outcome that should be measured? The answer lies in what the innovation is intended to do, what the possible adverse consequences could be, and what the organization can afford to measure. In evaluating a new method for caring for incontinent patients, for example, the nurse manager might identify as an intended outcome a reduction in the number of episodes of incontinence

Table 8-3 **Cost Estimation Example in a Hospital**

	Day of Stay	A	B	C	D	E	F
				Hours for Each Patient Served			
1. Apply workload measurement system	1	3	5	4	5	3	2.8
	2	2.8	5	4	4.9	3	2.8
	3	2.5	4.8	4	4.9	2	2
	4	2.5	4.6	3	4.6	2.3	
	5	2.3	4.6	3			
2. Add hours of care for length of stay		13.1	24.0	18.0	19.4	10.3	7.6
3. Assign hourly cost of nursing care to individual patients (e.g., $16/hour)		× $16 $209.60	× $16 384.00	× $16 288.00	× $16 310.40	× $16 164.80	× $16 121.60
4. Add indirect costs (e.g., $20/patient day)		$309.60	484.00	388.00	390.40	244.80	181.60

5. Calculate average cost per case

   A. Add total cost for all relevant patients
$$\begin{aligned}&\$\ \ 309.60\\&\ \ \ \ 484.00\\&\ \ \ \ 388.00\\&\ \ \ \ 390.00\\&\ \ \ \ 244.80\\&\ \ \ \ \underline{181.60}\\&\$1{,}998.40\end{aligned}$$

   B. Divide sum by number of patients
$$\$1{,}998.40/6 = \$333.07$$

and incidence of skin breakdown. Outcome criteria would include the number of incontinent episodes per day and the degree of skin excoriation. Adverse consequences might include unsightly garments or decreased patient autonomy. Procedures for evaluating patients' emotional responses also could be used. In this example, each of the proposed outcomes could be measured at a relatively modest cost.

The nursing staff also may want to know the long-term outcome of their new care strategy. This implies that patients will need to be located after hospital discharge and outcome measurements made at that time, a potentially costly procedure. There are, however, several ways to do this with little cost to the unit. One approach might be to enlist a nurse researcher interested in the problem. Another would be for the unit

staff to apply for external grant funding to perform their own evaluation. Finally, information about patient outcome data may become more available as a network of care providers is formed and as patient records are kept on compatible computer files. Follow-up information from home-care or long-term care settings may then provide the needed outcome data.

Taxonomy for Nursing An area of current discussion in the nursing literature is the need for a standardized, global language for the description of essential nursing information (McCloskey & Bulechek, 1994). One collection of this type of information is referred to as the **Nursing Minimum Data Set** (Werley & Lang, 1988). McCloskey and Bulechek have developed a standardized taxonomy of nursing interventions (Table 8-4). For outcome information to become standardized, much research is still needed to identify what nursing assessments, diagnoses, and treatments must be included. Until the creation of such a database, data analysis for the purposes of outcomes research will be difficult to perform. Although nursing has not come to consensus as to what should be included,

KEY TERMS

Nursing Minimum Data Set A standardized taxonomy of nursing interventions.

Table 8-4   Nursing Interventions Classification Taxonomy

	Domain 1	Domain 2	Domain 3
Level 1 Domains	1. Physiological: Basic Care that supports physical functioning	2. Physiological: Complex Care that supports homeostatic regulation	3. Behavioral Care that supports psychosocial functioning and facilitates lifestyle changes
Level 2 Classes	A. Activity and Exercise Management: Interventions to organize or assist with physical activity and energy conservation and expenditure B. Elimination Management: Interventions to establish and maintain regular bowel and urinary elimination patterns and manage complications due to altered patterns C. Immobility Management: Interventions to manage restricted body movement and the sequelae D. Nutrition Support: Interventions to modify or maintain nutritional status E. Physical Comfort Promotion: Interventions to promote comfort using physical techniques F. Self-Care Facilitation: Interventions to provide or assist with routine activities of daily living	G. Electrolyte and Acid-Base Management: Interventions to regulate electrolyte acid base balance and prevent complications H. Drug Management: Interventions to facilitate desired effects of pharmacologic agents I. Neurologic Management: Interventions to optimize neurologic function J. Perioperative Care: Interventions to provide care prior to damage and immediately after surgery K. Respiratory Management: Interventions to promote airway patency and gas exchange L. Skin/Wound Management: Interventions to maintain or restore tissue integrity M. Thermoregulation: Interventions to maintain body temperature within a normal range N. Tissue Perfusion Management: Interventions to optimize circulation of blood and fluids to the tissue	O. Behavior Therapy: Interventions to reinforce or promote desirable behaviors or alter undesirable behaviors P. Cognitive Therapy: Interventions to reinforce or promote desirable cognitive functioning or alter undesirable cognitive functioning Q. Communication Enhancement: Interventions for delivering and receiving verbal and nonverbal messages R. Coping Assistance: Interventions to assist another to build on own strengths to adapt to a change in function or achieve a higher level of function S. Patient Education: Interventions to facilitate learning T. Psychological Comfort Promotion: Interventions to promote comfort using psychological techniques

Table continues on following page

Note: "Validation and coding of the NIC taxonomy structure: Iowa intervention project. Nursing interventions classification" by J. McCloskey and G. Bulechek, 1995, *Image, 27*, pp. 43–49.

there is general agreement that such a database is urgently needed.

Using Cost and Outcome Data   Once cost and outcome data are gathered, the two must be compared to determine whether the innovation was beneficial. A cost-effectiveness model is shown in Figure 8-2. Any option that produces equal or superior results and costs less, or any option that produces superior results for equal cost, should be chosen as the most cost effective. Similarly, any option that produces inferior results for equal or greater costs should be rejected. Ambiguity arises when a superior result costs more or when the costs and results are equal for the two options. In these cases, the choice is based on a value judgment about the importance of the goal in comparison to other organizational objectives. An ambiguous choice also may inspire the staff to identify

Table 8-4	Continued

Domain 4	Domain 5	Domain 6
4. Safety Care that supports protection against harm	5. Family Care that supports the family unit	6. Health System Care that supports effective use of the health care delivery system
U. Crisis Management: Interventions to provide immediate short-term help in both psychological and physiological crises V. Risk Management: Interventions to initiate risk reduction activities and continue monitoring risks over time	W. Childbearing Care: Interventions to assist in understanding and coping with the psychological and physiological changes during the childbearing period X. Lifespan Care: Interventions to facilitate family unit functioning and promote the health and welfare of family members throughout the lifespan	Y. Health System Mediation: Interventions to facilitate the interface between patient/family and the health care system a. Health System Management: Interventions to enhance environmental support services b. Information Management: Interventions to facilitate communication among health care providers

third and fourth options to achieve the same objective at a somewhat lower cost.

The evaluation strategy for assessing the effects of changes in the process of care described here is but one of several that could be used. Whichever evaluation method is selected, it is important that it be selected before an innovation or change begins so that the data to determine whether the change did or did not enhance productivity can be collected.

Overall, these are just a sampling of what nurses and nurse managers can do in concert with administrative staff and physicians to find ways to deliver quality care while meeting an organization's financial objectives. The American public demands and is entitled to information about the efficiency and effectiveness of the health care services provided to them. The nursing profession can do one of two things: (a) develop methods for demonstrating its own value as a

		Cost of program A relative to program B		
		A is less costly	A is as costly	A is more costly
Effectiveness of program A relative to program B	A is less effective	?	Choose B	Choose B
	A is as effective	Choose A	Either A or B	Choose B
	A is more effective	Choose A	Choose A	?

Figure 8-2 **Cost-effectiveness matrix.** *Note:* Adapted from *Development and testing of a cost-effectiveness methodology for CMHCs* by D. Fishman, 1975, NTIS Publication nos. PB 246-676 and PB 246-677, Springfield, VA: National Technical Information Service.

health care discipline or (b) wait for others to do that evaluation. The choice seems clear. The profession must move to define the product of nursing services, provide scientific evidence of the links between nursing intervention and patient outcome, and then use professional and scientific knowledge about productivity to influence health care policy.

Summary

- Effectiveness is the measure used to determine whether an intervention improves people's health under ordinary circumstances and in ordinary settings.
- Efficiency is the relationship between achieving objectives and consuming resources.
- Productivity describes the relationship between inputs and outputs; productivity refers to the resources used to produce a product or provide a service and the quantity and quality of that product or service.
- It has been difficult to measure productivity in health care because of the unique nature of the service provided and a lack of clarity about how best to measure output.
- Nursing productivity can be enhanced by making changes in the use of inputs and in the processes used to deliver care.
- Nurse managers can improve the use of inputs by matching the supply of staff with the demand for care, by carefully evaluating the consequences of staff substitutions, and by controlling the use of supplies and equipment.
- Demonstrating the relative productivity of nursing services is the responsibility of every nurse manager.
- Processes to ensure continuous quality improvement enhance both efficiency and effectiveness.

■ LEADERSHIP AND MANAGEMENT _in Action_

1. What is nursing productivity? How is it measured? Describe two ways productivity can be improved.
2. Define efficiency and effectiveness. How do the two differ?
3. What benefits would a taxonomy for nursing provide?

References

American Management Sciences, Inc. (AMSI). (1980). *Productivity and health.* DHHS Publication no. (HRA) 80-14028. Bethesda, MD: Office of the Assistant Secretary of Health.

American Nurses Association (1993). *Professional nurses and unlicensed assistive personnel.* Washington, DC: Author.

Avigne, G., Guin, P., Pittman, L., & Surdez, M. (1998). Moving from an hourly pay model to a professional salary model. *AORN Journal, 68*(3), 400–402, 405–408.

Baer, E. D. (1994). Money managers are unraveling the tapestry of nursing. *American Journal of Nursing, 94*(10), 38–40.

Brett, J. L. L., & Tonges, M. C. (1990). Restructured patient care delivery: Evaluation of the ProACT model. *Nursing Economics, 8,* 36–40.

Edwardson, S. R. (1986). The cost-quality tradeoff in productivity management. In F. A. Shaffer (Ed.), *Patients and purse strings—Patient classification and cost management* (pp. 259–271). New York: National League for Nursing.

Feldstein, M. S. (1971). *The rising cost of hospital care.* Washington, DC: Information Resources Press.

Fishman, D. (1975). *Development and testing of a cost-effectiveness methodology for CMHCs.* NTIS Publication nos. PB 246-676 and PB 246-677. Springfield, VA: National Technical Information Service.

Holzemer, W. L. (1990). Quality and cost of nursing care: Is anybody out there listening? *Nursing & Health Care, 11*(8), 412–415.

Hornbrook, M. C. (1982). Hospital case mix: Its definition, measurement and use. Part I. The conceptual framework. *Medical Care Review, 39*(1), 1–43.

Jelinek, R. C., & Dennis, L. C. (1976). *A review and evaluation of nursing productivity.* DHEW Publication no. (HRA) 77-15. Bethesda, MD: Health Resources Administration.

Jones, K. R. (1993). Outcomes analysis: Methods and issues. *Nursing Economics, 11*(3), 145–151.

Jones, K. R. (1989). Economics of the prospective payment system. Implications for nursing. *Nursing Economics, 7*(6), 299–305.

Jordan, S. D. (1994). Nursing productivity in rural hospitals. *Nursing Management, 25*(3), 58–62.

Kirby, K. K., & Garfink, C. M. (1991). The university hospital nurse extender program. Part I. An overview and conceptual framework. *Journal of Nursing Administration, 21*(1), 25–30.

Koerner, J. G., & Karpiuk, K. L. (1994). *Implementing differentiated practice: Transformation by design.* Gaithersburg, MD: Aspen.

Malloch, K. M., Milton, D. A., & Jobes, M. O. (1990). A model for differentiated nursing practice. *Journal of Nursing Administration, 20,* 20–26.

Massel, D. (1999). Evidence-based budgeting is now necessary. [Letter] *British Medical Journal, 319*(7206), 384.

McCloskey, J. C., & Bulechek, G. M. (1994). Standardizing the language for nursing treatments: An overview of the issues. *Nursing Outlook, 42*(2), 56–63.

McCloskey, J. C., & Bulechek, G. M. (1995). Validation and coding of the NIC taxonomy structure: Iowa intervention project. Nursing interventions classification. *Image, 27*(1), 43–49.

McIntosh, L. (1987). Hospital-based case management. *Nursing Economics, 5,* 232–236.

McVay, E. (1983). *Lost supply charges: Would visible price tags reduce their number?* Unpublished master's thesis. University of Minnesota, Minneapolis, Minnesota.

Morrow, K. L. (1994). Nursing staffing and scheduling information to support change. *Nursing Management, 25*(5), 78–80.

Pauly, M. V. (1970). Efficiency, incentives and reimbursement for health care. *Inquiry, 7,* 114–131.

Smalley, H. E., & Freeman, J. R. (1966). *Hospital industrial engineering.* New York: Reinhold.

Sovie, M. D. (1994). Nurse manager: A key role in clinical outcomes. *Nursing Management, 25*(3), 30–34.

Townsend, M. B. (1991). Creating a better work environment: Measuring effectiveness. *Journal of Nursing Administration, 21*(1), 11–14.

U.S. Congress, Office of Technology Assessment (September, 1994). *Identifying health technologies that work: Searching for evidence,* OTA-H-608. Washington, DC: Government Printing Office.

Werley, H. H., & Lang, N. M., (Eds.). (1988). *Identification of the nursing minimum data set.* New York: Springer.

C H A P T E R   9

Quality Management

History of Quality Management

Total Quality Management (TQM)

> TQM Characteristics
> Continuous Quality Improvement
>   (CQI)
> Comprehensive Components of
>   Quality Management
> CQI—How It Works: A Practical
>   Example

Risk Management

> A Risk Management Program
> Nursing's Role in Risk
>   Management
> Examples of Risk

Role of the Nurse Manager

> Key Behaviors for Handling
>   Complaints
> A Caring Attitude

Evaluation of Risk Management

Looking Ahead

We now move into a more specific discussion of the implementation of quality management in health care. Chapter 9 examines the role of nursing management in relationship to the concepts of quality and risk. The chapter describes the history of quality management and the evolution of Total Quality Management (TQM), a philosophy seeking to balance cost-effectiveness with quality patient care. TQM provides the initial framework for a discussion of techniques and programs that nurses can implement according to their organizational needs.

Objectives

After reading this chapter, you will be able to:

- Describe the characteristics of Total Quality Management (TQM).
- Discuss nursing's role in risk management.
- Describe the role of the incident report.
- Delineate the types of risks in health care.
- Describe key behaviors for handling complaints.

In today's highly competitive health care environment, each member of the health care organization must be accountable for the quality and cost of health care. If cost containment was the emphasis for the past decade, then quality care has become the focus of the next (National League for Nursing, 1993). A natural evolution of both quality and cost containment is found in the concept of total quality management (TQM). TQM and its principles of continuous quality improvement reduce costs and improve quality by improving system and process performance. TQM provides the nurse manager with a framework to manage both the costs and quality of patient care. It also provides the tools to organize, implement, and evaluate an integrated quality and risk management program.

History of Quality Management

The process of systematic evaluation of health care is not new. Quality management activities date back to Florence Nightingale, who urged that all nursing care be evaluated. During the Crimean War, Nightingale reported statistics on the mortality of British soldiers in comparison to that of civilians before and after the implementation of some of her innovative nursing practices. She reported that the patient mortality rate decreased from nearly 50% to 2% in a 6-month period at one military hospital (Nutting & Dock, 1907). As a result of her findings, the public's interest in the accountability of health care increased, resulting in the regular evaluation of hospital care. These efforts eventually contributed to an improvement in the quality of the health care delivered to both soldiers and civilians.

Patient outcomes also were evaluated by the medical profession in the early 20th century. Through the studies of Dr. Armory Grove, support for a classification system for different diseases developed, along with standards for assessing individuals with these conditions (Bull, 1985).

By the late 1940s and early 1950s, the public had become more aware of the importance of evaluating health care services. In 1952, the Joint Commission on Accreditation of Hospitals (JCAH) was founded to provide standards for accreditation of hospitals. (In 1987 the JCAH changed its name to the Joint Commission on the Accreditation of Healthcare Organizations [JCAHO]). Shortly thereafter, the American Nurses Association (ANA) in 1959 published its *Functions, Standards and Qualifications for Practice,* and the National League for Nursing published *What People Can Expect of a Modern Nursing Service.* In addition, the ANA created a division of the organization charged with developing standards of practice to ensure quality care. The ANA also developed a model for implementing the quality assurance process. The nursing profession assumed that its responsibility was to be accountable to patients for providing, evaluating, and improving patient care through the use of the ANA standards and model. All of these efforts helped form professional and public expectations about adequate care.

Several landmark decisions have forced hospitals and health care providers to be more accountable. In a 1965 case, *Darling v. Charleston Community Memorial Hospital,** the Illinois Supreme Court found the hospital liable for the care of a young athlete whose leg was amputated following complications from a fracture. The court found the hospital negligent in two areas: (a) by the nurses' failure to inform the physician or hospital regarding the onset of complications and (b) by the hospital's failure to protect the patient from incompetence of the physician. Decisions in similar cases have been based on this precedent of corporate responsibility for providing a system to monitor patient care and to correct deficiencies in quality. In addition, hospitals and other not-for-profit institutions (including schools and churches) lost their charitable immunity through a Supreme Court decision in 1969. Since that time, health care organizations have experienced a steady increase in litigation, insurance premiums, and the cost of settlements.

As a consequence of increasing litigation, malpractice insurance premiums have skyrocketed, pushing organizational costs even higher. Many insurance carriers now require organizations to develop risk management programs as a condition for coverage.

The federal government amended the Social Security Act in 1972 to mandate professional review of health care delivery through the Professional Standards Review Organization (PSRO). Replaced by Peer Review Organizations (PROs), one per state, in 1982, PROs evaluate the quality of existing health care, determine whether the health care offered meets professional standards, and determine whether it was provided in an appropriate health care setting.

In 1975, JCAH increased the number of multidisciplinary reviews required for the accreditation process, and nursing care became a major component

*211 N.E. 2d 53, 33 Ill. 2d, 326 (1965), cert. denied 383 U.S. 946, 16 L. Ed. 2d 209, 86 S.Ct. 1204 (1966).

of the evaluation of patient care. During the early 1980s, JCAH revised its standard of evaluating nursing care by stating that care needed to be evaluated objectively against preestablished standards and criteria. JCAH further required that results from the evaluation be analyzed to determine the problem areas in nursing practice and a plan be developed to correct practice deficiencies. A method to reevaluate the effectiveness of the corrective action was also necessary. In the late 1980s, the Joint Commission's "Agenda for Change" further emphasized this major shift in focus from individual performance to the performance of the health care organization's systems and processes (McLaughlin & Kaluzny, 1990). The more recent focus of JCAHO is to integrate performance measures into the accreditation process. This program, called ORYX, is intended for hospitals, long-term–care facilities, and behavioral health organizations (JCAHO, 1999).

With the increased interest in the cost-effectiveness and quality of all health care providers, a number of other organizations have begun to assess quality and outcomes in the health care industry. In 1979, the National Committee for Quality Assurance (NCQA) was formed. This organization accredits HMOs and assesses performance measures called HEDIS (Health Plan Employer Data and Information Set). Unfortunately, HMOs are not required to disclose HEDIS scores to the public (Bodenheimer, 1999).

The Health Care Financing Administration (HCFA) has instituted several initiatives in the past few years to set standards for agencies serving Medicare and Medicaid enrollees. OASIS (Outcome and Assessment Information Set) is an assessment program that forms the basis for outcome-based quality improvement (OBQI) in home health care (Simpson, 2000). QISMC (Quality Improvement System for Managed Care) was established in 1996 to set standards for managed care organizations. QISMC has the authority to publish data regarding its constituent HMOs (Bodenheimer, 1999). HCQIP (Health Care Quality Improvement Program) is another HCFA program designed to improve the quality of care of Medicare recipients (Simpson, 2000).

In 1986, the Health Care Quality Improvement Act created a federal data bank, the National Practitioner Data Bank (NPDB), to identify incompetent practitioners and restrict movement between states without discovery. Legislation in 1987 expanded the NPDB to include nurses and other health care practitioners. A second database was created by the Health Insurance Portability and Accountability Act of 1996. This database, the Healthcare Integrity and Protection Data Bank (HIPDB), was developed to combat fraud and abuse in both health care insurance and health care delivery.

Professional organizations also are identifying ways to improve quality of care. In 1997, the AMA established the National Patient Safety Foundation to identify system inadequacies leading to medical errors (Bodenheimer, 1999). In 1994, the ANA launched a safety and quality initiative that resulted in the identification of ten quality indicators for acute-care settings (Box 9-1). Data on these indicators are being maintained in a database intended to facilitate standardization of information on nursing quality and patient outcomes (ANA, 1999).

Total Quality Management (TQM)

Total quality management (TQM) is a management philosophy that emphasizes a commitment to excellence throughout the organization. The creation of Dr. W. Edwards Deming, TQM was adopted by the Japanese and helped transform their industrial development after World War II. Dr. Deming developed 14 points that provide the foundation for the Deming

| Box 9-1 | Nursing-Sensitive Quality Indicators for Acute Care Settings |

- **Mix of RNs, LPNs, and Unlicensed Staff Caring for Patients in Acute Care Settings**
  Recommended Definition: The percent of registered nursing care hours as a total of all nursing care hours. This measure would include only those staff on acute care units. A secondary measure would be the percent of RN contracted hours of total nursing care hours.

- **Total Nursing Care Hours Provided per Patient Day**
  Recommended Definition: Total number of productive hours worked by nursing staff with direct patient care responsibilities on acute care units per patient day. Secondary measures would be RN contracted hours, total contracted hours, RN nursing care hours per 1000 patient days.

  Box continues on following page

Box 9-1 Continued

- **Pressure Ulcers**
  Recommended Definition: This measure would be defined and calculated as:

$$\frac{\text{Total number of patients with NPUAP-AHCPR stage I, II, III, or IV ulcers}}{\text{Number of patients in a prevalence study}}$$

A secondary measure should explore the relationship between nursing assessments using a standardized tool and the development of pressure ulcers. The secondary measure would be collected on a "look-back" basis by auditing the charts of patients. Use of the Braden or Norton scales is required. (These can be obtained at a local health services library.)

- **Patient Falls**
  Recommended Definition: The rate per 1000 patient days at which patients experience a fall during the course of their hospital stay. The measure would be computed as:

$$\frac{\text{Total number of patient falls leading to injury} \times 1000}{\text{Total number of patient-days}}$$

A secondary measure should explore the relationship between nursing assessments performed and falls. The measure would be defined, for those patients who fell, as the number of patients who had nursing fall assessments as compared to the total number of patients who fell. This secondary measure would be collected on a "look-back" basis by auditing the charts of patients.

- **Patient Satisfaction with Pain Management**
  Recommended Definition: Patient opinion of how well nursing staff managed their pain as determined by scaled responses to a uniform series of questions designed to elicit patient views regarding specific aspects of pain management. The questions would be administered to a sample of all patients admitted to the hospital for acute care service.

- **Patient Satisfaction with Educational Information**—A measure of patient perception of the hospital experience related to satisfaction with patient education.
  Recommended Definition: Patient opinion of nursing staff efforts to educate them regarding their conditions and care requirements as determined by scaled responses to a uniform series of questions designed to elicit patient views regarding specific aspects of

patient education activities. The questions would be administered to a sample of all patients admitted to the hospital for acute care services.

- **Patient Satisfaction with Overall Care**—A measure of patient perception of the hospital experience related to satisfaction with overall care.
  Recommended Definition: Patient opinion of the care received during the hospital stay as determined by scaled responses to a uniform series of questions designed to elicit patient views regarding global aspects of care. The questions would be administered to a sample of all patients admitted to the hospital for acute-care services.

- **Patient Satisfaction with Nursing Care**—A measure of patient perception of the hospital experience related to satisfaction with nursing care.
  Recommended Definition: Patient opinion of care received from nursing staff during the hospital stay as determined by scaled responses to a uniform series of questions designed to elicit patient views regarding satisfaction with key elements of nursing care services. The questions would be administered to a sample of all patients admitted to the hospital for acute care services.

- **Nosocomial Infection Rate**
  Recommended Definition: This measure would be defined and calculated as:

$$\frac{\text{Number of laboratory-confirmed bacteremia associated with sites of central lines}}{\text{1000 patient-days per unit}}$$

[This indicator is under investigation for its usefulness. For purposes of this effort, infection would be defined according to parameters established by the Centers for Disease Control and Prevention.]

- **Nursing Staff Satisfaction**
  Recommended Definition: Job satisfaction expressed by nurses working in hospital settings as determined by scaled responses to a uniform series of questions designed to elicit nursing staff attitudes toward specific aspects of their employment situation. The questions would be administered to all RNs in direct patient care or middle management roles at the institution. The six SNAs funded to implement the indicators are using either the Kramer & Schmalenberg or Stamps & Piedmont tools. (These can be obtained at a local health services library.)

Note: American Nurses Association (ANA). (1999). *Nursing sensitive quality indicators for acute care settings and ANA's safety and quality initiative.* Washington, DC: Author.

management method (Koch & Fairly, 1993) (Box 9-2). These principles of quality management were originally applied to improve quality and performance in the manufacturing industry. They are now widely used to improve quality and customer satisfaction in a number of service industries, including health care.

TQM Characteristics

Four core characteristics of total quality management are customer/client focus, total organizational involvement, the use of quality tools and statistics for measurement, and the identification of key processes for improvement.

Customer/Client Focus   An important theme of quality management is to address the needs of customers. There are both internal and external customers of health care organizations. Internal customers include employees and departments within the organization, such as the laboratory, admitting office, and environmental services. External customers of a health care

---

Box 9-2   Deming's 14 Points

1. *Create constancy of purpose for improvement of product and service.* A company must develop a plan to become competitive and to stay in business through research, innovation, continuous improvement, and maintenance of improvement.

2. *Adopt the new philosophy.* Americans must not tolerate poor service and workmanship. Americans must religiously reject mistakes and negativism.

3. *Cease dependence on mass inspection.* American companies must eliminate need for inspection after the product is produced. When products are defective, the company pays for workers who made the products that must be either reworked or discarded. Quality comes from improving the production process, enlisting the workers involved when properly trained, rather than from inspection.

4. *End the practice of awarding business on the basis of price tag.* Instead, industry leaders should depend on meaningful measures of quality, along with price. Seek the best quality supplier and build a long-term relationship to improve the quality.

5. *Improve constantly and forever the system of production and service.* It is management's job to work continuously on the system to reduce waste and improve quality. Quality improvement is not a one-time effort or "program."

6. *Institute training.* Management must invest in training and not ask another worker who has never been trained to be the trainer. Workers cannot do the job because they have not been properly trained.

7. *Institute leadership.* The role of the supervisor is to lead, not tell workers what to do. Leading means the supervisor helps the worker do better work and objectively evaluates who is in need of individual assistance.

8. *Drive out fear.* Fear has a great economic loss. When people are afraid to ask questions or express their thoughts, the job may continue to be done wrong. To improve quality and productivity, the people must feel secure with management.

9. *Break down barriers between staff areas.* When departments, units, or areas have conflicting goals, competition may occur. This stops any teamwork toward finding opportunities for improvement.

10. *Eliminate slogans, exhortations, and targets for the workforce.* Quality is not a program with management-defined slogans. Let the people write their own slogans.

11. *Eliminate numerical quotas.* Quotas are only numbers and do not take quality or process methods into account. Quotas may be counterproductive because people will meet quotas to maintain a job although the company may suffer damage.

12. *Remove barriers to pride of workmanship.* People are eager to do a good job and want to do so. Management must remove barriers such as faulty equipment and defective materials, so the people can improve the quality of the product and process.

13. *Institute a vigorous program of education and retraining.* Management and workers must be educated and retrained in statistical techniques and teamwork for quality improvement to take place.

14. *Take action to accomplish the transformation.* It takes a dedicated team of top management with a defined action plan to lead the quality mission.

Note: From *Integrated Quality Management: The Key to Improving Nursing Care Quality* (pp. 25–28) by M. W. Koch and T. M. Fairly, 1993, St. Louis: Mosby.

KEY TERMS

PDCA cycle Plan, do, check, act; a model developed by Deming based on the scientific method that is used in total quality management.

Continuous quality improvement A process used to systematically investigate ways to improve patient care.

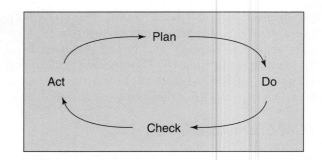

Figure 9-1 **PDCA cycle.** *Note:* **From *Improving quality performance* by P. Schroeder, 1994, St. Louis: Mosby.**

organization include patients, visitors, physicians, managed care organizations, insurance companies, and regulatory agencies, such as the JCAHO and public health departments. Under the principles of TQM, it is important for the nurse manager to know who the customers are and to endeavor to meet their needs. Providing flexible schedules for employees, adjusting routines for A.M. care to meet the needs of patients, extending clinic hours beyond 5 P.M., and putting infant changing tables in restrooms are some health care examples. Putting the customer first requires creative and innovative methods to meet the ever-changing needs of internal and external customers.

Total Organizational Involvement The goal of quality management is to involve all employees and empower them with the responsibility to make a difference in the quality of service they provide. This means all employees must have knowledge of the TQM philosophy as it relates to their job and the overall goals and mission of the organization. Knowledge of the TQM process breaks down barriers between departments. The phrase "That's not my job" is eliminated. Departments work together as a team. On occasion, nursing personnel might clean a bed for a new admission from the emergency room or a physician might transport a patient to the radiology department.

Use of Quality Tools and Statistics for Measurement Measurement is a key component to improving quality: "If you measure it and post it, you will improve it" (Covey, 1992, p. 232). There are many tools, formats, and designs that can be used to build knowledge, make decisions, and improve quality. Tools for data analysis and display can be used to identify areas for process and quality improvement, and then to benchmark the progress of improvements. (See Chapter 10 for a description of these tools.) Deming applied the scientific method to the concept of TQM to develop a model he called the **PDCA cycle** (**Plan, Do, Check, Act**) depicted in Figure 9-1.

Identification of Key Processes for Improvement All activities performed in an organization can be described in terms of processes. Processes within a health care setting can be systems-related (e.g., admitting, discharging, and transferring patients), clinical (e.g., administering medications, managing pain), or managerial (e.g., risk management and performance evaluations) (Schroeder, 1994). Processes can be very complex and involve multidisciplinary or interdepartmental actions. Processes involving multiple departments must be investigated in detail by members from each department involved in the activity so that they can proactively seek opportunities to reduce waste and inefficiencies and develop ways to improve performance and promote positive outcomes.

Continuous Quality Improvement (CQI)

TQM is the overall philosophy, whereas **continuous quality improvement** (CQI) is the process used to improve quality and performance. TQM and CQI often are used synonymously. In health care organizations, CQI is the process used to investigate systematically ways to improve patient care. As the name implies, continuous quality improvement is a never-ending endeavor. CQI means more than just meeting standards, thresholds, or solving problems. It involves evaluation, actions, and a mind-set to strive constantly for excellence. This concept is sometimes difficult to grasp because patient care involves the synchronization of activities in multiple departments. Therefore, the importance of developing and implementing a well-thought-out process is key to a successful CQI implementation. Figure 9-2 shows an example of how CQI can be implemented organizationally in a health care setting.

There are four major players in the CQI process: the resource group, CQI coordinator, team leader, and

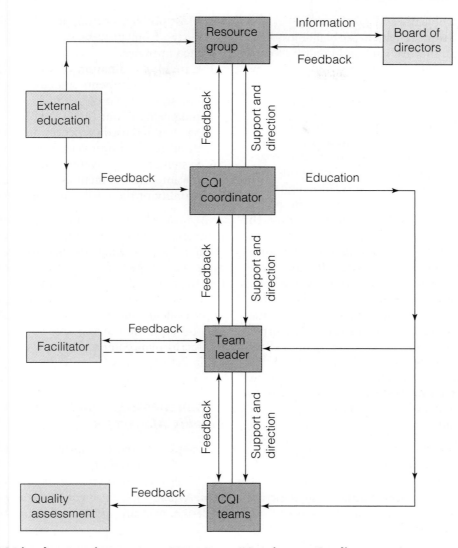

Figure 9-2   CQI implementation process. *Note:* **From "Continuous Quality Improvement: Improving Quality in Your Home Health Organization" by N. Bohnet et al., 1993,** *Journal of Nursing Administration, 23*(2), 42–48.

CQI team. The *resource group* is made up of senior management (e.g., CEO, vice presidents, department directors). It establishes overall CQI policy, vision, and values for the organization and actively involves the board of directors in this process, thereby ensuring that the CQI program has sufficient emphasis and is provided with the training resources needed. The CQI *coordinator* is often appointed by the CEO to provide day-to-day management of the CQI process and related activities (e.g., training programs). CQI *teams* are designated to evaluate and improve select processes. They are formally established and supported by the resource group.

CQI teams range in size from 5 to 10 people, representing all major functions of the process being evaluated. Each CQI team is headed by a *team leader* who is familiar with the process being evaluated. The leader organizes team meetings, sets the agenda, and guides the group through the discussion, evaluation, and implementation process. Each group also has a facilitator to ensure the group remains focused, and that diverse opinions are considered (Bohnet, Ilcyn, Milanovich, Ream, & Wright, 1993).

CQI in Health Care   Continuous quality improvement moved health care from a mode of identifying failed standards, problems, and problem people to a proactive organization in which problems are prevented and ways to improve care and quality of care are sought. This paradigm shift involved all in the organization and promoted problem solving and experimentation (Koch & Fairly, 1993).

JCAHO and Performance Improvement Standards

The Joint Commission on the Accreditation of Healthcare Organizations (JCAHO) assists health care organizations by providing guidelines and standards that help focus quality improvement efforts. Although these standards are broad-based and subject to interpretation, their intent is to provide a framework for each health care organization to customize the process to meet its unique conditions. It is essential for the nurse manager to become familiar with JCAHO standards for both nursing and the organization as a whole. Nursing is an integral player in improving the quality of patient care throughout the organization. It is the one area that truly integrates the functions of all other systems in the health care organization as they affect the patient/customer.

The JCAHO does not require an organization to specifically adopt CQI or TQM programs or tools to structure its improvement process. However, sections of the JCAHO standards focus heavily on improving performance. Examples of CQI concepts incorporated into the standards include the following (JCAHO, 1995):

1. The organization's leaders institute systematic assessment and improvement of performance.

2. Most problems or opportunities for improvement derive from process weaknesses, not individual incompetence.
3. Careful coordination of work and collaboration among departments and professional groups is necessary.
4. Judgments about quality should be sought from patients and used to identify areas of improvement.
5. Priorities for improvement should be set.
6. Systematic improvement of the performance of the important functions and maintenance of the stability of these functions are necessary.

A flow chart depicting important actions and processes in improving organizational performance (Figure 9-3), known as the **performance improvement cycle**, has evolved from JCAHO's previous method, the 10-step model. As the term *cycle* conveys, never-ending improvement is the central theme. The four improvement models (Deming's PDCA, JCAHO 10-step process, the nursing process, and JCAHO's current performance improvement cycle) are compared in Table 9-1.

Comprehensive Components of Quality Management

The steps required to implement quality management in a health care setting follow.

1. *Develop a comprehensive quality management plan.* A quality management plan is a systematic method to design, measure, assess, and improve organizational

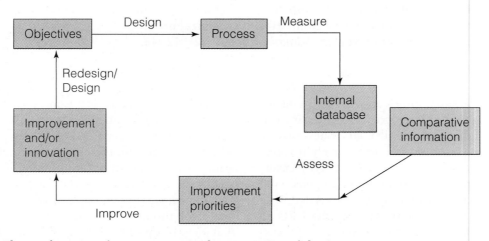

Figure 9-3   **The performance improvement cycle. Note. Copyright © 1996**
Comprehensive Accreditation Manual for Hospitals. **Oakbrook Terrace, IL: Joint Commission on Accreditation of Healthcare Organizations, 1996, p. 35. Reprinted with permission.**

Table 9-1   Comparison of Improvement Models

PDCA	10-Step Process	Nursing Process	Performance Improvement Cycle
Plan	1. Responsibility	Assess	Design
	2. Scope of care	Diagnose	
	3. Important aspects of care	Plan	
	4. Indicators		
	5. Thresholds		
Do	6. Collect data	Intervene	Measure
Check	7. Evaluate	Evaluate	Assess
Act	8. Take actions		Improve
	9. Reassess		Redesign
	10. Communicate findings		

Note: Adapted from *Improving quality performance*, by P. Schroeder, 1994, St. Louis: Mosby.

performance. Using a multidisciplinary approach, this plan identifies processes and systems that represent the goals and mission of the organization, identifies the customers, and specifies opportunities for improvement. Critical paths, which are described in Chapter 3, are an example of a quality management plan. Critical paths identify expected outcomes within a specific time frame. Then variances are tracked and accounted for.

2. *Set standards and benchmarking.* **Standards** are written statements that define a level of performance or a set of conditions determined to be acceptable by some authority (Smith-Marker, 1988). Standards relate to three major dimensions of quality care: structure, process, or outcome (Berstein & Hilborne, 1993). **Structure standards** relate to the physical environment, organization, and management of an organization. **Process standards** are those connected with the actual delivery of care. **Outcome standards** involve the end results of care that has been given (Smith-Marker, 1988). An **indicator** is a tool used to measure the performance of structure, process, and outcome standards. It is measurable, objective, and based on current knowledge. Once indicators are identified, **benchmarking**, or comparing data with other reliable sources internally and externally, is the key to quality improvement. In nursing, both generic and specific standards are available from the American Nurses Association and specialty organizations; however, each organization and each patient care area must designate standards specific to the patient population being served. These standards are the foundation on which all other measures of quality are based. An example

of a standard is: Every patient will have a written care plan within 12 hours of admission.

3. *Conduct performance appraisals.* Based on requirements of the job, employees are evaluated on their performance. This feedback is essential for employees to be professionally accountable. (See Chapter 19 for more on performance appraisals.)

KEY TERMS

Performance improvement cycle A model developed by JCAHO that evolved from the 10-step model and depicts important actions and processes in improving organizational performance.

Standards Written statements that define a level of performance or a set of conditions determined to be acceptable by some authority.

Structure standards Standards that relate to the physical environment, organization, and management of an organization.

Process standards Standards connected with the actual delivery of care.

Outcome standards Standards that reflect the desired result or outcome of care.

Indicator A tool used to measure the performance of structure, process, and outcome standards.

Benchmarking The process of comparing data with reliable internal and external sources.

4. *Focus on intradisciplinary assessment and improvement.* There will always be a need for groups to assess, analyze, and improve their own performance (Schroeder, 1994). Methods to assess performance should, however, focus on the CQI philosophy, which involves group or intradisciplinary performance. Peer review is an example of intradisciplinary assessment. (Peer review is discussed later in the chapter.)

5. *Focus on interdisciplinary assessment and improvement.* Multidisciplinary, patient-focused teamwork emphasizing collaboration, communication, coordination, and integration of care is the core of CQI in health care. It is important not to disband departmental quality functions, such as patient satisfaction, utilization review, or infection control, but rather to refocus information on improving the process.

CQI—How it Works: A Practical Example

The following example describes how one hospital used quality assessment activities to provide feedback information into the CQI process. Reduction in the length of stay for breast surgeries was the goal. A team consisting of physicians, surgeons, and nurses was formed to examine the feasibility of reducing length of stay. The idea initially met much resistance. Surgeons were concerned about the potential for postoperative infection, while nurses were concerned with the effective management of pain. An investigation of infection rates revealed, however, that no infections had occurred for the past 5 years, thus negating that argument. Furthermore, the team determined that pain management could be effectively managed with oral medications administered by the patient.

Another concern was continuity of care. Operating room nurses were consulted to determine whether a preoperative visit and postoperative follow-up system could be implemented. The nurses proposed and implemented a system whereby the same nurse would see the patient before surgery and for postoperative follow-up visits. During the follow-up visit, the nurse also would give the patient a satisfaction survey to identify ways to improve the process from a patient's perspective (Quality Review Bulletin, 1993).

This example shows how CQI can work interdepartmentally to improve the process in a specific area of health care. It also shows how resources within the hospital are used to collect data, such as the number of postoperative infections, to guide the decision-making process. Throughout the evaluation and implementation process, the team's focus was the patient. Implementation was continually evaluated using a patient satisfaction survey, which is just one of the methods used to monitor nursing care. Other methods include the nursing audit, peer review, and utilization review.

Nursing Audits A nursing audit can be retrospective or concurrent. A **retrospective audit** is conducted after a patient's discharge and involves examining records of a large number of cases. The patient's entire course of care is evaluated and comparisons made across cases. Recommendations for change can be based on the experiences of many patients with similar care problems as well as on the spectrum of care considered.

A **concurrent audit** is conducted during the patient's course of care; it examines the care being given to achieve a desired outcome in the patient's health and evaluates the nursing care activities being provided. Changes can be made if patient outcomes so indicate.

Peer Review Peer review occurs when practicing nurses determine the standards and criteria that indicate quality care and then assess performance against these. In this case, nurses are the experts at determining what the indicators of quality care are and when such care has been provided. Their expertise is especially useful in complicated cases; sometimes, more than one expert's opinion is used for comparisons.

Utilization Review Utilization reviews are based on the appropriate allocation of resources and are mandated by the JCAHO. Such a review is not specifically directed toward nursing care, but it may provide information on nursing practices that require further investigation.

Once standards have been set, criteria established, and methods for evaluating adherence to the standards determined, the organization is prepared to examine its risk in relation to its accountability. Risk management programs in health care organizations involve two important areas: patient and/or family incident review, and employee and visitor safety.

Outcomes Management **Outcomes management** is a new technology in which costs and quality are concurrently and retrospectively measured and evaluated in order to improve clinical practice (Luquire & Houston, 1997). Internal or external data from the literature or other health care providers are used as benchmarks against which process, quality, and financial goals can be set and achieved. Collaborative practice teams consisting of physicians, nurses, dietitians, pharmacists, social workers, and finance experts develop research-based standardized practice models such as

KEY TERMS

Retrospective audit A nursing audit conducted after a patient's discharge that involves examining records of a large number of cases.

Concurrent audit A nursing audit conducted during the patient's course of care.

Peer review An evaluation by practicing nurses who have determined the standards and criteria that indicate quality care.

Utilization reviews JCAHO-mandated reviews based on the appropriate allocation of resources.

Outcomes management A system in which costs and quality are concurrently and retrospectively measured and evaluated in order to improve clinical practice.

Risk management A program directed toward the identifying of, evaluating of, and taking corrective action against potential risks that could lead to injury.

order sets or critical pathways. These models are implemented and patient outcomes measured. The outcomes are statistically analyzed. Care is redesigned based on the outcomes analysis and the new processes implemented. The cycle continues, constantly evaluating whether desired outcomes have been achieved (Luquire & Houston, 1997).

Risk Management

Risk management is a program directed toward identifying of, evaluating of, and taking corrective action against potential risks that could lead to injury of patients, staff, or visitors. Historically, risk management has focused on incompetence, informed consent, and the right to refuse treatment. Risk management is problem-focused, whereas CQI is a prevention-focused approach. Today, risk management programs are not outdated, but they should be integrated into the organization's overall CQI program.

A Risk Management Program

Risk management follows the current trend of adapting business strategies to health care; it is the organizational parallel to product liability prevention in industry. Risk management is a planned program of loss prevention and liability control. Its purpose is to identify, analyze, and evaluate risks and then to develop a plan for reducing the frequency and severity of accidents and injuries. Risk management is a continuous daily program of detection, education, and intervention.

Risk management involves all departments of the organization. It must be an organization-wide program, with the board of director's approval and input from all departments. The program must have high-level commitment, including that of the chief executive officer and the chief nurse. A risk management program includes the following activities.

1. Identifying potential risks for accident, injury, or financial loss. Formal and informal communication with all organizational departments and inspection of facilities are essential to identifying problem areas.
2. Reviewing current organization-wide monitoring systems (incident reports, audits, committee minutes, oral complaints, patient questionnaires), evaluating completeness, and determining additional systems needed to provide the factual data essential for risk management control.
3. Analyzing the frequency, severity, and causes of general categories and specific types of incidents causing injury or adverse outcomes to patients. To plan risk intervention strategies, it is necessary to estimate the possible loss associated with the various types of incidents.
4. Reviewing and appraising safety and risk aspects of patient care procedures and new programs.
5. Monitoring laws and codes related to patient safety, consent, and care.
6. Eliminating or reducing risks as much as possible.
7. Reviewing the work of other committees to determine potential liability and recommend prevention or corrective action. Examples of such committees are infection, medical audit, safety/security, pharmacy, nursing audit, and productivity. In many organizations, quality and risk management committees and programs have been combined.
8. Identifying needs for patient, family, and personnel education suggested by all of the foregoing and implementing the appropriate educational program.
9. Evaluating the results of a risk management program.
10. Providing periodic reports to administration, medical staff, and the board of directors.

The establishment of a risk management program starts at the top. The board of directors commits the necessary resources and directs the administrator to establish the program. The administrator then appoints a risk management committee, whose members are responsible for the overall planning and decision making that are involved in risk management. A risk manager should be appointed to manage the day-to-day operation of the program.

Nursing's Role in Risk Management

In the organizational setting, nursing is the one department involved in patient care 24 hours a day; nursing personnel are therefore critical to the success of a risk management program. The chief nursing administrator must be committed to the program. Her or his attitude will influence the staff and their participation. After all, it is the staff, with their daily patient contact, who actually implement a risk management program.

High-risk areas in health care fall into five general categories: (a) medication errors, (b) complications from diagnostic or treatment procedures, (c) falls, (d) patient or family dissatisfaction with care, and (e) refusal of treatment or refusal to sign consent for treatment. Nursing is involved in all areas, but the medical staff may be primarily responsible in cases involving refusal of treatment or of consent to treatment.

Medical records and incidence reports serve to document organizational, nurse, and physician accountability. However, it has been estimated that for every reported occurrence, 35 are unreported. If records are faulty, inadequate, or omitted, the organization is more likely to be sued and more likely to lose. Incident reports are used to analyze the severity, frequency, and causes of occurrences within the five risk categories. Such analysis serves as a basis for intervention.

Incident Reports   Accurate and comprehensive reporting on both the patient's chart and in the incident report is essential to protect the organization and caregivers from litigation. Incident reporting is often the nurse's responsibility. Reluctance to report incidents is usually due to fear of the consequences. This fear can be alleviated by (a) staff education programs that emphasize objective reporting, omitting inflammatory words and judgmental statements; and (b) a clear understanding that the purposes of the incident reporting process are documentation and follow-up and that the report will not be used, *under any circumstances*, for disciplinary action.

> ### KEY TERMS
>
> *Incident report*   An accurate and comprehensive report on unplanned or unexpected occurrences that could potentially affect a patient, family member, or staff.

A reportable incident should include any unexpected or unplanned occurrence that affects or could potentially affect a patient, family member, or staff. The report is only as effective as the form on which it is reported, so attention should be paid to the adequacy of the form as well as to the data it calls for (Duran, 1980). See Figure 9-4 for a sample incident report form.

Reporting incidents involves the following steps.

1. *Discovery.* Nurses, physicians, patients, families, or any employee or volunteer may report actual or potential risk.
2. *Notification.* The risk manager receives the completed incident form within 24 hours after the incident. A telephone call may be made earlier to hasten follow-up in the event of a major incident.
3. *Investigation.* The risk manager or representative investigates the incident immediately.
4. *Consultation.* The risk manager consults with the referring physician, risk management committee member, or both to obtain additional information and guidance.
5. *Action.* The risk manager should clarify any misinformation to the patient or family, explaining exactly what happened. The patient should be referred to the appropriate source for help and, if needed, be assured that care for any necessary service will be provided free of charge.
6. *Recording.* The risk manager should be sure that all records, including incident reports, follow-up, and actions taken, if any, are filed in a central depository.

Examples of Risk

The following are some examples of actual events in the various risk categories.

Medication Errors, Including Administration of Intravenous Fluids   A reportable incident occurs when a medication or fluid is omitted, the wrong medication

Figure 9-4 **Sample incident report.**   ➤

Privileged and Confidential
–Not a part of Hospital Record–
Hospital Report of Incident to Counsel

Complete this report in the event of an accident, discovery of a hazardous condition, or any occurrence which is not consistent with the routine operation of the hospital or routine care of a patient.

1. Name:
   Address:

Unit #:

(Use addressograph if available)

2. ☐ Inpatient ☐ Outpatient ☐ Visitor ☐ Employee ☐ Other ___

3. Sex ☐ M ☐ F

4. Age

5. If patient admission date

6. Occurrence information: ☐ am ☐ pm
   Date: _____ Time: _____
   Location: Bldg. _____ Floor ____
   Room ____

7. Reason for being in hospital: _____

8. Type of occurrence and/or related factors:
   ☐ Fall ☐ Blood transfusion ☐ Equipment ☐ Patient behavior
   ☐ Medication ☐ Diagnostic procedure ☐ Communication ☐ Visitor: faint/fall (Circle one)
   ☐ IV Therapy ☐ Therapeutic procedure ☐ Support services ☐ Other: _____

9. If fall from bed, siderails position: ☐ One up—full ☐ Two up—full ☐ One up—1/2 ☐ None up
   Bed position: ☐ Locked ☐ Fixed ☐ High ☐ Low

10. Were any of the following medications given in the past four (4) hours: ☐ No ☐ Yes
    ☐ Sedative ☐ Laxative ☐ Diuretic ☐ Insulin ☐ Narcotic ☐ Other: _____

11. Ambulation privilege:
    ☐ Unlimited ☐ Limited w/o assistance ☐ Limited w/assistance ☐ Bed rest ☐ Not specified

12. Description of incident (state significant facts in chronological order): _____

13. Physician of record: _____ Dept.: _____
    R.N. or L.P.N. assigned to patient at time of occurrence: _____ N.C./Charge nurse: _____
    Resident (year): _____
    Others present during the time of occurrence:
    Name: _____ Status: _____

14. Pertinent findings by examining physician: _____

15. Patient/family aware of incident ☐ Yes ☐ No   Examination or follow-up refused ☐ Yes ☐ No

16. Follow-up treatment ☐ Yes ☐ No   X-rays ☐ Yes ☐ No

                Print last name   Signature   Date
17. Examining physician _____

Reported by _____
Staff member present at time of incident (if other than above) _____

or fluid is administered, or a medication is given to the wrong patient, given at the wrong time, in the wrong dosage, or by the wrong route. Here are some examples.

Patient A. *Weight was transcribed incorrectly from emergency room sheet. Medication dose was calculated on incorrect weight; therefore, patient was given double the dose required. Error discovered after first dose and corrected. Second dose omitted.*

Patient B. *Tegretol dosage written in Medex as "Tegretol 100 mg chewable tab—50 mg po BID." Tegretol 100 mg given po at 1400. Meds checked at 1430 and error noted. 50 mg Tegretol should have been given. Doctor notified. Second dose held.*

Patient C. *During rounds at 3:30 P.M. found .9% sodium chloride at 75 c.c.'s per hour hanging. Order was D$_5$W. Fluids last checked at 2:00 P.M. Changed to correct fluid. Doctor notified.*

Diagnostic Procedure   Any incident occurring before, during, or after such procedures as blood sample stick, biopsy, X-ray examination, lumbar puncture, or other invasive procedure is categorized as a diagnostic procedure incident. Examples follow.

Patient A. *When I checked the IV site, I saw that it was red and swollen. For this reason, I discontinued the IV. When removing the tape, I noted a small area of skin breakdown where the tape had been. There was also a small knot on the medial aspect of the left antecubital above the IV insertion site. Doctor notified. Wound dressed.*

Patient B. *Patient found on the floor after lumbar puncture. Right side rail down. Examined by a physician, BP 120/80, T 98.6, P 72, R 18. No injury noted on exam.*

Medical-Legal Incident   If a patient or family refuses treatment as ordered and prescribed or refuses to sign consent forms, the situation is categorized as a medical-legal incident.

Patient A. *After a visit from a member of the clergy, patient indicated he was no longer in need of medical attention and asked to be discharged. Physician called. Doctor explained potential side effects if treatment was discontinued. Patient continued to ask for discharge. Doctor explained "against medical advice" (AMA) form. Patient signed AMA form and left at 1300 without medications.*

Patient B. *Patient refused to sign consent for bone marrow biopsy. States side effects not understood. Doctor reviewed reasons for test and side effects*

three different times. Doctor informed the patient that without consent he could not perform the test. Offered to call in another physician for second opinion. Patient agreed. After doctor left, patient signed consent form.

Patient or Family Dissatisfaction with Care   When a patient or family indicates general dissatisfaction with care and the situation cannot be or has not been resolved, then an incident report is filed.

Patient A. *Mother complained that she had found child saturated with urine every morning (she arrived around 0800). Explained to mother that diapers and linen are changed at 0600 when 0600 feedings and meds are given. Patient's back, buttocks, and perineal areas are free of skin breakdown. Parents continue to be distressed. Discussed with primary nurse.*

Patient B. *Mr. Smith obviously very angry. Greeted me at the door complaining that his wife had not been treated properly in our emergency room the night before. Wanted to speak to someone from administration. Was unable to reach the administrator on call. Suggested Mr. Smith call administrator in the morning. Mr. Smith thanked me for my time and assured me that he would call the administrator the next day.*

Role of the Nurse Manager

The nurse manager plays a key role in the success of any risk management program. Nurse managers can reduce risk by helping their staff view health and illness from the patient's perspective. Usually, the staff's understanding of quality differs from the patient's expectations and perceptions. By understanding the meaning of the course of illness to the patient and the family, the nurse will manage risk better because that understanding can enable the nurse to individualize patient care. This individualized attention produces respect and, in turn, reduces risk.

A patient incident or a patient's or family's expression of dissatisfaction regarding care indicates not only some slippage in quality of care but also potential liability. A distraught, dissatisfied, complaining patient is a high risk; a satisfied patient or family is a low risk. A risk management or liability control program should therefore emphasize a personal approach. Many claims are filed because of a breakdown in communication between the health care provider and the patient. In many instances, after an incident or bad outcome, a quick visit or call from an organization's representative to the patient or family can soothe tempers and clarify misinformation.

In the examples given, prompt attention and care by the nurse manager protected the patients involved and may have averted a potential liability claim. Once an incident has occurred, the important factors in successful risk management are recognition of the incident, quick follow-up and action, personal contact, and immediate restitution (where appropriate). It is estimated that 90% of patients' concerns can and should be handled at the unit level. When that first line of communication breaks down, however, the nurse manager needs a resource—usually the risk manager or nursing service administrator.

Key Behaviors for Handling Complaints

Handling a patient's or family member's complaints stemming from an incident can be very difficult. These confrontations are often highly emotional; the patient or family member must be calmed down, yet have their concerns satisfied. Sometimes just an opportunity to release the anger or emotion is all that is needed. Box 9-3 shows a set of key behaviors that may be used to defuse a complaint from a patient or family member.

The first three key behaviors have to do with *listening* to the person to hear concerns and to help defuse the situation. Arguing or interrupting only increases the person's anger or emotion. After the patient or family member has had his or her say, the nurse manager can then attempt to solve the problem by asking what is expected in the form of a solution. The nurse manager or other organizational representative should then explain what can and cannot be done and try to negotiate with the injured party an agreement or a solution. It is important to be specific. Offering vague solutions (e.g., "everything will be taken care of") may only lead to more problems later on if expectations as to solution and timing differ.

All incidents must be properly documented. Information on the incident form should be detailed and include all the factors relating to the incident, as demonstrated in the previous examples. The documentation in the chart, however, should be only a statement of the *facts* and of the patient's physical response; no reference to the incident report should be made, nor should words like *error* or *inappropriate* be used. When a patient receives 100 mg of Demerol instead of 50 mg as ordered, the proper documentation in the chart is, "100 mg of Demerol administered. Physician notified." The remainder of the documentation should include any reaction the patient has to the dosage, such as "Patient's vital signs unchanged." If there is an adverse reaction, a follow-up note should be written in the chart, giving an update of the patient's status. A note related to the patient's reaction should be written as frequently as the status changes and should continue until the patient returns to his or her previous status.

The chart must never be used as a tool for disciplinary comments, action, or expressions of anger. Notes such as "Incident would never have occurred if Doctor X had written the correct order in the first place" or "This carelessness is inexcusable" are totally inappropriate and serve no meaningful purpose. Carelessness and incorrect orders do indeed cause errors and incidents, but the place to address and resolve these issues is in the risk management committee or in the nurse manager's office, not on the patient chart.

A Caring Attitude

It is also the nurse manager who sets the tone with employees that contributes to a safe and low-risk environment. One of the most important ways to reduce risk is to instill a sense of confidence in both patients and families by emphasizing and recognizing that they will receive personalized attention and that their needs will be attended to with competence. This confidence is created environmentally and professionally. Examples

---

Box 9-3	Key Behaviors for Handling Complaints

- Listen openly.
- Do not speak until the person has had his or her say.
- Avoid reacting emotionally (don't get defensive).
- Ask for his or her expectations about a solution to the problem.
- Explain what you can and cannot do to solve the problem (if appropriate).
- Agree on specific steps to be taken and specific deadlines.

Note: Adapted from *Health care management microtraining* by P. J. Decker, 1982, St. Louis: Decker & Associates.

of environmental factors include cleanliness, attention to patients' privacy, an orderly looking unit, and minimal social conversations in front of patients. One example of portraying professional confidence is to provide patients and families with the name of the person in charge. A sincere visit by that person is re-assuring. Also, a thorough orientation creates independence for the patient and confidence in an efficient unit. The nurse manager needs to foster the attitude that any mistake that does occur is perceived as an opportunity to improve a system or a process rather than to punish an individual. If the nurse manager has developed a patient-focused atmosphere in which patients believe their best interests are a priority, the potential for risk will be reduced.

Evaluation of Risk Management

Identifying and reducing risks involves close monitoring and analysis of incident reports (see Figure 9-4). Incident reports that include statements of blame should be discussed. A risk management program needs support and participation from all staff. To elicit their commitment, the nurse manager must limit the use of incident reports to risk reduction only. This policy must be emphasized and practiced.

A risk management program requires resources. In times of budget reductions, it may be one of the first programs to be cut, but the purpose of risk management is to reduce losses; it is a case of spending money to save it. Return on the investment takes time, however, and it is difficult to estimate what might have been lost had risk management activities not been in place. Most organizations are convinced that a risk management program is cost-effective and provides a safer environment for patients, visitors, and employees.

An additional benefit of a risk management program may be an increase in positive attitudes toward the organization from employees, physicians, insurers, and the community. When implemented in a spirit of concern and responsibility, a risk management program can be a visible means of responding to patient needs. Health care organizations, physicians, and nurses have had their share of negative press in the past—sometimes with good reason. The courts, insurance carriers, and legislative action have mandated that organizations respond to patient demands. Risk management helps meet this obligation.

Risk management makes sense. It improves the quality of patient care and reduces liability claims. It represents the outstanding characteristic of health care professionals: care and concern for people. It provides the best care possible at the most reasonable cost.

Summary

- Accountability in health care organizations has prompted the recent development of standardized data sets and report cards.
- Quality management is the method by which performance of care is evaluated and improved.
- The principles of total quality management (TQM) include a focus on the customer (patient), empowerment of employees, and the collective work of the team.
- Standards define an acceptable level of performance.
- Benchmarking is a method to track the progress of improvements.
- A continuous quality improvement program is a prevention-focused approach that provides the basis for managing risk.
- Outcomes management develops research-based models that are implemented, analyzed, and adapted based on identified benchmarks.
- The key ingredients in a successful risk management program are an organized program of incident reporting; review and follow-up; a risk manager and committee with well-defined objectives; nurse managers who support the risk management program; and, most important, an environment that the patient and family perceive as friendly and caring.
- Risk management programs help reduce costs and demonstrate the organization's concern for its patients, visitors, and employees.

■LEADERSHIP AND MANAGEMENT
in Action

1. Describe how continuous quality improvement differs from quality assurance.
2. What is nursing's role in addressing the various types of health care risks?
3. Why are incident reports important to a risk management program? Why are nurses reluctant to report incidents?

References

American Nurses Association [ANA] (1999). *Nursing sensitive quality indicators for acute care settings and ANA's safety and quality initiative.* Washington, DC: Author.

Anonymous. (1993). The role of quality management in health care today and tomorrow. *Quality Review Bulletin, 19*(5), 158–164.

Berstein, S., & Hilborne, L. (1993). Clinical indicators: The road to quality care. *Journal on Quality Improvement, 19,* 501–509.

Bodenheimer, T. (1999). The American Health Care System—the movement for improved quality in health care. *The New England Journal of Medicine, 340*(6), 488–492.

Bohnet, N. L., Ilcyn, J., Milanovich, P. S., Ream, M. A., & Wright, K. (1993). Continuous quality improvement improving quality in your home health organization. *Journal of Nursing Administration, 23*(2), 42–48.

Bull, M. (1985). Quality assurance: Its origins, transformation and prospects. In C. G. Meisenheimer (Ed.), *Quality assurance.* Rockville, MD: Aspen.

Covey, S. R. (1992). *Principle-centered leadership.* New York: Simon & Schuster.

Decker, P. J. (1982). *Health care management microtraining.* St. Louis: Decker & Associates.

Duran, G. S. (1980). On the scene: Risk management in health care. *Nursing Administration Quarterly, 5,* 19.

Joint Commission on Accreditation of Healthcare Organizations (JCAHO). (1999). ORYX: The next evolution in accreditation. http://www.jcaho.org/perfmeas/oryx_qa.html. Accessed June 28, 2000.

Joint Commission on Accreditation of Healthcare Organizations (JCAHO). (1995). *Comprehensive accreditation manual for hospitals.* Chicago: Author.

Koch, N. W., & Fairly, T. M. (1993). *Integrated quality management: The key to improving nursing care quality.* St. Louis: Mosby.

Luquire, R., & Houston, S. (1997). Outcomes management: Getting started. *Outcomes Management for Nursing Practice, 1*(1), 5–7.

McLaughlin, L., & Kaluzny, A. (1990). Total quality management in health: Making it work. *Healthcare Management Review, Summer,* 7–13.

National League for Nursing. (1993). *TQM: A context for change.* New York: Author.

Nutting, M. A., & Dock, L. L. (1907). *A history of nursing.* New York: Putnam.

Schroeder, P. (1994). *Improving quality performance.* St. Louis: Mosby.

Simpson, R. L. (2000). Minding the store: How IT impacts outcomes measurement. *Nursing Administration Quarterly, 24*(2), 87–90.

Smith-Marker, C. (1988). *Setting standards for professional nursing: The Marker model.* St. Louis: Mosby.

 Additional on-line resources for this chapter can be found on the World Wide Web at http://www.prenhall.com/sullivan_decker. Select Chapter 9 from the drop-down menu.

Problem Solving and Decision Making

Critical Thinking

Problem Solving

> Problem-Solving Methods
> The Problem-Solving Process
> Group Problem Solving

Decision Making

> Types of Decisions
> Decision-Making Conditions
> The Decision-Making Process
> Decision-Making Techniques
> Group Decision Making
> Stumbling Blocks

Creativity in Decision Making

> Characteristics of Creative Persons
> Managing Creativity in Health
>   Care Settings

Looking Ahead

Nurses constantly face numerous decisions to make and problems to solve; problem solving and decision making are the very core of nursing, but they are not easy tasks. Developing critical-thinking, problem-solving, and decision-making skills allows nurses to see all sides of an issue, look for creative alternatives and approaches to problems, and make well-thought-out decisions. The effect is a stronger organization and more competent leader. This chapter introduces you to the ways you can become a more critical thinker.

Objectives

After reading this chapter, you will be able to:

- Differentiate critical thinking, creative thinking, problem solving, and decision making.
- Relate aspects of the nursing process to critical thinking.
- Describe various methods for solving problems and making decisions.
- Describe the creative process and methods for encouraging creativity.

Nurse managers are expected to use knowledge from various disciplines to solve problems with patients, staff, and the organization, as well as problems in their own personal and professional lives. They also must make decisions in dynamic situations. For example, do the advantages of the primary nursing care delivery system outweigh proposed advantages of expanded use of unlicensed personnel? Would a new model of differentiated practice be more useful? Is the present policy requiring 12-hour shifts adequate for both patients and nurses? Which is the best staffing pattern to prevent turnover and ensure quality patient care? Critical thinking helps nurse managers examine all aspects of an issue and look for different and exciting ways to solve new and old problems. This chapter explains and differentiates critical thinking, problem solving, and decision making and describes processes and techniques for using each.

Critical Thinking

Critical thinking is the process of examining underlying assumptions, interpreting and evaluating arguments, imagining and exploring alternatives, and developing a reflective criticism for the purpose of reaching a reasoned conclusion that can be justified. Critical thinking is not the same thing as criticism, though it does require inquiring attitudes, knowledge about evidence and analysis, and skills to combine them (Brookfield, 1987). Critical-thinking skills can be used to resolve problems rationally. Identifying, analyzing, and questioning the evidence and implications of each problem stimulate and illuminate critical thought processes. Critical thinking is also an essential component of decision making. However, compared to problem solving and decision making, which involve seeking a single solution, critical thinking is broader and encompasses an aspect of feeling and emotion that increases awareness of values, meaning, and personal relationships (Kurfiss, 1988). Critical thinking is a higher-level cognitive process that includes creativity, problem solving, and decision making (Figure 10-1).

The critical-thinking process seems abstract unless it can be related to practical experiences. One way to develop this process is to consider a series of questions when examining a specific problem or making a decision. The following questions are suggested.

1. *What are the underlying assumptions?* Underlying assumptions are unquestioned beliefs that influence an individual's reasoning. They are perceptions that may or may not be grounded in reality.

For example, some people believe the AIDS epidemic is punishment for homosexual behavior. This attitude toward people with AIDS could alter one's approach to care for an AIDS patient.

2. *How is evidence interpreted? What is the context?* Interpretation of information also can be value-laden. Is the evidence presented completely and clearly? Can the facts be substantiated? Are the people presenting the evidence using emotional or biased information? Are there any errors in reasoning?

3. *How are the arguments to be evaluated?* Is there objective evidence to support the arguments? Have all value preferences been determined? Is there a good chance that the arguments will be accepted? Are there enough people to support decisions? For example, many health care institutions changed to a smoke-free environment when it was found that passive smoking was harmful to people's health. In addition, the value system of society favored nonsmokers, and a strong majority supported the movement.

4. *What are possible alternative perspectives?* Using different basic assumptions and paradigms can

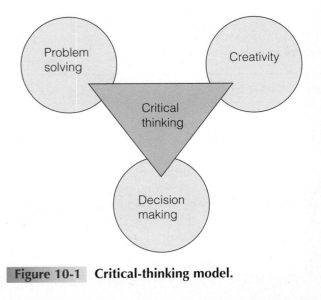

Figure 10-1   Critical-thinking model.

help the critical thinker develop several different views of an issue. For instance, a nurse manager who assumes that high proportions of RN staffing are necessary to provide high-quality patient care will have a different alternative solution to a mandated budget cut than a manager who is committed to using assistive personnel. What ideas are reported in the nursing literature? What solutions do staff members, patients, physicians, and others propose? What would be the ideal alternative?

Managers need to build on the knowledge base they began laying in school to make the critical-thinking process a conscious one in daily activities. Managers also should view identifying problems and analyzing the variety of alternatives as positive opportunities, not negative obligations.

The label *problem solving* is used inconsistently and often interchangeably with *decision making* in organizational literature. Although the two processes appear similar and may in some instances depend on one another, they are not synonymous. The main distinctions between the two are that **problem solving** involves diagnosing a problem and solving it, which may or may not entail deciding on one correct solution, whereas **decision making** may or may not involve a problem, but it always involves selecting one of several alternatives, each of which may be appropriate under certain circumstances.

Most of the time, decision making is a subset of problem solving. However, some decisions are not of a problem-solving nature, such as decisions about scheduling, equipment, inservices, or other matters that do not involve problem solving as a deliberate process. Also, habit and tradition may be modes of decision making, such as holding onto the wall when walking down a wet hospital corridor or scheduling patient care activities in traditional ways (e.g., giving every patient a bath every morning).

Problem Solving

People use problem solving when they perceive a gap between an existing state (what is going on) and a desired state (what should be going on). How one perceives the situation influences how the problem is identified or solved. Therefore, perceptions need to be clarified before problem solving can occur (Lowry, 1999). *Questioning* also is central to problem solving. Questioning identifies central issues, examines reasoning, clarifies ambiguities in defining the problem, explores value conflicts and challenges assumptions

Table 10-1 Overview of Critical Thinking Throughout the Nursing Process

The Nursing Process	Critical Thinking Skills
Assessment	Observing
	Distinguishing relevant from irrelevant data
	Distinguishing important from unimportant data
	Validating data
	Organizing data
	Categorizing data
Diagnosis	Finding patterns and relationships
	Making inferences
	Stating the problem
	Suspending judgment
Planning	Generalizing
	Transferring knowledge from one situation to another
	Developing evaluative criteria
	Hypothesizing
Implementation	Applying knowledge
	Testing hypotheses
Evaluation	Deciding whether hypotheses are correct
	Making criterion-based evaluations

Note: From *Nursing process in action: A critical thinking approach* (p. 29) by J. Wilkinson, 1992, Redwood City, CA: Addison-Wesley Nursing.

(Boychuk, 1999). This type of reflection allows problems to become opportunities to enhance professional growth and organizational efficiency and effectiveness. The scientific problem-solving process requires searching for information to clarify the nature of the problem and to discover a variety of solutions. These solutions are carefully evaluated and the best is chosen for implementation. The implemented solution is maintained over time to ensure its immediate and continued effectiveness. If difficulties are encountered, some or all of the process is repeated.

The nursing process is an example of a problem-solving method. Table 10-1 demonstrates the critical-thinking skills used in the nursing process.

Problem-Solving Methods

A variety of methods can be used to solve problems. People with little management experience tend to use the **trial-and-error method**, applying one solution after another until the problem is solved or appears to be improving. These managers often cite lack of experience and of time and resources to search for alternative solutions.

For example, in a step-down unit with an increasing incidence of medication errors, Nancy, the nurse manager, uses various strategies to decrease errors, such as asking nurses to use calculators, having the charge nurse check medications, and posting dosage and medication charts in the unit. After a few months, by which time none of the methods has worked, it occurs to Nancy that perhaps making nurses responsible for their actions would be more effective. Nancy develops a point system for medication errors: When nurses accumulate a certain amount of points, they are required to take a medication test; repeated failure of the test may eventually lead to termination. Nancy's solution is effective, and a low level of medication errors is restored. As this example shows, a trial-and-error process can be time-consuming and may even be detrimental. Although some learning can occur during the process, the nurse manager risks being perceived as a poor problem solver who has wasted time and money on ineffective solutions.

Experimentation, another type of problem solving, is more rigorous than trial and error. Pilot projects or limited trials are examples of experimentation. Experimentation involves testing a theory (hypothesis) or hunch to produce knowledge, understanding, or prediction. A project or study is carried out in either a controlled setting (e.g., in a laboratory) or an uncontrolled setting (e.g., in a natural setting such as an outpatient clinic). Data are collected and analyzed and results interpreted to determine whether the solution

tried has been effective. For example, Lin, a nurse manager of a pediatric floor, has received many complaints from mothers of children who think the nurses are short-tempered. Lin has a hunch that 12-hour shifts, which have been recently implemented on her floor, are contributing to the problem; she believes that nurses who must interact frequently with families would perform better on 8-hour shifts. She can test her theory by setting up a small study comparing the two staffing patterns with patient satisfaction.

Experimentation may be creative and effective or uninspired and ineffective, depending on how it is used. As a major method of problem solving, experimentation may be inefficient because of the amount of time and control involved. However, a well-designed experiment can be persuasive in situations in which an idea or activity, such as a new staffing system or care procedure, can be tried in one of two similar groups and results objectively compared.

Still other problem-solving techniques rely on *past experience* and *intuition*. Everyone has various and countless experiences. Individuals build a repertoire of these experiences and base future actions on what they considered successful solutions in the past. If a particular course of action consistently resulted in positive outcomes, the person will try it again when similar circumstances occur. In some instances, an individual's past experience can determine how much risk he or she will take in present circumstances. The nature and frequency of the experience also contribute significantly to the effectiveness of this problem-solving method. How much the person has learned from these experiences, positive or negative, can affect the current viewpoint and can result in either subjective and narrow judgments or very wise ones. This is especially true in human relations problems. A nurse manager who has an unfortunate experience with a nurse recovering from chemical dependency may, in the future, judge negatively the performance of all nurses with acknowledged chemical dependency problems. Intuition relies heavily on past experience and trial and error. The extent to which past experience is related to intuition is difficult to determine, but nurses' wisdom, sensitivity, and intuition are known to be valuable in solving problems.

Some problems are self-solving: If permitted to run a natural course, they are solved by those personally involved. This is not to say that a uniform laissez-faire management style solves all problems. The nurse manager must not ignore managerial responsibilities, but often difficult situations become more manageable when participants are given time, resources, and support to discover their own solutions. This typically happens, for example, when a newly graduated BSN joins a unit where most of the staff are diploma RNs who resent the new nurse's level of education as well as the nurse's lack of experience. If the nurse manager intervenes, a problem that the staff might have worked out on their own becomes an ongoing source of conflict. The important skill required here is knowing when to do nothing. Chapter 11 discusses this issue further.

The Problem-Solving Process

Many nursing problems require immediate action. Nurses don't have time for formalized processes of research and analysis specified by the scientific method. Therefore, learning an organized method for problem solving is invaluable. One practical method for problem solving is to follow this seven-step process, which is also outlined in Box 10-1.

1. *Define the problem.* The most important part of problem solving is defining the problem. How the problems are perceived determines the solutions or identifies needed changes. The nurse manager identifies a problem as a departure from what he or she perceives to be a desirable state of affairs. The nurse manager is responsible not only for dealing with the situation, but also for dealing with it with foresight.

Suppose a nurse manager reluctantly implements a self-scheduling process and finds that each time the schedule is posted, evenings and some weekend shifts are not adequately covered. The manager might identify the problem as the immaturity of the staff and their inability to function under democratic leadership. The causes may be lack of interest in group decision making, minimal concern over providing adequate patient coverage, or, perhaps more correctly, a few

nurses' lack of understanding of the process. The definition of a problem should be a descriptive statement of the state of affairs, not a judgment or conclusion. If one begins the statement of a problem with a judgment, the solution may be equally judgmental, and critical descriptive elements could be overlooked. If the nurse manager defines the above problem as immaturity and reverts to making out the schedules without further fact-finding, a minor problem could develop into a full-blown crisis. Sometimes the problem is not easily identified. In this case, tools may be helpful. One such tool is the **affinity map**. Lepley (1998) describes six steps to the process. (See Figure 10-2 for an example.)

a. A problem is acknowledged and a thoughtful question is raised to stimulate ideas.

b. Without talking among the group, ideas about the problem are generated and recorded on individual slips of paper or cards.

c. Then, again without talking, the group is asked to organize similar ideas into no more than six categories.

d. The group facilitator names the categories, explains the rationale used for the naming process, and ensures agreement on category names.

e. The group is allowed an opportunity to explain their thinking. In doing so, perceptions about the problem are discovered and consensus is built. One rule during this step is that there are no right or wrong answers, therefore, none of the ideas should be criticized.

f. Finally, the affinity map can be used to determine cause-and-effect relationships. The name of each category is written down in a circular format to create a diagram. The relationships between categories are identified and directional arrows used. The category with the most number of outgoing arrows is considered the root cause of the problem. The category with the most incoming arrows is the effect.

Premature interpretation can alter one's ability to deal with facts objectively. For example, are there other explanations for the apparent behavior that do not entail negative assumptions about the maturity of

Box 10-1   Seven Steps to Problem Solving

1. Define the problem.	5. Make a decision.
2. Gather information.	6. Implement the decision.
3. Analyze the information.	7. Evaluate the solution.
4. Develop solutions.	

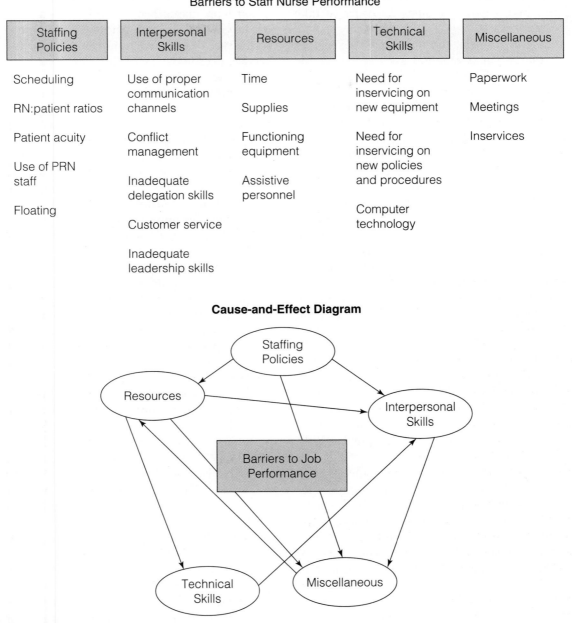

Affinity Map

Barriers to Staff Nurse Performance

Staffing Policies	Interpersonal Skills	Resources	Technical Skills	Miscellaneous
Scheduling	Use of proper communication channels	Time	Need for inservicing on new equipment	Paperwork
RN:patient ratios		Supplies		Meetings
Patient acuity	Conflict management	Functioning equipment	Need for inservicing on new policies and procedures	Inservices
Use of PRN staff	Inadequate delegation skills	Assistive personnel		
Floating	Customer service		Computer technology	
	Inadequate leadership skills			

Cause-and-Effect Diagram

Staffing Policies

Resources

Interpersonal Skills

Barriers to Job Performance

Technical Skills

Miscellaneous

Figure 10-2 **The affinity map and cause-and-effect diagram.** *Note:* **From Lepley, C. J. (1998). Problem-Solving Tools for Analyzing System Problems.** *Journal of Nursing Administration,* **28(2), 44–50.**

the staff? Premature interpretations can be avoided by using *reflective inquiry*. Schmieding (1999) describes four characteristics of reflective inquiry. First, objective data are tested against one's thoughts and feelings. Second, past experiences and knowledge are used to evaluate the situation. Next, ideas about the problem are validated or refuted based on empirical

evidence through a serial rather than a linear process. Finally, the facts and ideas generated are verified through deliberate investigation.

Accurate assessment of the scope of the problem also determines whether the manager needs to seek a lasting solution or just a stopgap measure. Is this just a situational problem requiring only intervention with a simple explanation, or is it more complex, involving the leadership style of the manager? The manager must define and classify problems in order to take action.

In defining a problem, the nurse manager should determine the area it covers and ask: Do I have the authority to do anything about this myself? Do I have all the information? The time? Who else has important information and can contribute? What benefits could be expected? A list of potential benefits provides the basis for comparison and choice of solutions. The list also serves as a means for evaluating the solution.

2. *Gather information.* Problem solving begins with collecting facts. This information gathering initiates a search for additional facts that provides clues to the scope and solution of the problem. A careful, systematic, complete search facilitates the accomplishment of goals and evaluates the possible effects of the solution. Information gathered will probably be a combination of facts and feelings. The manager should obtain relevant, valid, accurate, and detailed descriptions from appropriate people or sources and put the information in writing. This step encourages people to report facts accurately. The nurse manager or team may choose to have everyone involved provide information. Although this may not always provide objective information, it reduces misinformation and allows everyone an opportunity to tell what he or she thinks is wrong with a situation. Lack of time, of course, may prevent gathering written data.

Experience is another source of information—one's own experience as well as the experience of other nurse managers and staff. Everyone involved usually has ideas about what should be done about a problem, and many of these ideas provide good information and valuable suggestions. Yet information gathered may never be complete. Some data will be useless, some inaccurate, but some will be useful to develop innovative ideas worth pursuing.

3. *Analyze the information.* The manager should analyze the information only when all of it has been sorted into some orderly arrangement. The following is suggested:

a. Categorize information in order of reliability.

b. List information from most important to least important.

c. Set information into a time sequence. What happened first? Next? What came before what? What were the concurrent circumstances?

d. Set up information in terms of cause and effect. Is A causing B, or vice versa?

e. Classify information into categories: human factors, such as personality, maturity, education, age, relationships among people, and problems outside the organization; technical factors, such as nursing skills or the type of unit; temporal factors, such as length of service, overtime, type of shift, and double shifts; and policy factors, such as organizational procedures or rules applying to the problem, legal issues, and ethical issues.

f. Consider how long the situation has been going on.

Because no amount of information is ever complete or comprehensive enough, critical-thinking skills are important to the manager's ability to examine the assumptions, evidence, and potential value conflicts.

4. *Develop solutions.* As the nurse manager or group analyzes information, numerous possible solutions will suggest themselves. These should be written down and plans made to immediately start developing the best of them. It is not wise to limit consideration only to simple solutions, because doing so may constrain creative thinking and cause overconcentration on detail. Developing alternative solutions makes it possible to combine the best parts of several solutions into a superior one. Also, alternatives are valuable in case the first-order solutions prove impossible to implement.

When exploring a variety of solutions, the nurse manager should maintain an uncritical attitude toward the way the problem has been handled in the past. Some problems have had a long-standing history by the time they reach the nurse manager, and attempts may have been made to resolve them over a long period of time. "We tried this before and it didn't work," is often said and may apply—or more likely, may not apply—in a changed situation.

Past experience may not always supply an answer, but it can aid the critical-thinking process and help prepare for future problem solving. Nurse managers and others can review the literature, attend relevant seminars, and brainstorm ideas. Sometimes others have solved similar problems and those methods can be applied to a comparable problem.

5. *Make a decision.* After reviewing the list of potential solutions, the nurse manager should select the one that is most feasible and satisfactory and has the fewest undesirable consequences. Some solutions have to be put into effect quickly; matters of discipline or compromises in patient care delivery, for example, need immediate intervention. Nurse managers should have, in advance, the authority to act in an emergency and know the penalties to be imposed for various infractions.

If the problem is a technical one and its solution brings about a change in the method of doing work (or using new equipment), there may be resistance. All people become disturbed by changes that reorder their habit patterns and threaten personal security or status. Many solutions fail because the manager does not recognize the change process that must be initiated before solutions can be implemented. If the solution involves change, the manager should fully involve those who will be affected by it, if possible, or at least inform them of the process. (See Chapter 16 for discussion of the change process.)

6. *Implement the decision.* The manager implements the decision after selecting the best course of action. If unforeseen new problems emerge after implementation, the manager must evaluate these impediments as carefully as any other problem. Nurse managers must be careful, however, not to abandon a workable solution just because a few people object. A minority always will. If the previous steps in the problem-solving process have been followed, the solution has been carefully thought out, and potential problems have been addressed, implementation should move forward. Nurses must remember that no solution is perfect and that regardless of the benefits, all change is stressful.

Most employees cooperate only with solutions that fit into their "zone of acceptance." Some solutions are clearly unacceptable, some are neutral, others are barely acceptable, and some are fully acceptable. This last group lies within the zone of acceptance. Thus, if the nurse manager chooses a solution that he or she knows may not be accepted, the manager must take steps to educate or motivate the staff to comply with it. For example, the nurse manager may decide that when the census is low, nurses will "float" to other units. The unit's own staff, however, has negative ideas about floating and do not wish to cooperate. If the nurse manager cannot educate or motivate staff to see floating as an acceptable solution to fluctuating census problems, the solution, no matter how good, will fail because it is not within the staff's zone of acceptance. Participative management techniques, which are discussed throughout this book, help identify acceptable solutions to problems.

7. *Evaluate the solution.* After the solution has been implemented, nurses should review the plan instituted and compare the actual results and benefits to those of the idealized solution. People tend to fall back into old patterns of habit, only giving lip service to change and carrying out the same old behavior. The nurses must ask, Is the solution being implemented? If

so, are the results better or worse than expected? If they are better, what changes have contributed to its success? How can we ensure that the solution continues to be used and to work? Such a periodic checkup gives the nurse manager valuable insight and experience to use in other situations and keeps the problem-solving process on course.

The nurse manager should study outcomes of the solution somewhat as a football coach studies videotapes of a football game. Where were mistakes made? How can they be avoided in the future? What decisions were successes? Why? Many ineffective solutions are never challenged once they are implemented. If the nurse manager evaluates the outcome to ensure that the problem has indeed been solved and builds on that experience, problem solving becomes an expert skill that the nurse can use throughout a management career.

Group Problem Solving

Traditionally, managers solved most problems in isolation. This practice, however, is outdated. Both the complexity of problems and the staff's desire for meaningful involvement at work create the impetus for using group approaches to problem solving. Quality-oriented approaches used in total quality management are being applied widely in health care and emphasize consensus-based problem solving (see Chapter 9).

Advantage of Group Problem Solving   Groups collectively possess greater knowledge and information than any single member and may access more strategies to solve a problem. Under the right circumstances and with appropriate leadership, groups can deal with more complex problems than a single individual, especially if there is no one right or wrong solution to the problem. Individuals tend to rely on a small number of familiar strategies; a group is more likely to try several approaches. Group members may have a greater variety of training and experiences and approach problems from more diverse points of view. Together, a group may generate more complete, accurate, and less biased information than one person. Groups may deal more effectively with problems that cross organizational boundaries or involve change that requires support from all departments affected. Participative problem solving has additional advantages: It increases the likelihood of acceptance and understanding of the decision, and it enhances cooperation in implementation.

Disadvantages of Group Problem Solving Group problem solving also has disadvantages: It takes time and resources and may involve conflict. Group problem solving also can lead to the emergence of benign tyranny within the group. Members who are less informed or less confident may allow stronger members to control group discussion and problem solving. A disparity in participation may contribute to a power struggle between the nurse manager and a few assertive group members.

Group problem solving also can be affected by groupthink. **Groupthink** is a negative phenomenon that occurs in highly cohesive groups that become isolated. Through prolonged close association, group members come to think alike and have similar prejudices and blind spots, such as stereotypical views of outsiders. They exhibit a strong tendency to seek concurrence, which interferes with critical thinking about important decisions. In addition, the leadership of such groups suppresses open, free-wheeling discussion and controls what ideas will be discussed and how much dissent will be tolerated. The phenomenon of groupthink was studied in depth by Janis (1982), who cited the problem-solving process of the Kennedy administration's ad hoc committee on the Bay of Pigs invasion as a classic illustration.

Two phenomena are associated with groupthink (Forsyth, 1983): premature concurrence seeking, and illusions and misperceptions. **Premature concurrence** seeking is evidenced in several features of groupthink: (a) high pressure to conform and taboos against expressing dissent or criticizing ideas presented by the majority, a leader, or some other powerful member; (b) self-censorship of dissenting opinions, in which members with questions or concerns remain silent; (c) **mindguards**, who use "gate keeping" to protect the group from controversial information and discourage dissent by diverting doubts about the group's decisions or beliefs; and (d) apparent unanimity, reflected in the illusion that the group is in concurrence despite objections and concerns.

Misperceptions and illusions are also characteristic of groupthink. They may include the following: (a) a belief that the group is morally correct, which encourages members to ignore the ethical and moral consequences of their decisions; (b) rationalization of warnings and other forms of negative feedback; (c) biased perceptions of the out-group; and (d) collective rationalization of contradictory information (Janis, 1982). Groupthink seriously impairs critical thinking and can result in erroneous and damaging decisions.

KEY TERMS

Groupthink A negative phenomenon occurring in highly cohesive, isolated groups in which group members come to think alike, which interferes with critical thinking.

Premature concurrence A result of groupthink caused by pressure to conform, self-censorship, mindguards, and apparent unanimity.

Mindguards A feature of groupthink in which the group is "protected" from controversial information.

Dialectical inquiry A technique used to minimize groupthink through the use of a formal debate format.

Risky shift A phenomenon seen in groups in which riskier, more controversial decisions are made.

Leaders and group members may use the following tactics to prevent groupthink in cohesive groups (Janis, 1982):

1. Leaders should promote open inquiry by assigning the crucial evaluator role to each member. Encourage the group to give high priority to airing objections and doubts. Reinforce by accepting criticism.
2. The leader initially should delay stating his or her preferences and expectations until others' views have been fully disclosed.
3. The leader may set up several independent work groups to tackle the same issue. The groups then reconvene to explore a variety of approaches to problem solving and to hammer out differences.
4. Each member of the decision-making group should discuss periodically the group's deliberations with trusted associates in his or her own unit of the organization and report back nonmembers' views and reactions.
5. One or more outside experts within the organization who are not core members of the problem-solving group should be invited to each meeting on a rotating basis to challenge the views of the core members.
6. At every problem-solving meeting, at least one group member should be assigned the role of "devil's advocate" by attempting to find fault with any argument that might be considered valid.

7. Whenever problem solving involves relations with a rival, all warning signals from the rivals should be analyzed and possible interpretations of the rivals' intentions examined.

8. After reaching a preliminary consensus (agreement that everyone can support, arrived at without formal voting) about the best alternative, the problem-solving group should hold a second chance meeting at which every member is expected to express as vividly as possible all residual doubts and to rethink the entire issue before making a final choice.

Managers must recognize that although managing dissent may be complicated, time-consuming, and at times unpleasant, conflict is not always dysfunctional, and it is often necessary for quality decision making.

Dialectical inquiry is another technique to minimize groupthink. In dialectical inquiry, advocates of a plan and a counterplan undertake a formal debate. This technique formalizes conflict by allowing disagreement, encourages the exploration of alternative solutions, and reduces the emotional aspects of conflict. This approach can be used regardless of a manager's feelings. The benefits from this method come from the presentation and debate of the basic assumptions underlying proposed courses of action. Any false or misleading assumptions become apparent, and the process promotes better understanding of problems and leads to higher levels of confidence in a decision, but the method has some potential drawbacks. It can lead to an emphasis on who won the debate rather than what the best decision is, or it can lead to inappropriate compromise (Cosier & Schwenk, 1990).

Risky Shift Groups tend to make riskier decisions than individuals. Groups are more likely to support unusual or unpopular positions (e.g., public demonstrations). Groups tend to be less conservative than individual decision makers and frequently display more courage and support for unusual or creative solutions to problems. This phenomenon is referred to as **risky shift** (Napier & Gershenfeld, 1981).

Several factors contribute to this phenomenon. Individuals who lack information about alternatives may make a safe choice, but after group discussion they acquire additional information and become more comfortable with a less secure alternative. The group setting also allows for the diffusion of responsibility. If something goes wrong, others also can be assigned the blame or risk. In addition, leaders may be greater risk takers than individuals, and group members may attach a social value to risk taking because they identify it with leadership. Risky shift may be less of a problem in health care organizations because society discourages risk about health matters. However, nurse managers should be aware of this phenomenon, especially in relation to organizational decisions (e.g., starting or terminating a service).

When to Use Groups for Problem Solving Vroom and Jago (1974, 1988) developed a model for determining when to use a group for problem solving. In practice, several factors determine the degree of participation in group problem solving: (a) who initiates ideas, (b) how much support from subordinates is required to implement a solution, (c) how completely an employee is involved in each phase of problem solving (identifying the problem, analyzing the problem, finding alternatives, estimating consequences, and making choices), (d) how much weight the nurse manager attaches to the ideas received, and (e) how much the nurse manager knows about the issue.

Generally, groups should be used for problem solving when time and deadlines allow for a group decision; the problem is complex or unstructured; the group members share the organization's goals; there is need for acceptance, or at least understanding, of the decision if it is to be implemented properly; and the process will not lead to unacceptable conflict.

Decision Making

Considering all the practice individuals get in making decisions, it would seem they might become very good at it. However, the number of decisions a person makes does not correspond to his or her skill at making them. The assumption is that decision making comes naturally, like breathing. It does not. The decision-making process described in this chapter provides nurses with a system for making decisions that is applicable to any decision. It is a useful procedure for making practical choices. A decision not to solve a problem is also a decision.

Research has discredited the early belief that all decisions are choices people make after extensive evaluation of all options in order to find an optimal solution. Simon (1955) and others recognized that evaluation is seldom extensive and virtually never exhaustive. In the 1970s it was recognized that decision makers have a variety of strategies for making choices and a variety of aims in addition to utility. Most often, past experiences provide ways of dealing with problems. Some researchers have found that making a deliberate choice is relatively rare and usually is done by screening out the unacceptable options and choosing the best option from the remainders (Beach & Potter, 1992).

Types of Decisions

The types of problems nurse managers encounter and decisions they must make vary widely and determine the problem-solving or decision-making methods they should use. Relatively well defined, common problems can usually be solved with **routine decisions**, often using established rules, policies, and procedures. For instance, when a nurse makes a medication error, the manager's actions are guided by policy and the report form. Routine decisions are more often made by first-level managers than by top administrators. **Adaptive decisions** are necessary when both problems and alternative solutions are somewhat unusual and only partially understood. Often they are modifications of other well-known problems and solutions. As an example, a nurse manager may decide to adapt a negotiating strategy that was successful in a previous job to a present conflict with pharmacy. Managers must make **innovative decisions** when problems are unusual and unclear and when creative, novel solutions are necessary. In today's health care environment, many nurse managers are participating in a major redesign of the way patient care is given on their units. Such innovative decisions typically require a number of small decisions that involve many people over time and are difficult to implement in an orderly way.

Decision-Making Conditions

The question is often asked whether decision making is an individual or an organizational process: Do nurse managers or organizations make decisions? In this chapter, managerial decision making is treated as both individual and group processes that occur in an organizational context. The conditions surrounding decision making can vary and change dramatically. It is essential for the manager to consider the total system, realizing that whatever solutions are created will succeed only if they are compatible with other parts of the system. Organizational culture also is an important influence on decision making (VanEss-Coeling & Wilcox, 1988). As organizations decentralize, decision making is delegated to more individuals and groups who are most familiar with issues and problems. Within the organization, decisions must be made under conditions of certainty, risk, or uncertainty.

KEY TERMS

Routine decisions The type of decisions made when problems are relatively well defined and common and when established rules, policies, and procedures can be used to solve them.

Adaptive decisions The type of decisions made when problems and alternative solutions are somewhat unusual and only partially understood.

Innovative decisions The type of decisions made when problems are unusual and unclear and creative solutions are necessary.

Probability The likelihood that an event will or will not occur.

Probability analysis A calculation of the expected risk made to accurately determine the probabilities of each alternative.

Objective probability The likelihood that an event will or will not occur based on facts and reliable information.

Subjective probability The likelihood that an event will or will not occur based on a manager's personal judgment and beliefs.

Decision Making under Certainty When nurse managers know the alternatives and the conditions surrounding each alternative, a state of *certainty* is said to exist. Suppose a nurse manager on a unit with acutely ill patients wants to decrease the number of venipunctures a patient experiences when an IV is started, as well as reduce costs resulting from failed venipunctures. Three alternatives exist: (a) establish an IV team on all shifts, which is known to minimize IV attempts and reduce costs; (b) establish a reciprocal relationship with the anesthesia department to start IVs when nurses experience difficulty; and (c) set a standard of two insertion attempts per nurse per patient. Although this last method reduces the number of times an IV is started, it does not substantially lower equipment costs. The manager, however, knows the alternatives (IV team, anesthesia department, standards) and the conditions associated with each (reduced costs, assistance with starting IVs, minimum attempts and some cost reduction). A condition of strong certainty is said to exist and the decision can be made with full knowledge of what the payoff probably will be.

Table 10-2	Decision Making under Risk

	Probability Analysis
Agency A	60% Filling shifts
	100% Fixed wages
Agency B	50% Filling shifts
	70% Fixed wages

Decision Making Under Conditions of Risk In organizational settings, few decisions are made under certainty. The complexity of health care problems makes such situations rare. The more common decision-making condition is that of risk. The nurse manager does not always know the state of the situation. If the weather forecaster predicts a 40% chance of snow, the nurse manager is operating in a situation of risk when trying to decide how to staff the unit for the next 24 hours. In a risk situation, availability of each alternative, potential successes, and costs are all associated with probability estimates. **Probability** is the likelihood, expressed as a percentage, that an event will or will not occur. If something is certain to happen, its probability is 100%. If it is certain not to happen, its probability is 0%. If there is a 50–50 chance, its probability is 50%.

Suppose a nurse manager decides to use agency nurses to staff a unit during heavy vacation periods. Two agencies look attractive, and the manager must decide between them. Agency A has had modest growth over the past 10 years and offers the manager a 3-month contract, freezing wages during that time. In addition, the unit will have first choice of available nurses. Agency B is much more dynamic and charges more but explains that the reason they have had a high rate of growth is that their nurses are the best and the highest paid in the area. The nurse manager can choose Agency A, which will provide a safe, constant supply of nursing personnel, or B, which promises better care but at a higher cost.

The key element in decision making under conditions of risk is to determine the probabilities of each alternative accurately. The nurse manager can use a probability analysis, whereby expected risk is calculated or estimated. Using the **probability analysis** shown in Table 10-2, it appears as though Agency A offers the best outcome. However, if the second agency had a 90% chance of filling shifts and a 50% chance of fixing costs, a completely different situation would exist. The nurse manager might decide that the potential for increased costs was a small tradeoff for having more highly qualified nurses and the best probability of having the unit fully staffed during vacation periods. **Objective probability** is the likelihood that an event will or will not occur based on facts and reliable information. **Subjective probability** is the likelihood that an event will or will not occur based on a manager's personal judgment and beliefs (Figure 10-3).

Decision Making under Conditions of Uncertainty Most critical decision making in organizations is done under the condition of *uncertainty*. The individual or group making the decision does not know all the alternatives, attendant risks, or likely consequences of each option. Uncertainty is inevitable because of the complex and dynamic nature of health care organizations. Consider the problem of increased technology in health care. John, a nurse manager of a specialized cardiac intensive care unit, faces the task of

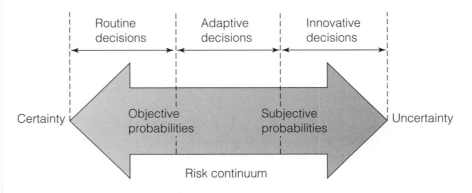

Figure 10-3 **Types of decisions based on risk and probability.** *Note:* **From** *Management*, **5th ed., by D. Hellriegel and J. W. Slocum, 1989, p. 196. Reading, MA: Addison-Wesley.**

recruiting scarce and highly skilled nurses to care for coronary bypass patients. The obvious alternative is to offer a salary and benefit package that rivals that of all other institutions in the area. However, this means John will have costly specialized nursing personnel in his budget who are not easily absorbed by other units in the organization. The probability that coronary bypass procedures will become obsolete in the future is unknown. In addition, other factors (e.g., increased competition, government regulations regarding reimbursement) may contribute to conditions of uncertainty.

The Decision-Making Process

The management literature describes decisions as discrete events made by an individual manager or a group using an orderly, rational process. This process, the **rational, or normative, decision-making model**, is a series of steps that managers take in an effort to make logical, well-grounded rational choices that maximize the achievement of objectives (Figure 10-4). The rationality of the decision made depends on the manager's ability to use information and analysis and on his or her values, beliefs, and objectives. The decision-making process is a sequence of the basic steps in the problem-solving process. However, not every step is used in every decision. In making adaptive and innovative decisions, managers rarely use these steps in sequence.

An application of the normative decision-making method is the optimizing strategy. The decision maker first identifies all possible outcomes, examines the probability of each alternative, and then takes the action that yields the highest probability of achieving the most desirable outcome. The rational or normative decision-making model is thought of as the ideal but often cannot be fully used.

Individuals seldom make major decisions at a single point in time and often are unable to recall when a decision was finally reached. Some major decisions are the result of many small actions or incremental choices the person makes without regarding larger strategic issues. In addition, decision processes are likely to be characterized more by confusion, disorder, and emotionality than by rationality. For these reasons, it is essential that the nurse manager develop appropriate technical skills and the capacity to find a good balance between lengthy processes and quick, decisive action.

The **descriptive, or bounded, rationality model**, developed by Simon in 1955 and supported by research in the 1990s (Simon, 1993), emphasizes the limitations of the rationality of the decision maker and the situation. It recognizes three ways in which decision makers depart from the rational decision-making model. First, the decision maker's search for possible objectives or alternative solutions is limited because of time, energy, and money. Second, managers frequently lack adequate information about problems and cannot

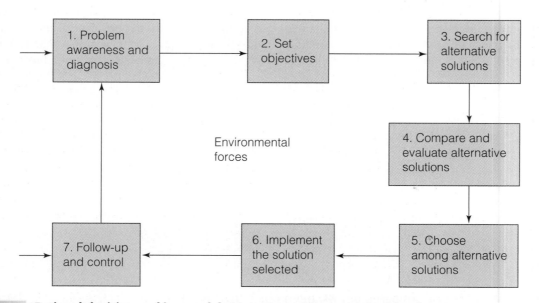

Figure 10-4 Rational decision-making model. *Note:* From *Management*, 5th ed., by D. Hellriegel and J. W. Slocum, 1989, p. 211. Reading, MA: Addison-Wesley.

control the conditions under which they operate. Finally, managers often use a satisficing strategy.

Satisficing is not a misspelled word; it is a decision-making strategy whereby the individual chooses an alternative that is not ideal but either is good enough (suffices) under existing circumstances to meet minimum standards of acceptance or is the first acceptable alternative.

Nursing management situations present a multitude of problems that are ineffectively solved with satisficing strategies. For example, Sue, a nurse manager in charge of a busy neurosurgical floor with high turnover rates and high patient acuity levels, uses a satisficing alternative when hiring replacement staff. She hires all nurse applicants in order of application until no positions are open. A better approach would be for Sue to replace staff only with nurse applicants who possess the skills and experiences required to care for neurosurgical patients, regardless of the number of applicants or desire for immediate action. Sue also should develop a plan to promote job satisfaction, the lack of which is the real reason for the vacancies.

Nurse managers who solve problems using satisficing may lack specific training in problem solving and decision making. They may view their units or floors as drastically simplified models of the real world and be content with this simplification because it allows them to make decisions with relatively simple rules of thumb or from force of habit. However, *optimizing techniques*, where the best of all possible alternatives is chosen, make demands on managers' willingness and ability to collect information, analyze it, and choose the best alternative.

The **political decision-making model** describes the process in terms of the particular interests and objectives of powerful stakeholders, such as hospital boards, medical staffs, corporate officers, and regulatory bodies. Power is the ability to influence or control how problems and objectives are defined, what alternative solutions are considered and selected, what information flows, and, ultimately, what decisions are made.

The decision-making process begins when the nurse manager perceives a gap between what is actually happening and what should be happening, and it ends with action that will narrow or close this gap. The simplest way to learn decision-making skills is to integrate a model into one's thinking by breaking the components down into individual steps. The seven steps of the decision-making process (Box 10-2) are as applicable to personal problems as they are to nursing

KEY TERMS

Rational (normative) decision-making model A decision-making process based on logical, well-grounded rational choices that maximize the achievement of objectives.

Descriptive (bounded) rationality model A decision-making process that emphasizes the limitations of the rationality of the decision maker and the situation.

Satisficing A decision-making strategy whereby the individual chooses a less than ideal alternative that meets minimum standards of acceptance.

Political decision-making model A decision-making process in which the particular interests and objectives of powerful stakeholders influence how problems and objectives are defined.

Artificial intelligence Computer technology that can diagnose problems and make limited decisions.

Expert systems Computer programs that provide complex data processing, reasoning, and decision making.

management problems. Each step is elaborated by pertinent questions clarifying the statements, and they should be followed in the order in which they are presented.

Decision-Making Techniques

Decision-making techniques vary according to the nature of the problem or topic, the decision maker, the context or situation, and the decision-making method or process. For routine decisions, choices that are tried and true can be made for well-defined, known situations or problems. Well-designed policies, rules, and standard operating procedures can produce satisfactory results with a minimum of the manager's time. **Artificial intelligence,** including programmed computer systems such as **expert systems** that can store, retrieve, and manipulate data, can diagnose problems and make limited decisions.

For adaptive decisions involving moderately ambiguous problems and modification of known and well-defined alternative solutions, there are a variety of techniques. Many types of decision grids or tables can be used to compare outcomes of alternative solutions.

Box 10-2   Steps in the Decision-Making Process

1. Identify the purpose:	Why is a decision necessary? What needs to be determined? State the issue in the broadest possible terms.
2. Set the criteria:	What needs to be achieved, preserved, and avoided by whatever decision is made? The answers to these questions are the standards by which solutions will be evaluated.
3. Weight the criteria:	Rank each criterion on a scale of values from 1 (totally unimportant) to 10 (extremely important).
4. Seek alternatives:	List all possible courses of action. Is one alternative more significant than another? Does one alternative have weaknesses in some areas? Can these be overcome? Can two alternatives or features of many alternatives be combined?
5. Test alternatives:	First, using the same methodology as in step 3, rank each alternative on a scale of 1 to 10. Second, multiply the weight of each criterion by the rating of each alternative. Third, add the scores and compare the results.
6. Troubleshoot:	What could go wrong? How can you plan? Can the choice be improved?
7. Evaluate the action:	Is the solution being implemented? Is it effective? Is it costly?

Decisions about units or services can be facilitated, with analyses comparing output, revenue, and costs over time or under different conditions. Analyzing the costs and revenues of a proposed new service is an example.

Making innovative decisions requires both discovering and diagnosing unfamiliar and ambiguous problems and developing unique and creative solutions. These decisions involve considerable uncertainty and, often, risk. One example of a situation requiring innovative decisions is the addition of home care to the services offered by a hospital maternity nursing unit.

Regardless of the decision-making model or strategy chosen, data collection and analysis are essential. In many health care organizations, quality teams are using a variety of tools to gather, organize, and analyze data about their work. Based on the work of Deming (Walton, 1988), nurses are using tools such as cause-and-effect diagrams, flow charts, Pareto charts, run charts, histograms, control charts, and scatter diagrams to help understand facts and relationships in processes they are examining. (See Figure 10-5 for examples.) Figure 10-6 illustrates a cause-and-effect diagram that a team of nurses created to help them improve the documentation process for their ambulatory oncology unit.

Group Decision Making

The widespread use of participative management, quality improvement teams, and shared governance in health care organizations requires every nurse manager to determine when group, rather than individual, decisions are desirable and how to use groups effectively. A number of studies have shown that professional people do not function well under micromanagement. As an alternative, group problem solving of substantial issues casts the manager in the role of facilitator and consultant. Compared to individual decision making, groups can provide more input, often produce better decisions, and generate more commitment. The nurse manager must understand the group decision-making process, troubleshoot, and be a positive role model. Several group decision-making techniques can be used.

Nominal Group Technique   The **nominal group technique (NGT)**, developed by Delbecq, VandeVen, & Gustafen (1975) is a structured and precise method of eliciting written questions, ideas, and reactions from group members. NGT is a group process in name only because no direct exchange occurs among members. NGT consists of (a) silently generating ideas in writing, (b) round-robin presentation by group members of their individual ideas in a terse phrase on a flip

KEY TERMS

Nominal group technique (NGT)   A decision-making approach that elicits written questions, ideas, and reactions from group members.

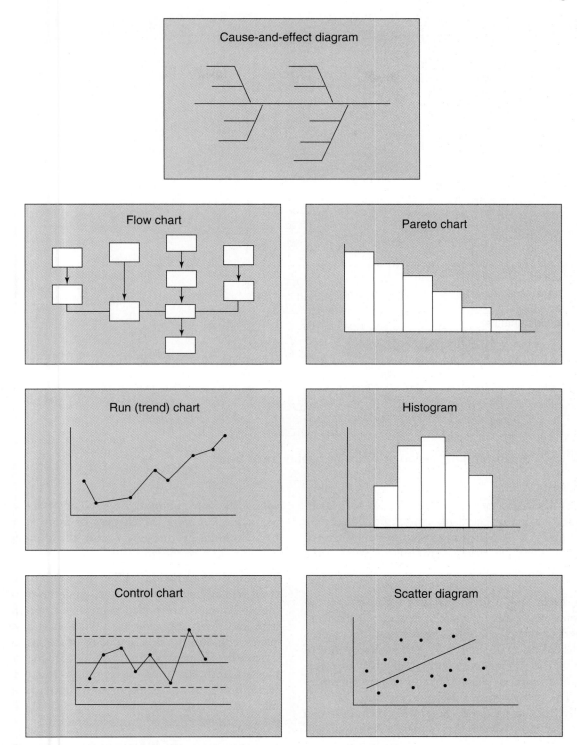

Figure 10-5   **Decision-making tools.** *Note:* From *The Deming management method* by M. Walton, 1988, Northbrook, IL: Dodd, Mead.

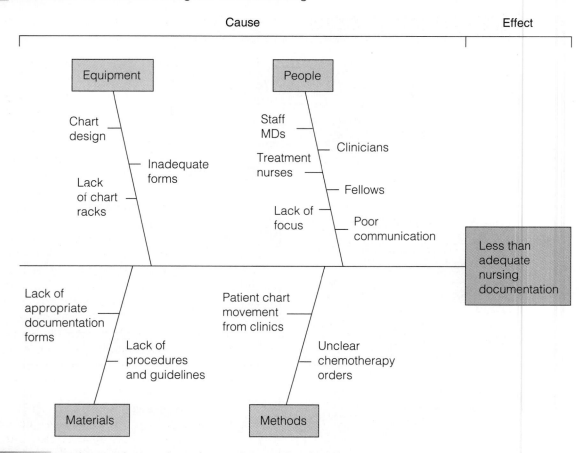

Figure 10-6 Brainstorming session of a nursing quality focus team.

chart, (c) discussion of each recorded idea for clarification and evaluation, and (d) voting individually on priority ideas, with the group solution being derived mathematically through rank ordering or rating using the group's decision rule.

Delphi Technique In the **Delphi technique**, judgments on a particular topic are systematically gathered from participants who do not meet face-to-face. Ideas are collected through a carefully designed sequence of questionnaires interspersed with summaries of information and opinions derived from previous questionnaires. The process may involve many iterations but normally does not exceed three. This technique can rely on the input of experts widely dispersed geographically. It can be used to evaluate the quality of research proposals or to make predictions about the future based on current scientific knowledge. This technique is useful when expert opinions are needed and expense would prohibit bringing them together.

For fact-finding problems with no known solution, the NGT and the Delphi technique are superior to other group techniques. Both NGT and the Delphi technique minimize the chances of more vocal members dominating discussion and allow independent consideration of ideas.

Statistical Aggregation Like the Delphi technique, **statistical aggregation** does not require a group meeting. Individuals are polled regarding a specific problem, and their responses are tallied. It is a very efficient technique, but it is limited to problems for which a quantifiable answer can be obtained. One disadvantage of both statistical aggregation and the Delphi technique is that no opportunity exists for group members to strengthen their interpersonal ties or for the generative effect of group interaction.

Brainstorming In **brainstorming**, group members meet together and generate many diverse ideas about the nature, cause, definition, or solution to a problem without consideration of their relative value. A premium is placed on generating lots of ideas as quickly as possible and on coming up with unusual ideas. (The wilder the idea, the better.) Most importantly,

Delphi technique   A decision-making technique in which judgments on a particular topic are systematically gathered from participants who do not meet face-to-face.

Statistical aggregation   A decision-making technique in which individuals are polled regarding a specific problem and their responses are tallied.

Brainstorming   A decision-making method in which group members meet and generate diverse ideas about the nature, cause, definition, or solution to a problem.

members do not critique ideas as they are proposed. Evaluation takes place after all the ideas have been generated. Members are encouraged to improve on each other's ideas. These sessions are very enjoyable but are often unsuccessful because members inevitably begin to critique ideas, and as a result, meetings shift to the ordinary interacting group format. Criticisms of this approach are the high cost factor, the time consumed, and the superficiality of many solutions.

Stumbling Blocks

Personality traits, inexperience, lack of adaptability, and preconceived ideas are several obstacles to problem solving and decision making.

Personality   The nurse manager's personality can and often does affect how and why certain decisions are made. Many nurse managers are selected because of their expert clinical, not management, skills. Inexperienced in management, they may resort to various unproductive activities. On the one hand, a nurse manager who is insecure may base decisions primarily on approval seeking. When a truly difficult situation arises, the manager, rather than face rejection from the staff, makes a decision that will placate people rather than one that will achieve the larger goals of the unit and organization. On the other hand, a nurse manager who demonstrates an authoritative type of personality might make unreasonable demands on the staff, fail to reward staff for long hours because he or she has a "workaholic" attitude, or give the staff no control over patient-care activities. Similarly, an inexperienced manager may cause a unit to flounder because the manager is not inclined to act on new ideas or solutions to problems. Managerial traits of optimism, humor, and a positive approach are crucial to energizing staff and promoting creativity.

Rigidity   Rigidity, an inflexible management style, is another obstacle to problem solving. It may result from ineffective trial-and-error solutions, fear of risk taking, or inherent personality traits. As discussed previously, the nurse manager can avoid ineffective trial-and-error problem solving by gathering sufficient information and determining a means for early correction of wrong or inadequate decisions. Also, to minimize risk in problem solving, the manager should know and understand alternative risks and expectations.

The nurse manager who uses a rigid style in problem solving easily develops *tunnel vision*—the tendency to look at new things in old ways and from established frames of reference. It then becomes very difficult to see things from another perspective, and problem solving becomes a process whereby one person makes all of the decisions with little information or data from other sources. In the current changing health care setting, rigidity can at times be a nurse manager's greatest barrier to effective problem solving.

Preconceived Ideas   Effective nurse managers do not start out with the preconceived idea that one proposed course of action is right and all others wrong. Nor do they assume that only one opinion can be voiced and others will be silent. They start out with a commitment to find out why staff members or others disagree. If the staff, other professionals, or patients see a different reality or even a different problem, nurse managers need to integrate this information into a database to develop additional problem-solving alternatives.

Most people have preconceived ideas about the nature of problems and their solutions. Those who are certain that only their perception is accurate may never accept the final decision. Nurse managers, however, have formal responsibility for problem solving and decision making and must put personal ideas on hold until they have gathered enough information to view the situation objectively and in the widest possible perspective.

Pederson (1993) identified qualities that staff nurses most consistently attributed to excellent head nurses. Excellent head nurses were characterized as positive, happy, energetic, authentic, sincere, honest, and open. They develop relationships that are supportive, caring, sensitive, and appreciative. Effective head nurses also are forward-thinking, courageous, creative, and willing to take risks. They advocate for others and support professional standards and growth. They do not avoid conflict but are skilled in resolving it and solving problems. In a nationwide survey of nurse administrators and managers in academic health centers, human management skill was ranked as the most important criterion of nurse manager effectiveness; the characteristics of flexibility, negotiation, and compromise were second (Patz, Biordi, & Holm, 1991). A successful nursing administrator, Dr. Maryann Fralic (1993), suggests that personality characteristics of the nurse executive in the new era include caring, credibility, creativity, equanimity, sense of humor, futuristic perspective, and confidence.

Creativity in Decision Making

A realistic, supportive management climate and an environment conducive to critical thinking and evaluation are all important for creative decision making. What turns a mediocre problem-solving team into an excellent one is the quality and originality of thinking. Creativity is an essential part of the critical-thinking process. *Creativity* is the ability to develop and implement new and better solutions. Maintaining a certain level of creativity is the only way to keep an organization alive. One that functions by the rule stifles creativity, is inflexible, and is on the way to oblivion.

Creativity has four stages: preparation, incubation, insight, and verification (Wallas, 1945). Even people who think they are not naturally creative can learn this process (Figure 10-7). First, the individual must acquire information necessary to understand the situation. Anyone can do this through hard work and observation. Consider Jeffrey, who was just promoted to manager. He has identified that staff nurses are reluctant to sign up and do quality chart audits. He gathers information about quality improvement, reviews the literature on motivation and incentives, and discusses the issue with other nurse managers (*preparation*). He continues to manage the unit, thinking about the information he has gathered but does not consciously make a decision or reject new ideas (*incubation*). When working on a new problem, self-scheduling, he realizes a connection between the two problems. Many nurses complain that by the time they receive the schedule the desirable shifts are filled. Jeffrey states that he will review the chart audits and that those nurses who regularly participate in quality improvement projects will receive a "perk." They will be allowed, on a rotating basis, first choice at

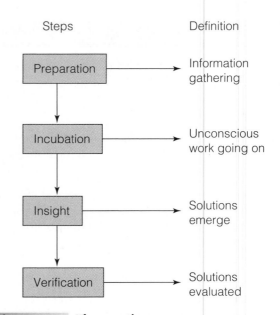

Steps   Definition

Preparation ────────────▶ Information gathering

Incubation ────────────▶ Unconscious work going on

Insight ────────────▶ Solutions emerge

Verification ────────────▶ Solutions evaluated

Figure 10-7 **The creative process.**

selecting the schedule they want to work (this is the insight stage). He discusses the plan with the staff and proposes a 2-month trial period to determine whether the solution is effective (*verification*).

In a survey of organizational scientists, Campbell, Daft, and Hulin (1982) found that the first three stages of the creative process were most important. Significant exposure to the topic as well as intuition and chance were the main contributors to creativity. The more knowledge, skill, and ability the individual acquires about a potential problem or issue, the more likely that a creative solution will result.

Characteristics of Creative Persons

Steiner (1965) found general agreement among top managers regarding many of the intellectual and personality characteristics of creative persons. In general, they are people who

1. Generate ideas rapidly.
2. Are flexible, can discard one frame of reference for another, and/or can change approaches spontaneously.
3. Have a tendency to provide original solutions to problems.
4. Prefer complex thought processes to simple and easily understood ones.
5. Are independent in judgment and more able to believe in themselves, even when under pressure.
6. Exhibit distinct individualistic characteristics, seeing themselves as different from their peers.

7. View authority as conventional rather than absolute, which means they accept authority as a matter of expedience rather than personal allegiance or moral obligation.

8. Are willing to entertain and express personal whims or impulses, exhibit a more diverse fantasy life on clinical tests, and inject humor into situations.

Creative people are unlikely to view authority as absolute, make few black-and-white distinctions, have a less dogmatic view of life, show more independence of judgment and less conformity, are more willing to give consideration to their own impulses, have a sense of humor, and are less rigid and freer though less effectively controlled.

Managing Creativity in Health Care Settings

For creativity to be of value to the nurse manager, it must be useful to solve problems and make decisions. Using the four stages of creativity, the following steps can help stimulate the generation of new ideas.

1. *Preparation.* A carefully designed planning program is essential. For example, the nurse manager can plan creativity conferences in which participants will question all work methods. A method of work simplification, built on the premise that most people can increase productivity not by working harder but by eliminating certain steps and creating new services or solutions, can be used at these conferences. Some organizations have instituted such conferences on a monthly or bimonthly basis, involving all employees. The focus is on problems any member of the group chooses to bring up that are creating difficulties for the unit or individual. This is not a gripe session, but a setting where problem solving is done in a creative manner. A skillful group leader is important to facilitate progress at these conferences. The process follows this sequence: (a) pick a specific task to improve, (b) gather relevant facts, (c) challenge every detail, (d) develop preferred solutions, and (e) implement improvements.

2. *Incubation.* The nurse manager also needs to meet with new employees routinely as part of the orientation process, at which time everyone seeks information about solutions to problems. New employees are not encumbered with details of accepted practices and can offer suggestions based on their prior experiences or insights before they get set in their ways or have their innovative ideas "turned off." The advantages offered by new employees should be explored because all staff gain from such use of valuable human resources.

3. *Insight.* Most nurse managers are employed in bureaucratic settings that do not foster creativity.

Control is exercised over staff, and rigid adherence to formal channels of communication jeopardizes innovation. In addition, there is little room for failure, and when failures do occur they are not tolerated very well. When staff are afraid of the consequences of failure, their creativity is inhibited and innovation does not take place. If risk cannot be accepted, special ground rules need to be established that permit innovative managers and staff to function without fear of reprisals or termination if they fail. In addition, nurse managers must realize, as other organizations do, that innovative people may not fit the organizational mold. Innovative people generally avoid highly structured and controlled situations and at times may appear disorganized or lackadaisical. The challenge for nurse managers is to know when, for whom, and to what extent control is appropriate. If creativity does have a priority in the health care setting, then the reward system should be geared to and commensurate with that priority.

4. *Verification.* Creativity demands a certain amount of exposure to outside contacts, receptiveness to new and seemingly strange ideas, proper research assistance, a certain amount of freedom, and some permissive management. The climate must promote the survival of potentially useful ideas. Many good new ideas go unused because they arise in an environment grown cold to creativity. A new idea is extremely perishable, and its creator is likely to be its sole supporter, after which it may have none, because the usual reaction is either to ignore it or to look for defects in the new idea. The nurse manager can build an attitude favorable to giving new ideas a fair and proper hearing and thereby reduce the tendency to destroy the creative process in individuals and within groups. The major limitation on creativity stems from the initial cost. The greater the creativity sought and the greater the departure from present practice, the greater the investment will be. In the long run, however, creative ideas may turn out to be highly cost-effective. The challenge is to determine if and when they are important, how important they are, and to encourage the creative exchange of such ideas broadly so there is a visible effect of the nurse manager's leadership, measurable in enhanced vitality and productivity.

Summary

- Critical thinking requires examining underlying assumptions about current evidence, interpreting information, and evaluating the arguments presented to reach a new and exciting conclusion.

- Problem-solving and decision-making processes use critical-thinking skills.
- Methods of problem solving include trial and error, intuition, experimentation, past experience, tradition, and recognizing problems that are self-solving.
- The problem-solving process involves (a) defining the problem, (b) gathering information, (c) analyzing information, (d) developing solutions, (e) making a decision, (f) implementing the decision, and (g) evaluating the solution.
- The decision-making process may employ several models: (a) rational or normative; (b) descriptive or bounded rationality; (c) satisficing; and (d) political.
- Decision-making techniques vary according to the nature of the problem and the degree of risk and uncertainty in the situation.
- The creative process involves preparation, incubation, insight, and verification, which can be learned by individuals and used in groups.

■ LEADERSHIP AND MANAGEMENT
in Action

1. What is the difference between creative thinking and critical thinking?
2. Describe the steps in the problem-solving process. How do problem solving, decision making, and the nursing process differ?
3. Can creativity be encouraged in others? Why or why not?

References

Beach, L. R., & Potter, R. E. (1992). The pre-choice screening of options. *Acta Psychologica, 81,* 115–126.

Benner, P. (1984). *From novice to expert.* Menlo Park, CA: Addison-Wesley Nursing.

Boychuk, J. E. D. (1999). Catching the wave: Understanding the concept of critical thinking. *Journal of Advanced Nursing, 29*(3), 577–583.

Brookfield, S. D. (1987). *Developing critical thinkers.* San Francisco, CA: Jossey-Bass.

Campbell, J. P., Daft, R. L., & Hulin, C. L. (1982). *What to study: Generating and developing research questions.* Beverly Hills, CA: Sage Publications.

Connolly, L. (1994). Encouraging critical thinking in staff development. *Kansas Nurse, 69*(5), 1–2.

Cosier, R. A., & Schwenk, C. R. (1990). Agreement and thinking alike: Ingredients for poor decisions. *Academic Management Extract, 4*(1), 69–74.

Delbecq, A. L., VandeVen, A. H., & Gustafson, D. H. (1975). *Group Techniques for Program Planning.* Glenview, IL: Foresman.

Forsyth, D. R. (1983). *An introduction to group dynamics.* Monterey, CA: Brooks/Cole.

Fralic, M. (1993). The new era nurse executive: Centerpiece characteristics. *Journal of Nursing Administration, 23*(1), 7–8.

Gordon, W. J. (1968). *Synectics.* New York: Collier.

Hellriegel, D., & Slocum, J. W. (1989). *Management,* 5th ed. Reading, MA: Addison-Wesley.

Janis, I. L. (1982). *Groupthink: Psychological studies of policy decisions and fiascos,* 2nd ed., Boston: Houghton Mifflin.

Jenks, J. M. (1993). The pattern of personal knowing in nurse clinical decision-making. *Journal of Nursing Education, 32*(9), 399–405.

Kurfiss, J. G. (1988). *Critical thinking: Theory, research, practice, and possibilities.* College Station, TX: Association for the Study of Higher Education.

Lepley, C. (1998). Problem-solving tools for analyzing system problems: The affinity map and the relationship diagram. *Journal of Nursing Administration, 28*(12), 44–50.

Lowry, M. (1999). Dealing with problems in clinical practice. *Nursing Standard, 13*(48), 43–45.

Napier, R. W., & Gershenfeld, M. K. (1981). *Groups: Theory and experience.* Boston: Houghton Mifflin.

Osborn, A. F. (1953). *Applied imagination.* New York: Scribner's.

Patz, J., Biordi, D., & Holm, K. (1991). Middle nurse manager effectiveness. *Journal of Nursing Administration, 21*(1), 15–24.

Pederson, A. (1993). Qualities of the excellent head nurse. *Nursing Administration Quarterly, 18*(1), 40–50.

Schmieding, N. J. (1999). Reflective inquiry framework for nurse administrators. *Journal of Advanced Nursing, 30*(3), 631–639.

Simon, H. A. (1955). A behavioral model of rational choice. *Quarterly Journal of Economics, 69,* 99–118.

Simon, H. A. (1993). Decision making: Rational, nonrational, and irrational. *Education Administration Quarterly, 29*(3), 392–411.

Steiner, G. (1965). *The creative organization.* Chicago: University of Chicago Press.

VanEss-Coeling, H., & Wilcox, J. (1988). Understanding organizational culture: Key to management decision making. *Journal of Nursing Administration, 18*(11), 16–23.

Vroom, V. H., & Jago, A. G. (1974). Decision making as a social process: Normative and descriptive models of leader behavior. *Decision Sciences, 5,* 743–769.

Vroom, V. H., & Jago, A. G. (1988). *The new leadership.* Englewood Cliffs, NJ: Prentice Hall.

Wallas, G. (1945). *The art of thought.* London: C. A. Watts.

Walton, M. (1988). *The Deming management method.* Northbrook, IL: Dodd, Mead.

Wilkinson, J. (1992). *Nursing process in action: A critical thinking approach.* Redwood City, CA: Addison-Wesley Nursing.

Communication and Conflict

Communication

Modes of Communication
Directions of Communication
Factors Influencing
Communication

Assertiveness

The Role of Communication in Leadership

Communicating with Different Populations

Subordinates
Superiors
Peers
Medical Staff
Other Health Care Personnel
Patients and Families
Difficult People

Conflict

Conflict Process Model

Conflict Management

Goals of Conflict Management
Conflict Management Modes
Other Conflict Management
Techniques

Looking Ahead

As one of the most fundamental components of society and one of the most basic tools of management, communication encompasses so much that it nearly defies definition. We communicate to relay information, and the methods, implications, and results vary immensely. This chapter provides an overview of communication skills and techniques, including conflict management, that you can use to be more effective within your organization.

Objectives

After reading this chapter, you will be able to:

- Describe the factors influencing communication.
- Discuss the role of assertiveness in communication.
- Delineate ways to communicate with different populations.
- Discuss the positive and negative aspects of conflict.
- Compare and contrast different ways of managing conflict.

Successful and effective management and leadership depend on well-developed interpersonal skills. Communicating clearly and effectively is critical because managers report spending 80 to 90% of the day communicating (Bass, 1990). Communication skills are needed to facilitate team building, manage conflict, and demonstrate insight, empathy, caring, and trustworthiness. This chapter discusses the use of communication in management and leadership. Communication skills are essential to handle conflict, which also is included in this chapter.

Communication

Communication is a complex, ongoing dynamic process in which the participants simultaneously create shared meaning in an interaction. The goal of communication is to approach, as closely as possible, a common understanding of the message sent and the one received. At times, this can be difficult because both participants are influenced by past conditioning, the present situation, each person's purpose in the current communication, and each person's attitudes toward self, the topic, and each other. In addition, the level of knowledge and speaking skills affects the structure, style, and channels used by the participants

(Ehninger, Gronbeck, McKerrow, & Monroe, 1986). Therefore, it is important that participants construct messages as clearly as possible, listen carefully, monitor each other's response, and provide feedback (Figure 11-1).

Modes of Communication

Messages may be written (handwritten, typed, electronically mailed, faxed), oral (face-to-face, one-on-one, or in groups; by telephone; on voice mail), or interactive video. The purpose of the message is one characteristic that helps determine the best mode to use. In general, the more important or delicate the issue, the more intimate the mode should be. Levels of personal intimacy in communication are influenced, in descending order, *in person, telephone, voice mail, electronic mail,* and *written mail.* For example, any difficult issue should be communicated face to face,

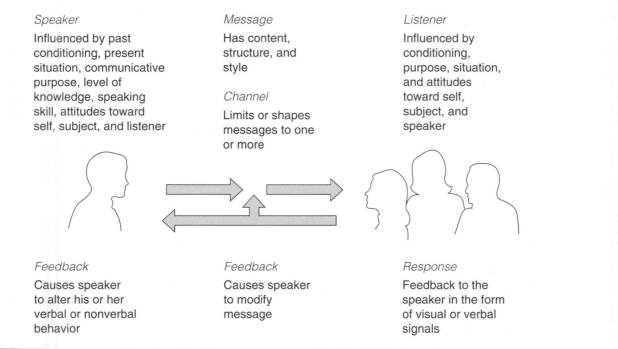

Speaker
Influenced by past conditioning, present situation, communicative purpose, level of knowledge, speaking skill, attitudes toward self, subject, and listener

Message
Has content, structure, and style

Channel
Limits or shapes messages to one or more

Listener
Influenced by conditioning, purpose, situation, and attitudes toward self, subject, and speaker

Feedback
Causes speaker to alter his or her verbal or nonverbal behavior

Feedback
Causes speaker to modify message

Response
Feedback to the speaker in the form of visual or verbal signals

Figure 11-1 The process of communication. *Note:* From *Principles and types of speech communications,* edited by D. Ehninger, B. E. Gronbeck, R. E. McKerrow, and A. H. Monroe, Glenview, IL: Scott, Foresman, p. 13. Used by permission.

such as terminating an individual's employment. Conflict or confrontation also is usually best handled in person so that the individual's response can be seen and answered appropriately.

Oral messages are accompanied by a number of nonverbal messages known as **metacommunications**. These behaviors include head or facial agreement or disagreement; eye contact; tone, volume, and inflection of the voice; gestures of the shoulders, arms, hands, or fingers; body posture and position; dress and appearance; timing; and environment.

Bass (1990) also notes that nonverbal behaviors are trusted more than verbal messages. Therefore, people need to pay close attention to their nonverbal behaviors to make sure they convey an accurate message.

When a verbal message is incongruent with the nonverbal message, the recipient has difficulty interpreting the intended meaning; this results in **intrasender conflict**. For example, a manager who states, "Come talk to me anytime," but keeps the office door closed at all times, sends a conflicting message to the staff. **Intersender conflict** occurs when a person receives two conflicting messages from differing sources. For example, the risk manager may encourage a nurse to report medication errors, while the nurse manager follows up with discipline over the error. The nurse is caught between conflicting messages from the two.

The telephone is slightly less intimate than in-person communication. Tone of voice, for instance, can be conveyed and may facilitate cooperation. Voice mail is the next level of communication. Voice mail is useful to convey information that is not necessarily sensitive and may or may not require a reply. The time and place of an upcoming meeting, for example, can be communicated by voice mail, which has the added advantage of avoiding "phone tag." Electronic mail (e-mail) is useful for information similar to that conveyed by voice mail and has the added advantage of being able to broadcast messages to large groups via a listserv. The dates and times for a blood drive are a good example of a broadcast e-mail message. Conveying complicated information that may require thought before the receiver replies is another use of e-mail.

The level of formality of the communication also affects the mode used. An application for a position in a health care organization requires a written letter, usually mailed, although some organizations accept faxed applications today. Also, the relationship between the sender and receiver also affects the mode. If a staff nurse, for example, wants to nominate a co-worker for an award given by the hospital board of directors, a written letter is required.

KEY TERMS

Metacommunications   Nonverbal messages in communication, including body language and environmental factors.

Intrasender conflict   Difficulty in interpreting the intended meaning of a message due to incongruity between verbal and nonverbal communication.

Intersender conflict   Difficulty in interpreting the intended meaning of a message due to two conflicting messages received from differing sources.

Downward communication   Communication, generally directive, given from an authority figure or manager to staff.

Upward communication   Communication, generally reporting, that occurs from staff to management.

Lateral communication   Communication that occurs between individuals at the same hierarchical level.

Diagonal communication   Communication involving individuals at different hierarchical levels.

Distortion can arise in any type of communication. Common causes are inadequate reasoning; the use of strong, judgmental words; speaking too fast or too slowly; using unfamiliar words; or spending too much time on details. Distortion also occurs when the recipient is busy or distracted, bases understanding on previous experiences with the sender, or has a biased perception of the meaning of the message or the messenger. Consider the example of distortion of written communication provided in Box 11-1.

Directions of Communication

Formal or informal communication may be downward, upward, lateral, or diagonal. **Downward communication** (manager to staff) is often directive. The staff is *told* what needs to be done or given information to facilitate the job to be done. **Upward communication** occurs from staff to management or from lower management to middle or upper management. Upward communication often involves *reporting* pertinent information to facilitate problem solving and decision making. **Lateral communication** occurs between

Box 11-1 Distortion in Written Communication

There is ample opportunity for distortion in the complicated process of sending, receiving, and responding to messages, as demonstrated by the following correspondence between a plumber and an official of the National Bureau of Standards (Donaldson & Scannell, 1979).

Bureau of Standards
Washington, D.C.
Gentlemen:
   I have been in the plumbing business for over 11 years and have found that hydrochloric acid works real fine for cleaning drains. Could you tell me if it's harmless?
                                    Sincerely,
                                    Tom Brown, Plumber

Mr. Tom Brown, Plumber
Yourtown, U.S.A.
Dear Mr. Brown:
   The efficacy of hydrochloric acid is indisputable, but the chlorine residue is incompatible with metallic permanence!
                                    Sincerely,
                                    Bureau of Standards

Bureau of Standards
Washington, D.C.
Gentlemen:
   I have your letter of last week and am mightily glad you agree with me on the use of hydrochloric acid.
                                    Sincerely,
                                    Tom Brown, Plumber

Mr. Tom Brown, Plumber
Yourtown, U.S.A.
Dear Mr. Brown:
   We wish to inform you we have your letter of last week and advise that we cannot assume responsibility for the production of toxic and noxious residues with hydrochloric acid and further suggest you use an alternate procedure.
                                    Sincerely,
                                    Bureau of Standards

Bureau of Standards
Washington, D.C.
Gentlemen:
   I have your most recent letter and am happy to find you still agree with me.
                                    Sincerely,
                                    Tom Brown, Plumber

Mr. Tom Brown, Plumber
Yourtown, U.S.A.
Dear Mr. Brown:
   Don't use hydrochloric acid, it eats the hell out of pipes!
                                    Sincerely,
                                    Bureau of Standards

For communication among more than two people, the chance of distortion increases proportionally.

individuals or departments at the same hierarchical level (e.g., nurse managers, department heads). **Diagonal communication** involves individuals or departments at different hierarchical levels (e.g., staff nurse to chief of the medical staff). Both lateral and diagonal communication involve information sharing, discussion, and negotiation.

   An informal channel commonly seen in organizations is the grapevine (i.e., rumors and gossip). Grapevine communication is usually rapid, haphazard, and prone to distortion. Ribiero and Blakely (1998) identify three reasons distortion occurs through the grapevine. One, is that the original message is elaborated on as it is passed. A second reason is that the message is deliberately or unintentionally distorted. The third reason is a contradictory message is started due to disagreement with the original message. The problem with grapevine communication is that no one is accountable for the misinformation relayed.

Factors Influencing Communication

Many factors affect communication. Three important factors are gender, cultural background, and organizational culture and climate.

Gender   Studies indicate that gender has an impact on many aspects of communication (Table 11-1). For example, men and women become socialized through communication patterns that reflect their societal roles. Men tend to talk more, longer, and faster, whereas women are more descriptive, attentive, and perceptive. Women tend to use tag questions (e.g., "I

Table 11-1 Gender Differences in Communication

Males	Females
Concentrate on individual performance.	Use descriptive language (e.g., adjectives, intensifiers).
Talk more, longer, and faster.	Relate personal experience.
Focus on content.	Use open communication techniques to seek and clarify information.
Are more responsive to superiors.	Attend to message and messenger.
Express views more.	Are more responsive to subordinates.
Disagree more.	Perceive verbal and nonverbal messages.
Withdraw when stressed	Promote harmony and cooperation.
	Use tag questions.
	Withdraw from conflict.
	Seeks to be heard.
	Requires validation.

Note: Developed from "The influence of gender on communication for nurse leaders" by J. B. Edwards and C. L. Lenz, 1990, *Nurse Administration Quarterly, 15*(1), 49–55; "Relationships among perceived supervisor communication, nurse morale, and sociocultural variables" by C. W. Kennedy, C. T. Camden, and G. M. Timmerman, 1990, *Nursing Administration Quarterly, 14*(4), 38–46; and J. Gray (1992). *Men are from Mars, women are from Venus.* New York: HarperCollins.

can take off this weekend, can't I?") and tend to self-disclose more than men (Edwards & Lenz, 1990).

In addition, the communication of female managers fulfills a socioemotional or expressive function; women tend to ask more questions and solicit more input than their male counterparts. In general, female communication behaviors are attentive, friendly, and open, characteristics that improve productivity and morale (Kennedy, Camden, & Timmerman, 1990).

The communication of male managers fulfills a task or instrumental function; the focus is on content. Men express their opinion and disagree more than women managers. In unpleasant situations, men talk more while women withdraw.

Although females are identified as having better communication skills, males are stereotyped as more knowledgeable and more experienced speakers and clearer writers (Fine, Johnson, & Foss, 1991). These researchers believe that expectations are higher for women than for men performing the same communication behavior; therefore, men tend to be perceived to have more "expertise." Leet-Pellegrini (1980) noted that men who talked longer, dominating the conversation, were perceived to be influential. However, when females adopt these male speech patterns, they are criticized as overbearing. As a result, some speculate that women avoid "power behaviors," which lowers their prestige but increases perceptions of their credibility, goodwill, and fairness (Kenton, 1989).

Blanchard and Sargent (1986) contend that the best managers are "androgynous"—a combination of the best of male and female characteristics. This con-

tention was confirmed in a study by Jurma and Powell (1994); subordinates rated androgynous managers as better handlers of conflict. Recommendations to overcome gender weaknesses are listed in Table 11-2.

Cultural Background The workforce has increasingly become more diverse. Women currently constitute 58% of the workforce; minorities, one-third (U.S. Bureau of the Census, 1993). Ethnic minorities include African Americans, Asian Americans, Hispanic Americans, and Native Americans. Each group has unique cultural characteristics.

Cultural attitudes, beliefs, and behaviors all affect communication. Such elements as body movement, gestures, tone, and spatial orientation are culturally defined. A great deal of misunderstanding results from people's lack of understanding of each other's cultural expectations. For example, Asians take great care in exchanges with superiors so that there is no conflict or "loss of face" for either person.

Understanding the cultural heritage of employees and learning to interpret cultural messages is essential for the nurse manager to communicate effectively with staff from diverse backgrounds. Personal and professional cultural enrichment training is recommended. This includes reading the literature and history of the culture; participating in open, honest, respectful communication; and exploring the meaning of behavior (Ingram & Siantz, 1991). It is important to recognize, however, that subcultures exist within all cultures; therefore, what applies to one individual may not be true for another individual of that same culture.

Table 11-2 Recommendations to Overcome Gender Weaknesses

In order to be androgynous . . .

Men need to	Women need to
1. Give evidence of how and why their lives are men's lives.	1. Be powerful and forthright and have a direct visible impact on others.
2. Understand that men value women as validators of masculinity, as a haven from the competitive male world, and as the expressive partner in the relationship.	2. Be entrepreneurial.
3. Beware of how physical and political power determines behavior.	3. State their own needs and refuse to back down.
4. Openly express feelings of love, fear, anger, pain, joy, loneliness, and dependence.	4. Recognize the equal importance of accomplishing the task as well as being concerned about relationships.
5. Personalize experience as opposed to relying on objectivity and rationality.	5. Build support systems with other women.
6. Build support systems with other men, sharing competencies without competition, feelings, and needs.	6. Be able to intellectualize and generalize.
7. Learn how to fail at a task without feeling one has failed as a man.	7. Deal directly with anger and blame, thereby rejecting feelings of suffering and victimization; be vulnerable to destructive feedback.
8. Value an identity that is not so totally defined by work.	8. Talk and cry at the same time.
9. Assert the right to work for self-fulfillment, rather than to play the role of provider.	9. Respond directly with "I" statements rather than "you" statements.
10. Listen empathetically and actively without feeling responsible for problem solving.	10. Be analytic, systematic, and share abstract models.
11. Enjoy friendships with both men and women.	11. Take more risks with power.
	12. Continue to be supportive and compassionate, as well as becoming more autonomous and independent.

Note: From Blanchard, K. H. & Sargent, A. G. (1986). "The one minute manager is an androgynous manager." *Nursing Management,* 17(5), pp. 44–45.

Organizational Culture and Climate   As discussed in Chapter 2, the customs, norms, and expectations within an organization are powerful forces that shape behavior. Focusing on relevant issues regarding the organizational culture can identify failures in communication. Communication is a frequent source of job dissatisfaction as well as a powerful determinant of an organization's effectiveness. Just as violation of other norms within the organization results in repercussions, so does violation of communication rules. Farley (1989) has identified six critical components of formal organizational communication systems based on the formal and informal, explicit or implicit rules that affect interactions and govern the conditions under which information exchange occurs.

1. *Accessibility of information.* Information is necessary for all employees to perform their jobs. Where can they find details about the job? How easy or difficult is it to access information? Do employees know whom to contact?

2. *Communication channels.* Communication channels describe the formal and informal links within the system through which information normally passes. How long does it take for information to travel through the system? Is it primarily formal or informal? Which is more effective? Who are the key people? Who initiates or distributes information? Does information travel as well up as down?

3. *Organizational structures.* Groups with a centralized structure communicate more effectively than those with other types of organizational structures. Sharing space and physical proximity also facilitates both formal and informal communication because it diminishes territoriality (Bass, 1990).

4. *Clarity of message.* Clear messages are important to prevent misunderstandings and promote trust and confidence. Clear messages adhere to established grammatical rules and avoid words with multiple meanings. Sending dual messages or

messages that rely on personal interpretation also affects clarity. Also, concise messages are more likely to be heard and retained.

5. *Flow control and information load.* Controlling what information is disseminated and the amount of information shared influences employees' comprehension, as well as their trust and satisfaction. Job satisfaction increases when appropriate information is shared with employees, but unrestricted release of information (low flow control) produces information overload. Overload limits information processing and increases errors. Excessively restricting the amount of information released (high flow control), conversely, results in information underload, threatens productivity, and encourages rumors. Sharing appropriate information with employees in a timely fashion enhances the success of the organization.

6. *Communicator effectiveness.* Effective communication promotes productivity, satisfaction, and commitment to the organization. To communicate effectively, the sender must organize ideas and select a medium and style appropriate to the message and the receiver. Active listening encourages others to express their views and conveys concern. Active listening also allows the listener to check how others interpret messages; that is, actively listening fulfills a feedback function.

Organizational policies, norms, and managerial pressures influence the type of medium (face to face, telephone, memo, meeting) chosen, but there are some general guidelines to use in deciding which method of communication to use (Fulk & Boyd, 1991).

1. Face to face verbal communication is considered the most effective method of communication, followed, in diminishing order, by the telephone, voice mail, electronic mail, and finally, written documents.
2. Difficult communication should be relayed face to face.
3. Routine and simple communication may be sent via memos or letters.
4. Multiple forms of media should be used to clarify critical issues. For example, follow up a telephone communication with a memo.
5. As new technologies are developed, they should be critically evaluated before they are assumed to be appropriate for the full range of management tasks.

Style also affects how a message is interpreted, retained, and acted on. Speaking softly helps to calm and defuse anger; speaking deliberation can facilitate control of a situation. Conversely, using direct and piercing eye contact or loud and confident speech may be either persuasive, alienating, or even intimidating (Davidhazar & Shearer, 1993).

Assertiveness

Assertive communication techniques help to identify problems and facilitate problem solving and decision making. Although participants may not agree with each other's responses, each participant's position is clarified, and each accepts the other's right to be heard.

Assertive behavior is specific to the situation and can be differentiated from nonassertive and aggressive behavior, in which participants respond in a certain manner regardless of the situation. As nurses develop skill in expressing ideas and feelings clearly, accurately, and honestly, others are encouraged to respond in kind. Consider the following example.

As Jeanine, the nurse manager, enters Mr. Wilson's room, she finds him scowling. He promptly states, "That stupid nurse forgot my medicine *again*!" Jeanine could respond in one of the following ways:

1. "There now, don't worry, I'm sure it will be all right."
2. "Oh, really! Well, I'll take care of her!"
3. "Tell me what you missed, and I'll check on it."

If she uses the first response, Jeanine negates the patient's rights by patronizing him. She is responding nonassertively and accepting responsibility for her staff nurse's actions without finding out the facts. With the second response, she assumes the staff nurse is to blame and plans to chastise the nurse. This is aggressive behavior. The third response indicates she has heard the patient and is going to take action in his behalf, but without taking the blame herself or blaming others. She has accepted his emotional response without reacting to it.

People who learn assertive communication are able to respond to problems when they occur. The nonassertive person often attempts to avoid problems by remaining silent when he or she is angry; the aggressive person responds to the emotional aspect of the situation, thereby alienating others. The assertive person responds appropriately to the specific situation and at the appropriate time. Participants may not agree with each other's responses, but they clarify the other's position and accept the other's right to differ. Open, direct, and timely interactions between employees uncover problems and facilitate problem solving and decision making. Smith (1975) has identified seven rules to help people develop more assertive behavior:

1. Avoid overapologizing.
2. Avoid defensive, adverse reactions, such as aggression, temper tantrums, backbiting, revenge, slander, sarcasm, and threats.
3. Use body language that is appropriate to and matches the verbal message (e.g., eye contact, body posture, gestures, facial expression).
4. Accept manipulative criticism while maintaining responsibility for your decision.
5. Calmly repeat a negative reply without justifying it.
6. Be honest about feelings, needs, ideas. Use "I" statements.
7. Accept and/or acknowledge your faults calmly and without apology.

The Role of Communication in Leadership

Although communication is inherent in the manager's role, the manager's ability to communicate often determines his or her success as a leader. Leaders who engage in frank, open, two-way communication and whose nonverbal communication reinforces the verbal communication are seen as informative. Communication is even more enhanced when the manager listens carefully and is sensitive to others. The major underlying factor, however, is an ongoing relationship with the manager's employees.

Successful leaders are able to persuade others and enlist their support (Bass, 1990). A variety of techniques may be used. One approach is indirectness. Hints at, prompts, or teases about a need for action are given instead of a direct request. For example, "You don't seem to have enough file space in your office" may be more effective than "Please take some time to put away these files." Another indirect approach avoids responsibility for making a demand. "You might find it helpful to attend the inservice on communication," is an example. The third technique involves the use of palliatives or polite strategies—expressing admiration, claiming common viewpoints, displaying concern, and desiring cooperation in order to protect the other person from a loss of respect. However, the most effective means of persuasion is the leader's personal characteristics. Competence, emotional control, assertiveness, consideration, and

respect promote trustworthiness and credibility. Bass (1990) has noted a correlation between leadership style and communication style. For example, a participative leader is seen as a careful listener who is open, frank, trustworthy, and informative.

Communicating with Different Populations

Subordinates

Depending on the organization's policies, the nurse manager's responsibilities may include selecting, interviewing, evaluating, counseling, and disciplining employees; handling their complaints; and settling conflicts. The principles of effective communication are especially pertinent in these activities because good communication is the adhesive that builds and maintains an effective work group.

Giving direction is *not*, in itself, communication. If the manager receives an appropriate response from the subordinate, however, communication has occurred. To give directions and achieve the desired results, the nurse manager needs to develop a message strategy. The techniques that follow can help improve effective responses from others.

- *Know the context of the instruction.* Be certain you know exactly what you want done, by whom, within what time frame, and what steps should be followed to do it. Be clear in your own mind what information a person needs to carry out your instruction, what the outcome will be if the instruction is carried out, and how that outcome can or will be evaluated. When you have thought through these questions, you are ready to give the proper instruction.
- *Get positive attention.* Avoid factors that interfere with effective listening. Informing the receiver(s) that the instructions will be given is one simple way to try to get positive attention. Highlighting the background, giving a justification, or indicating the importance of the instructions also may be appropriate.
- *Give clear, concise instructions.* Use an inoffensive and nondefensive style and tone of voice. Be precise, and give all the information receivers need to carry out your expectations. Follow a step-by-step procedure if several actions are needed.
- *Verify through feedback.* Make sure the receiver has understood your specific request for action. Ask for a repeat of the instructions.

Negative inquiry A communication technique used to clarify objections and feelings (e.g., I don't understand . . .).

Fogging A communication technique in which one agrees with part of what was said.

Negative assertion A communication technique in which one accepts some blame for what was said.

- *Give follow-up communication.* Understanding does not guarantee performance. Follow up to determine the outcome of your instruction and give feedback to the receiver.

The nurse manager is responsible both for the quality of the work life of individual employees and for the quality of patient care in the entire unit. To carry out this job, the nurse manager should acknowledge the needs of individual employees, especially if the needs of one conflict with needs of the department; the manager should speak directly with those involved and state clearly and accurately the rationale for the decisions made.

Superiors

The manager's interaction with higher administration is comparable to the interaction between the manager and a subordinate, except that the manager is now the subordinate. The nurse manager must recognize that higher administration is responsible for the consequences of decisions made for a larger area, such as all of nursing service or the entire organization. The principles used in communicating with subordinates are equally appropriate. Managers must be organized and prepared to state their needs clearly, explain the rationale for requests, suggest benefits for the larger organization, and use appropriate channels. They also must be prepared to listen objectively to their supervisor's response and be willing to consider reasons for possible conflict with needs of other areas.

Working effectively with a supervisor is important because a supervisor directly influences personal success in a career and within the organization. Managing a supervisor, or managing upward, is a crucial skill for nurses. To manage upward, remember that the relationship requires participation from both parties. Managing upward is successful when power and influence move in both directions.

One aspect of managing upward is to understand the supervisor's position from her or his frame of reference. This will make it easier to propose solutions and ideas that the supervisor will accept. Understand that a supervisor is a *person* with even more responsibility and pressure. Learn about the supervisor from a personal perspective: What pressures, both personal and professional, does the supervisor face? How does the supervisor respond to stress? What previous experiences are liable to affect today's issues? This assessment will allow you to identify ways to help your supervisor with his or her job and for your supervisor to help you with yours.

Influencing a Supervisor Nurse managers need to approach their supervisor to exert their influence on a variety of issues and problems. Support for the purchase of capital equipment, for changes in staffing, or for a new policy or procedure all require communicating with your supervisor. Timing, rationale, choice of form or format and possible objections all are important factors to consider as you prepare to make such a request. Timing is critical; choose an opportunity when the supervisor has time and appears receptive. Also, consider the impact of your ideas on other events occurring at that time. Guidelines for influencing your supervisor are shown in Box 11-2.

Should ideas be presented in spoken or written form? Usually some combination is used. Even if you have a brief meeting about a relatively small request, it is a good idea to follow up with a memorandum detailing your ideas and the plans to which you both agreed. Sometimes the procedure works in reverse. If you provide the supervisor a written proposal prior to a meeting, both of you will be familiar with the idea at the start. In the latter case, careful preparation of the written material is essential.

What can be done if, in spite of careful preparation, your supervisor says no? First, make sure you have understood the objections and associated feelings. **Negative inquiry** (e.g., "I don't understand") is a helpful technique to use. Do not interrupt or become defensive or distraught; remain diplomatic. **Fogging**, agreeing with part of what was said, or **negative assertion**, accepting some blame, are two additional techniques that you can use. After diplomacy, the next step is confrontation (Umiker, 1990). Keep your voice low and measured; use "I" language; and avoid absolutes, why questions, put-downs, inflammatory statements, and threatening gestures. Finally, if you feel you have lost and compromise is unlikely, table the issue by saying, "Could we continue discussing this at another time?" Then, think through your supervisor's

Box 11-2 Guidelines for Influencing Your Supervisor

Capitalize on your supervisor's strengths.
- What strengths and limitations does she or he have?
- What information do you have that she or he needs?
- What help can the supervisor provide personally and organizationally?

Be prepared.
- Do you know your supervisor's overall professional priorities or goals?
- What concerns or difficulties may she or he be facing?
- What excites your supervisor? What turns her or him off?

Cite benefits.
- What's in it for the supervisor if she or he supports your idea, proposal, or plan?
- How will the organization benefit?
- What are the short-term and long-term advantages?

Build a strong case.
- What policies, precedents, or procedures support what you want to do?
- Which of your supporters are valued by your supervisor for their opinions?
- How can you trade on your own expertise or credibility?
- What will the consequences be if the proposed idea is not accepted?
- What will have to be done later as a result?

Avoid surprises.
- Do you need to lay some groundwork with a brief memo or phone call explaining the purpose and importance of the meeting?
- What are the risks or advantages of presenting the supervisor with your idea, proposal, or plan?

Anticipate resistance.
- What aspects of your plan are likely to prompt resistance, such as "costs too much," "takes too long," or "too risky"?
- How can you minimize or eliminate potential resistance by the way you manage the meeting?
- What data do you need to help overcome resistance?
- How will your idea affect morale, turnover, absenteeism? These cost money.

Separate need from "nice to have."
- What tradeoffs or compromises are you prepared to make?
- What part of your proposal is essential, what part merely desirable?
- "Half a loaf is better than none"; which half do you want?

Persist.
- How far and how hard are you willing to push to get your idea accepted?
- What does past experience tell you about the best timing or sequence for your attempts to influence your supervisor?
- Remember: The best ideas or changes seldom are accepted the first time they are proposed. If you learn from previously unsuccessful efforts and try again, you improve your chances of acceptance.

Note: Adapted from *Leadership and influence, part 3*, Development Dimensions International, 1986, Pittsburgh: Development Dimensions International.

reasoning and evaluate it. Ask yourself: "What new information did I get from the supervisor?" "What are ways I can renegotiate?" "What do I need to know or do to overcome objections?" Once you can answer these questions, approach your supervisor again with the new information. This behavior shows that the proposal is a high priority, and the new information may cause him or her to reevaluate.

Managers often succeed in influencing superiors through persistence and repetition, especially if supporting data and documentation are supplied. If the issue is important enough, you may want to take it to a higher authority. If so, tell your supervisor you would like an administrator at a higher level to hear the proposal. Keep an open mind, listen, and try to meet objections with suggestions of how to solve

Box 11-3 Key Behaviors for Taking a Problem to Your Supervisor

- State your desire to talk about a work-related problem and, if necessary, make an appointment to meet, identifying the approximate amount of time needed.
- If the suggested time is not convenient, ask when and where would be convenient.
- State the problem and explain its effect on work activities.
- Listen for a restatement of the problem or for an indication that the problem has been understood.
- State your willingness to cooperate in any solution to the problem and listen openly to your supervisor's comments.

If necessary, continue:

- State an alternative or your preferred solution.
- Agree on steps each of you will take to solve the problem.
- Ask if there is a need to follow up the problem. If so, plan and record a specific follow-up date.

Note: Adapted from *Health care management microtraining* by P. J. Decker, 1983, St. Louis: Decker and Associates. Used by permission.

problems. Be prepared to compromise, which is better than no movement at all, or to be turned down.

Taking a Problem to Your Supervisor When you take a problem to your supervisor, you should follow certain steps or key behaviors. You can also use these behaviors when staff come to you with problems. The behaviors are designed to facilitate problem solving. By solving the problem together and, if necessary, by taking active steps together, you and your supervisor are more likely to accept the decision and be committed to it. Setting a specific follow-up date can prevent a solution from being delayed or forgotten.

Box 11-3 summarizes the steps to use in discussing a work-related problem with your supervisor. By using these steps, you ensure that the problem is addressed at a time when both you and your supervisor are able to devote attention to it. This should maximize the exchange of relevant information, understanding, and ideas.

Other strategies for managing a supervisor follow:

- Give immediate positive feedback for good things that the supervisor does; positive feedback is a welcome change.
- Never let your supervisor be surprised; keep her or him informed.
- Always tell the truth.
- Find ways to compensate for weaknesses of your supervisor. Fill in weak areas tactfully. Volunteer to do something the supervisor dislikes doing.
- Be your own publicist. Don't brag, but keep your supervisor informed of what you achieve.

- Keep aware of your supervisor's achievements and acknowledge them.
- If your supervisor asks you to do something, do it well and ahead of the deadline if possible. If appropriate, add some of your own suggestions.
- Establish a positive relationship with the supervisor's secretary.

Peers

Relationships with peers can vary from comfortable and easy to challenging and complex. Because peers often have much in common with respect to authority and power, they can share similar concerns. Camaraderie may be present; peers can exchange ideas and address problems creatively. Peers can provide support, and the strengths of one can be developed in the other. Conversely, there may also be competition or conflicts (e.g., battles over territory, personality clashes, differences of opinion). Interactions with peers are inevitable. Even when there are conflicts, peers should interact on a professional level; tactics for communicating with difficult people and negotiating may be helpful. Both topics are discussed later in this chapter.

Medical Staff

Communication with the medical staff may be difficult for the nurse manager because of the nature of the relationship between physician and nurse: Historically, the relationship of physicians and nurses has been that of superior and subordinate. Moreover, in spite of recent changes in medical school admissions, a gender disparity still exists among practitioners in both professions; therefore, gender-based differences in communication may add to the difficulty. In addition, the medical staff may not be employees of the organization but still have considerable power in the health care setting because of their ability to attract patients to the organization, and, finally, the medical staff is in itself diverse, consisting of physicians who are organizational employees, residents, physicians in private practice, and consulting physicians. Obviously, principles of effective communication are very important in interactions with the medical staff.

Today's nurse managers are role models and leaders for establishing nurse–physician relationships on their units. Researchers are beginning to document the relationship of nurse–physician communication to patient outcomes. Knaus, Draper, Wagner, and Zimmerman (1986) found that lower-than-expected death rates in intensive care units were related to excellent coordination and communication among the nurse–physician staff. Likewise, Gavett, Drucker, McCrum, and Dickenson (1985) reported that lack of communication and coordination among health care providers was related to unnecessarily high-cost stays for patients. Nurse managers have important reasons, then, for setting a positive tone that fosters mutual respect among nurses and physicians on their units.

In today's competitive health care marketplace, it also is necessary to view the physician as a nursing service customer. Organizations are competing for patients, and physicians (as well as insurers) are sources of patients. The product of nursing service is patient care; physicians help provide the patients.

What do physicians want? Physicians first want quality staff—nurses, health care workers, and other physicians. They want up-to-date facilities and equipment, quality care, and adequately trained nursing personnel. Physicians also want respect (as do nurses and others who work in health care) and regard patient care as their primary concern (Spitzer, 1988). These are many of the same goals that nurses have.

To support greater collaboration between nurses and physicians and to improve the product of nursing service—patient care—the following strategies are offered.

- Respect physicians as persons, and expect them to respect you.
- Consider yourself and your staff equal partners with physicians in health care.
- Build your staff's clinical competence and credibility. Ensure that your staff has the clinical preparation necessary to meet required standards of care.

- Actively listen and respond to physician complaints as customer complaints. Create a problem-solving structure. Stop blaming physicians exclusively for communication problems.
- Use every opportunity to increase your staff's contact with physicians and to include your staff in meetings that include physicians. Remember that limited interactions contribute to poor communication.
- Establish a collaborative practice committee on your unit whose membership is composed equally of nurses and physicians. In the meetings, identify problems, develop mutually satisfactory solutions, and learn more about each other. Emphasize similarities and quality care. Begin with those physicians who have a positive attitude toward collaboration.
- Serve as a role model to your staff in nurse–physician communication.
- Support your staff in participating in collaborative efforts by words and by your actions.

But if you are confronted with power plays or intimidation, what is the best way to respond? Intimidation results from vulnerability and a threat to self-worth (Davidhazar & Bowen, 1990). Intimidation can be counteracted by increasing self-confidence and personal feelings of power. Umiker (1990) describes four ways to generate power.

1. With words:
   - Use the other person's name frequently.
   - Use strong statements.
   - Avoid discounters, such as "I'm sorry, but . . ."
   - Avoid clichés.
   - Avoid fillers (such as "ah," "uh," and "um").
2. Through delivery:
   - Be enthusiastic.
   - Speak clearly and forcefully.
   - Make one point at a time.
   - Do not tolerate interruptions.
3. By listening:
   - For facts.
   - For feelings.
   - For what is not being said (e.g., body language, mixed messages, hidden messages).
4. Through body posture and body language:
   - Sit next to your antagonist; turn 30 degrees toward the person when you address that person.
   - Lean forward.
   - Expand your personal space.
   - Use gestures.
   - Stand when you talk.

- Smile when you are pleased, not in order to please.
- Maintain eye contact, but do not stare.

Additional techniques to counteract intimidation and threat are included in the section on conflict management.

Other Health Care Personnel

The nurse manager has the overwhelming task of co-ordinating the activities of a number of personnel with varied levels and types of preparation and different kinds of tasks. The patient may receive regular care from a registered nurse, unlicensed assistive personnel, a respiratory therapist, a physical therapist, and a dietitian. The nurse manager must use considerable skill to communicate effectively with the diverse personnel and managers involved in health care. In interacting with personnel from other departments, the nurse manager must recognize and respond to differences between the goals of their departments and the nursing unit. Recognizing this helps both parties identify their commonalities and to deal with their differences.

Patients and Families

Nurse managers deal with many difficult issues. Patient or family complaints about the delivery of care (e.g., complaints about a staff member, violations of policy) are one example. When dealing with patient or family complaints, keep the following principles in mind:

- The patient (and family) are the principal customers of the organization. Treat patients and families with respect; keep communication open and honest. Dissatisfied customers fail to continue to use a service and also inform their friends and families about their negative experiences. Handle complaints or concerns tactfully and expeditiously. Many times, even lawsuits can be avoided if the patient or family feels that someone has taken the time to listen to their complaints. (See the section on risk management in Chapter 9.)
- Most individuals are unfamiliar with medical jargon. Use words that are appropriate to the recipient's level of understanding. However, take care not to be condescending or intimidating. It is just as important to assess the person's knowledge base and level of understanding as it is to know his or her vital signs or liver status.
- Maintain privacy and identify a neutral location for dealing with difficult interactions.

- Make special efforts to find interpreters if a patient or family does not speak English. Have readily available a list of individuals who are able to communicate in a variety of languages. The list also should include individuals experienced in sign language and Braille. Another resource is AT&T's language line service (1-800-752-6096), which provides interpreters for over 140 languages 24 hours a day.
- It is essential to recognize cultural differences in communication. People in some cultures do not ask questions for fear of imposing on others. Some cultures prefer interpreters from their own culture; others do not (Brooks, 1992). Cultural education for the staff can help identify some of these differences and teach them appropriate, culturally sensitive responses.

Difficult People

Difficult personalities exist in all groups of people—subordinates, superiors, physicians, other health care team members, patients, and family members alike. Strategies for coping with difficult people follow (Nations, 1990a, 1990b, 1990c):

1. *Put physical distance between you and the difficult person.* A common method to achieve physical distance is to limit the time you spend with the individual. Match the person's energy level in speed, pitch, and volume; this conveys awareness and empathy. This technique is particularly effective with hostile, aggressive individuals. However, negative behavior, such as yelling and tantrums, should not be mirrored; instead, remain calm but assertive.

2. *Psychologically distance yourself from the individual.* View the person from a different perspective; try "putting on his shoes." Also "lose the shoulds" (for example, "Who does he think he is? He shouldn't be allowed to talk to us like that.") Ask: What does this person's behavior accomplish? What type of personality trait is being exhibited?

3. *Identify the individual's feelings and information level.* Then validate those feelings and information as well as your relationship, but don't patronize. This technique is particularly successful with a "know-it-all" who may be under the illusion that only he or she is right.

4. *Ask extensional questions.* Questions that begin with "how" or "what" often help the person to focus on his or her concerns and rethink what has

just been said. Focusing on holes in the individual's argument provides an opportunity for a graceful retreat.

5. *Use physical movement.* Lead an upset individual to your office or another neutral location, or suggest the two of you go for a cup of coffee. Physical activity often diminishes stress and hostility.
6. *Try humor.* If the situation is not too serious, humor is an excellent method to defuse anger and frustration; however, be careful to avoid sarcasm or putdowns.

Conflict

A manager's communication often centers around conflict. A study by the American Management Association (McElheney, 1996) reports that nurse managers spend approximately 20 percent of their time dealing with conflict. Conflict is a natural, inevitable condition in organizations, and it is often a prerequisite to change in people and organizations. **Conflict** is defined as the consequence of real or perceived differences in mutually exclusive goals, values, ideas, attitudes, beliefs, feelings, or actions (a) within one individual (*intrapersonal conflict*), (b) between two or more individuals (*interpersonal conflict*), (c) within one group (*intragroup conflict*), or (d) between two or more groups (*intergroup conflict*). Conflict is dynamic. It can be positive or negative, healthy or dysfunctional.

A certain amount of conflict is beneficial to an organization. It can provide heightened sensitivity to an issue, further piquing the interest and curiosity of others. Conflict also can increase creativity by acting as a stimulus for developing new ideas or identifying methods for solving problems. Wheatley (1992, p. 116) states that order is created "when we invite conflicts and contradictions to rise to the surface, when we search them out, highlight them, even allowing them to grow large and worrisome." For example, disagreements over patient care help all parties become more aware of the tradeoffs, especially costs versus benefits, of a particular service or technique.

Conflict also helps people recognize legitimate differences within the organization or profession and serves as a powerful motivator to improve performance and effectiveness, as well as satisfaction. For example, during intergroup conflict, individual groups become more cohesive and task-oriented, while communication between groups diminishes.

Aggressive behavior can occur. Groups placed in "win–lose" competition have the tendency to increase

KEY TERMS

Conflict The consequence of real or perceived differences in mutually exclusive goals, values, ideas, attitudes, beliefs, feelings, or actions.

Competitive conflict A type of conflict that is resolved through competition, in which victory for one side and loss for the other side is determined by a set of rules.

Disruptive conflict A type of conflict in which winning is not emphasized and there is no mutually acceptable set of rules; parties involved are engaged in activities to reduce, defeat, or eliminate the opponent.

the in-group versus out-group bias between them. Scapegoating may occur, with each group viewing the other as an enemy. This may make it difficult for the groups to work together in the future.

Conflict may be covert and inappropriate. Anger may be displaced to innocent bystanders. Others may repress their frustration or anger, which may surface later in behavior (e.g., increased errors, accidents, or illness). Other inappropriate responses to conflict are retaliation, projection, rationalization, attention-seeking behaviors, repression, or escape tactics, such as resignation or flight into fantasy.

Competition, such as that which occurs between health care organizations, also is a frequent source of conflict. Competition occurs when two or more groups attempt the same goals and only one group can attain those goals. Filley (1975) defines **competitive conflict** as a victory for one side at a loss for the other side. The process by which the conflict is resolved is determined by a set of rules. The goals of each side are mutually incompatible, but the emphasis is on winning, not the defeat or reduction of the opponent. When one side has clearly won, competition is terminated.

Disruptive conflict, in contrast, does not follow any mutually acceptable set of rules and does not emphasize winning. The parties involved are engaged in activities to reduce, defeat, or eliminate the opponent. This type of conflict takes place in an environment charged with fear, anger, and stress. For example, a resident on night call may contribute to disruptive behavior by refusing to answer pages, turning off the beeper, or by belittling nurses for calling with "minor" problems. Nurses often react to this type of behavior with their own disruptive behavior: frequent, "by the book," middle-of-the-night phone calls to get back at the offending resident. An example of a more subtle disruptive behavior would be the failure to extend minor work-saving courtesies to an unpopular resident. Disruptive conflict can, in unusual circumstances, result in irrational, upsetting, or even violent behavior.

Conflict Process Model

Filley's model of conflict resolution provides a generalized format for examining conflict behavior in relation to the nurse manager's job. This model provides a framework that helps explain how and why conflict occurs and, ultimately, how one can minimize conflict or resolve it with the least amount of negative aftermath.

Filley suggests that conflict and its resolution develop according to a specific process. This process begins with certain preexisting conditions (antecedent conditions). The parties are influenced by their feelings or perceptions about the situation (perceived or felt conflict), which initiates behavior (manifest behavior). The conflict is either resolved or suppressed (conflict resolution or suppression), and in the aftermath (resolution aftermath), new attitudes and feelings between the parties evolve (Figure 11-2).

Antecedent Conditions   Antecedent conditions are associated with increases in conflict. Antecedent conditions propel a situation toward conflict; they may or may not be the cause. In nursing, antecedent conditions include incompatible goals, differences in values and beliefs, task interdependencies (especially asymmetric dependencies, in which one party is dependent on the other but not vice versa), unclear or ambiguous roles, competition for scarce resources, differentiation or distancing mechanisms, proximity, and unifying mechanisms.

Goals and Their Importance to Conflict   The most important antecedent condition to conflict is incompatible goals. As discussed in Chapter 3, goals are desired results toward which behavior is directed. Even though the common goal in health care organizations is to give quality patient care in a cost-effective manner, conflict in achieving these goals is inevitable because individuals often view this from different perspectives. In addition, individuals and organizations have multiple goals that change over time. A health care organization may have specific goals to achieve the best possible care for patients and control costs to stay within budget and, at the same time, to provide

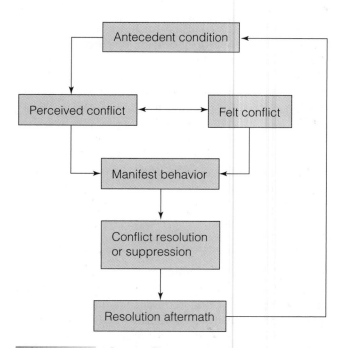

Figure 11-2   **The conflict process. *Note:* Adapted from *Managerial process and organizational behavior* by A. C. Filley, R. J. House, and S. Kerr, 1976, Madison, WI: A. C. Filley, University of Wisconsin, p. 72. Used by permission.**

intrinsically satisfying jobs for its employees. These multiple goals will frequently conflict with each other, so they will have to be prioritized. Priority setting can be one of the most difficult but important activities a health care manager must face. Goals are important because they become the basis for allocating resources and thus become an important source (antecedent) of conflict in the organization.

Similarly, individuals themselves have multiple goals, and those goals may also conflict. Individuals allocate scarce resources, such as their time, on the basis of priority and, therefore, might achieve one goal at the expense of others. The inability to attain multiple (and mutually incompatible) goals—whether those goals are personal or organizational—can cause conflict.

An example of goal conflict in nursing is the dichotomy between health care providers and third-party payers. This issue can best be described as a conflict between groups with differing goals. Health care providers want to maximize the quality of care, whereas payers are concerned with minimizing health care costs.

Other Antecedent Conditions   Roles are defined as other people's expectations regarding behavior and attitudes. Roles become unclear when one or more parties have related responsibilities that are ambiguous or overlapping. The nurse manager might experience conflict between his or her responsibilities as an administrator and responsibilities as a staff member. Similarly, unclear or overlapping job descriptions or assignments may lead to conflict. For example, there could be conflict over such mundane issues as who has responsibility to deliver a patient to the radiology department—the nurse or the transport staff?

Competition for scarce resources can be internal (among different units in the organization) or external (among different organizations). Internally, competition for resources may involve assigning staff from one unit to another or purchasing high-technology equipment when another unit is desperate for staff.

Externally, health care organizations compete for finite external resources (e.g., managed-care contracts). Organizations are using a variety of means, such as developing new services and advertising, to try to capture the market in health care. With increased numbers of nurse practitioners, competition between nurses and physicians for patients also has increased.

Differences in values and beliefs frequently contribute to conflict in health care organizations. Values and beliefs result from the individual's socialization experience. Conflicts between physicians and nurses, between nurses and administrators, or even between nurses with associate degrees versus those with baccalaureate degrees, often occur because of differences in values, beliefs, and experiences.

Task interdependence is another potential source of conflict in health care organizations. For example, an interdependence exists between nursing and housekeeping. Housekeeping cannot completely clean a room until nursing has discharged the patient. Other examples of interdependence are the relationships among shifts and those between physicians and nurses. Interdependent relationships have the potential to initiate conflict.

Distancing mechanisms or differentiation serve to divide a group's members into small, distinct groups, thus increasing the chance for conflict. This tends to lead to a "we–they" distinction. One of the more frequently seen examples is distancing between physicians and nurses. Opposition between intensive care nurses and nurses on medical floors, night versus day shifts, and unlicensed versus licensed personnel also are examples. Differentiation among subunits also occurs and is due to differences in structure. The

KEY TERMS

Perceived conflict   One's perception of the other's position in a conflict.

Felt conflict   The feelings of opposition within the relationship of two or more parties.

administrative unit may be bureaucratic, the nursing unit structured on a more professional basis, and staff physicians on an even different structure. Nonstaff physicians may be relatively independent of the health care organization.

Unifying mechanisms occur when greater intimacy develops or when unity is sought. All nurse managers might be expected to reach consensus over an issue, but they might experience internal conflict if they are forced to accept a group position even though individually they may not be wholly committed to the decision. A classic example of a unifying mechanism is the relationship between husband and wife. As intimacy increases, issues arise that would not normally cause conflict in a casual relationship but do affect closer relationships. A nurse manager's friendship with a staff member also may lead to this type of conflict.

One conflict commonly seen in the health care environment is structural conflict. Structured relationships (superior to subordinate, peer to peer) provoke conflict because of poor communication, competition for resources, opposing interests, or a lack of shared perceptions or attitudes. A nurse manager (superior) stimulates conflict with a staff member (subordinate) by reprimanding the staff member for some inappropriate act. If the nurse manager is unable to communicate to the staff member why the act was unacceptable, opposing interests develop, and the conflict is sustained. In this situation, positional power is often imposed. Positional power is the authority inherent in a certain position—for example, the nurse administrator has greater positional power than a nurse manager.

Other Aspects of the Conflict Process   Perceived and felt conflict are parts of the conflict process. These concepts account for the conflict that may occur when the parties involved view situations or issues from differing perspectives, when they misunderstand each other's position, or when positions are based on limited knowledge. **Perceived conflict** refers to each party's perception of the other's position. **Felt conflict** refers to the feelings of opposition within the relationship of two or more parties. It is characterized by mistrust, hostility, and fear.

To demonstrate how this process works, consider this situation. Nurse manager Jones and surgeon Smith have worked together for years. They have mutual respect for each other's ability and skills, and they communicate frequently. When their subordinates clash, they are left with conflicting accounts of a situation, in which the only agreed-upon fact is that a patient received less-than-appropriate care. Now consider the same scenario if the nurse and doctor have never dealt with each other or if one feels that the other will not approach the problem constructively.

In the first situation (perceived conflict), their positive regard for each other's abilities makes the nurse and physician believe they can constructively solve the conflict. The nurse does not feel the physician will try to dominate, and the physician respects the nurse manager's managerial ability. With these preexisting attitudes, the physician and nurse can remain neutral while helping their subordinates solve the conflict. If the nurse and physician were experiencing felt conflict, they might approach the situation differently. Each might assume the other will defend her or his subordinates at all costs and communication will be inhibited. The conflict is resolved by domination of the stronger person, either in personality or position. One wins; the other loses.

Manifest behavior is the outcome of conflict. Behaviors may be overt or covert. Overt behavior may take the form of aggression, competition, debate, or problem solving. Covert behavior may be expressed by a variety of indirect tactics, such as scapegoating, avoidance, or apathy.

The final stages of the conflict process are suppression or resolution and the resulting aftermath. **Suppression** occurs when one person or group defeats the

other. Only the dominant side is committed to the agreement, and the loser may or may not carry out the agreement. **Resolution** occurs when a mutually agreed-upon solution is arrived at and both parties commit themselves to carrying out the agreement.

The optimal solution is to manage the issues in a way that will lead to a solution wherein both parties see themselves as winners and the problem is solved. This leaves a positive aftermath that will affect future relations and influence feelings and attitudes. In the example of conflict between the nurse manager and the physician, consider the difference in the aftermath and how future issues would be approached if both parties felt positive about the outcome, as compared to future interactions if one or both parties felt they had lost.

Conflict Management

The management of conflict is an important part of the nurse manager's job. Nurse managers often are involved in conflict management on several different levels. They may be participants in the conflict as individuals, supervisors, or as representatives of a unit. In fact, they must often initiate conflict by confronting staff, individually or collectively, when a problem develops. They also may serve as mediators or judges to conflicting parties. There could be a conflict within the unit, between parties from different units, or between internal and external parties (for example, a nursing instructor from the university may have a conflict with staff on a particular unit).

It is important for the nurse manager and other participants in conflict management to be realistic regarding the outcome. Often those inexperienced in conflict negotiation expect unrealistic outcomes. When two or more parties hold mutually exclusive ideas, attitudes, feelings, or goals, it is extremely difficult, without the commitment and willingness of all concerned, to arrive at an agreeable solution that meets the needs of both.

Conflict management begins with a decision regarding if and when to intervene. Failure to intervene can allow the conflict to get out of hand, whereas early intervention may be detrimental to those involved, causing them to lose confidence in themselves and reduce risk-taking behavior in the future. Some conflicts are so minor, particularly if they are between only two people, that they do not require intervention and would be better handled by the two people involved. Allowing them to resolve their conflict might provide a developmental experience and improve their abilities to resolve conflict in the future. When there is potential that the conflict might result in considerable harm, however, the nurse manager must intervene.

Sometimes the nurse manager may postpone intervention purposely to allow the conflict to escalate, because increased intensity can motivate participants to seek resolution. The manager can escalate the conflict even further by exposing participants to each other more frequently without the presence of others and without an easy means of escape. Participants are then forced to face the conflict between them. Giving participants a shared task or shared goals not directly related to the conflict may help them understand each other better and increase their chances to resolve their conflicts by themselves. Using such a method is useful only if the conflict is not of high intensity, if the participants are not highly anxious about it, and if the manager believes that the conflict will not decrease the efficiency of the department in the meantime.

If a nurse manager decides to intervene in a conflict between two or more parties, he or she can apply mediation techniques, deciding when, where, and how the intervention should take place. Routine problems can be handled in either the superior's or subordinate's office, but serious confrontations should take place in a neutral location unless the parties involved are of unequal power. In this case, the setting should favor the disadvantaged participant, thereby equalizing their power.

The place should be one where distractions will not interfere and adequate time is available. Because conflict management takes time, the manager must be prepared to allow sufficient time for all parties to explain their points of view and arrive at a mutually agreeable solution. A quick solution that inexperienced managers often resort to is to impose positional power, making a premature decision. This results in a win–lose outcome, which leads to feelings of elation and eventual complacency for the winners and loss of morale for the losers.

Basic rules on how to mediate a conflict between two or more parties follow:

1. Protect each party's self-respect. Deal with a conflict of issues, not personalities.
2. Do not put blame or responsibility for the problem on the participants. The participants are responsible for developing a solution to the problem.
3. Allow open and complete discussion of the problem from each participant.

4. Maintain equity in the frequency and duration of each party's presentation. A person of higher status tends to speak more frequently and longer than a person of lower status. If this occurs, the mediator should intervene and ask the person of lower status for response and opinion.
5. Encourage full expression of positive and negative feelings in an accepting atmosphere. The novice mediator tends to discourage expressions of disagreement.
6. Make sure both parties listen actively to each other's words. One way to do this is to ask one person to summarize the comments of the other prior to stating her or his own.
7. Identify key themes in the discussion, and restate these at frequent intervals.
8. Encourage the parties to provide frequent feedback to each other's comments; each must truly understand the other's position.
9. Help the participants develop alternative solutions, select a mutually agreeable one, and develop a plan to carry it out. All parties must agree to the solution for successful resolution to occur.
10. At an agreed-upon interval, follow up on the progress of the plan.
11. Give positive feedback to participants regarding their cooperation in solving the conflict.

Conflict management is a difficult process, consuming both time and energy. Management and staff must be concerned and committed to resolving conflict by being willing to listen to others' positions and to find agreeable solutions.

Goals of Conflict Management

The system benefits when managers give attention to promoting the goals of the organization. Attending to the needs of only one party reflects a **partisan choice**. Attending to the well-being of both parties reflects a **joint-welfare choice**, which also optimizes the well-being of the organization (Thomas, 1992).

Filley (1975) identified three basic strategies for dealing with conflict according to the outcome: win–lose, lose–lose, and win–win. In the **win–lose strategy**, one party exerts dominance, usually by power of authority, and the other party submits and loses. Forcing, competing, and negotiation are techniques likely to lead to win–lose competition. Majority rule is another example of the win–lose outcome, especially within groups. It may be a satisfactory method of resolving conflict, however, if various factions vote differently on different issues and the group functions over time so that members win some and lose some. Win–lose outcomes often occur between groups. Frequent losing, however, can lead to the loss of cohesiveness within groups and diminish the authority of the group leader.

In the **lose–lose strategy**, neither side wins. The settlement reached is unsatisfactory to both sides. Avoiding, withdrawing, smoothing, and compromising may lead to lose–lose outcomes. One compromising strategy is to use a bribe to influence another's cooperation in doing something he or she dislikes. For example, the nurse manager may promise a future raise in an attempt to coerce a staff member to work an extra weekend. Using a third party as arbitrator can lead to a lose–lose outcome. Because an outsider may want to give something to each side, neither gets exactly what he or she desires, resulting in a lose–lose outcome. This is a common strategy in arbitration of labor–management disputes. Another strategy that may result in a lose–lose or win–lose outcome is resorting to rules. The outcome is determined by whatever the rules say, and confrontation is avoided.

The win–lose and lose–lose methods share some common characteristics (Filley, 1975):

1. The conflict is person-centered (we–they) rather than problem-centered. This is likely to occur when two cohesive groups that do not share common values or goals are in conflict.
2. Parties direct their energy toward total victory for themselves and total defeat for the other. This can cause long-term problems for the organization.
3. Each sees the issue from her or his own point of view rather than as a problem in need of a solution.
4. The emphasis is on outcomes rather than definition of goals, values, or objectives.
5. Conflicts are personalized.
6. Conflict-resolving activities are not differentiated from other group processes.
7. There is a short-run view of the conflict; the goal is to settle the immediate problem rather than resolve differences.

KEY TERMS

Win–lose strategy A strategy used during conflict in which one party exerts dominance and the other submits and loses.

Lose–lose strategy A conflict strategy in which neither side wins; the settlement reached is unsatisfactory to both sides.

Win–win strategy A conflict strategy that focuses on goals and attempts to meet the needs of both parties.

Consensus A conflict strategy in which a solution that meets everyone's needs is agreed upon.

Competing An all-out effort to win, regardless of the cost.

Collaboration All parties work together to solve a problem.

Compromise A conflict management technique in which the rewards are divided between both parties.

Avoiding A conflict management technique in which the participants deny that conflict exists.

Accommodating An unassertive, cooperative tactic used in conflict management when individuals neglect their own concerns in favor of others' concerns.

Suppression A technique used to manage conflict in which one party is eliminated through transfer or termination.

Withdrawal The removal of at least one party from the conflict, making it impossible to resolve the situation.

Smoothing Managing conflict by complimenting one's opponent, downplaying differences, and focusing on minor areas of agreement.

Forcing A conflict management technique that forces an immediate end to conflict but leaves the cause unresolved.

Win–win strategies focus on goals and attempt to meet the needs of both parties. Two specific win–win strategies are consensus and integrative decision making. **Consensus** involves attention to the facts and to the position of the other parties and avoidance of trading, voting, or averaging, where everyone loses something. The consensus decision is often superior to even the best individual one. This technique is most useful in a group setting because it is sensitive to the negative characteristics of win–lose and lose–lose outcomes. True consensus occurs when the problem is fully explored, the needs and goals of the involved parties are understood, and a solution that meets these needs is agreed upon.

Integrative decision-making methods focus on the means of solving a problem rather than the ends. They are most useful when the needs of the parties are polarized. Integrative decision making is a constructive process in which the parties jointly identify the problem and their needs. They explore a number of alternative solutions and come to consensus on a solution. The focus of this group activity is to solve the problem, not to force, dominate, suppress, or compromise. The group works toward a common goal in an atmosphere that encourages the free exchange of ideas and feelings. Using integrative decision-making methods, the parties jointly identify the value needs of each, conduct an exhaustive search for alternatives that could meet the needs of each, and then select the best alternative. Like the consensus methods, integrative decision making focuses on defeating the problem, not each other.

Conflict Management Modes

Thomas (1992) has described the following five conflict-handling modes in terms of two underlying dimensions: assertiveness (attempting to satisfy one's own concerns) and cooperativeness (attempting to satisfy others' concerns). These five modes are competing, collaborating, compromising, avoiding, and accommodating. **Competing** is an all-out effort to win, regardless of the cost. Competing may be needed in situations involving unpopular or critical decisions. Competing also is used in situations in which time does not allow for more cooperative techniques.

Collaboration implies mutual attention to the problem, in which the talents of all parties are used. In collaboration, the focus is on solving the problem, not defeating the opponent. The goal is to satisfy both parties' concerns. Collaboration is useful in situations in which the goals of both parties are too important to be compromised.

Compromise is used to divide the rewards between both parties. Neither gets what she or he wants. Compromise can serve as a backup to resolve conflict when collaboration is ineffective. It is sometimes the only

choice when opponents of equal power are in conflict over two or more mutually exclusive goals. Compromising also is expedient when a solution is needed rapidly.

In **avoiding**, the participants never acknowledge that a conflict exists. Avoidance is the conflict resolution technique often used in highly cohesive groups. The group avoids disagreement because they do not want to do anything that may interfere with the good feelings they have for each other.

Accommodating is an unassertive, cooperative tactic used when individuals neglect their own concerns in favor of others' concerns. Accommodating frequently is used to preserve harmony when one person has a vested interest in an issue that is unimportant to the other party.

Several researchers have looked at which modes nurse managers use most frequently. Compromising is the most common conflict management technique. Barton (1991) noted that the second most common conflict management technique differed with level of management: Nurse administrators used competing, whereas head nurses and their assistants used collaborating. Kiernan (1992) found that the most preferred conflict management style was compromising, with collaborating second, and avoiding third. Cavanaugh (1991) identified avoiding as the most common conflict management style used by staff nurses.

Other Conflict Management Techniques

In the early part of the century, when society discouraged conflict, a common technique used was suppression. **Suppression** could even include the elimination of one of the conflicting parties through transfer or termination. Other, less effective techniques for managing conflict include withdrawing, smoothing, and forcing, although each mode of response is useful in given situations. **Withdrawal** from the conflict simply removes at least one party, thereby making it impossible to resolve the situation. The issue remains unresolved, and feelings about the issue may resurface inappropriately.

Smoothing is accomplished by complimenting one's opponent, downplaying differences, and focusing on minor areas of agreement, as though little disagreement existed. Smoothing may be appropriate in dealing with minor problems, but in response to major problems, it produces the same results as withdrawing.

Forcing is a method that yields an immediate end to the conflict but leaves the cause of the conflict unresolved. A superior can resort to issuing orders, but

Negotiation A conflict management technique in which the conflicting parties give and take on various issues.

Confrontation The most effective means of resolving conflict, in which the conflict is brought out in the open and attempts are made to resolve it through knowledge and reason.

the subordinate will lack commitment to the demanded action. Forcing may be appropriate in life-or-death situations but is otherwise inappropriate. Negotiation and confrontation are generally more effective modes of responding to conflict.

Negotiation involves give and take on various issues among the parties. Its purpose is to achieve agreement even though consensus will never be reached. Therefore, the best solution is not often achieved. Negotiation often becomes a structured, formal procedure, as in collective bargaining. (See Chapter 20.) However, negotiation skills are important in arriving at an agreeable solution between any two parties. Staff learn to negotiate schedules, advanced practice nurses negotiate with third-party payers for reimbursement, insurance companies negotiate with vendors and hospitals for discounts, and clinic managers negotiate employment contracts with physicians. Although negotiation involves adept communication skills, its usefulness revolves around issues of conflict. Without differences in opinion, there would be no need for negotiation.

Levenstein (1984) lists ten commandments for negotiators:

1. Clarify the common purpose.
2. Keep the discussion relevant.
3. Get agreement on terminology.
4. Avoid abstract principles; concentrate on the facts.
5. Look for potential tradeoffs.
6. Listen.
7. Avoid debating tactics; use persuasive tactics.
8. Keep in mind the personal element.
9. Use logic logically.
10. Look for solutions that satisfy the other person's real interests.

Confrontation is similar to the collaboration technique and is considered the most effective means for resolving conflicts. This is a problem-oriented technique, in which the conflict is brought out into the open and attempts are made to resolve it through knowledge and reason. The goal of this technique is to achieve win–win solutions. Facts should be used to identify the problem. The desired outcome should be explicit. "This is the third time this week that you have not been here for report. According to hospital policy, you are expected to be changed, scrubbed, and ready for report in the lounge at 7:00 A.M.," is an example.

Confrontation is most effective when delivered in private as soon as possible after the incident occurs. Employee respect and manager credibility are two important considerations when a situation warrants confrontation. A more immediate confrontation also helps both the employee and manager sort out pertinent facts. In an emotionally charged situation, however, it may be best for the parties to wait. Regardless of timing, the message is usually more effective if the manager listens and is empathetic.

Many other techniques besides intervention can be used to resolve conflict and are consistent with the problem-solving approach. Some of these include changing or clarifying goals, making appeals to the hierarchy, providing cooling-off periods, using intermediaries, and dividing the resources so each party can partially achieve its goals.

Summary

- Communication is a complex, ongoing dynamic process in which participants simultaneously create meaning in an interaction.
- Information may be relayed by oral or written methods. Oral messages are accompanied by nonverbal messages that are often more trusted than verbal messages.
- Communication may be formal or informal and travel downward, upward, laterally, or diagonally in an organization.
- Intrasender conflict occurs when the verbal and nonverbal messages are incongruent to the recipient; intersender conflict occurs when two individuals give one person a different message about the same issue.
- Gender, cultural background, and the organizational culture influence communication and its outcome.
- Organizational culture is influenced by accessibility of information, communication channels, clarity of message, flow control and information load, and communicator effectiveness.
- Communication has an impact on leadership influence. Nurse managers can learn techniques to

improve communication with diverse groups under a variety of conditions.

- Conflict is a dynamic process, the consequence of real or perceived differences between individuals or groups. Conflict may be interpersonal, intrapersonal, intergroup, or intragroup.
- A number of conflict management techniques can be used to intervene when conflict is disruptive to the organization. The most common techniques are competition, collaboration, compromise, avoidance, accommodation, negotiation, and confrontation.

■ LEADERSHIP AND MANAGEMENT _in Action_

1. What types of problems can occur when verbal and nonverbal communication is incongruent?
2. How does assertive behavior differ from aggressive and passive behavior?
3. Describe two situations in which conflict would be positive.

References

Barton, A. (1991). Conflict resolution by nurse managers. *Nursing Management, 22*(5), 83–84, 86.

Bass, B. (1990). *Bass & Stodgdill's handbook of leadership: Theory, research, and managerial applications*, 3rd ed. New York: Free Press.

Blanchard, K. H., & Sargent, A. G. (1986). The one minute manager is an androgynous manager. *Nursing Management, 17*(5), 43–45.

Blake, R. R., Mouton, J. S., & Tapper, M. (1981). *Grid approaches for managerial leadership in nursing*. St. Louis: Mosby.

Brooks, T. R. (1992). Pitfalls in communication with Hispanic and African-American patients: Do translators help or harm? *Journal of the National Medical Association, 84*(11), 941–947.

Cavanaugh, S. J. (1991). The conflict management style of staff nurses and nurse managers. *Journal of Advanced Nursing, 16*, 1254–1260.

Davidhazar, R., & Bowen, M. (1990). Intimidation and the nurse manager. *Health Care Supervisor, 9*(1), 27–32.

Davidhazar, R., & Shearer, R. (1993). Soft-spoken managers: A blend of communication styles. *Nursing Management, 24*(7), 112L, 112P.

Decker, P. J. (1983). *Health care management microtraining*. St. Louis: Author.

Development Dimensions International. (1986). *Leadership and influence, part 3*. Pittsburgh: Author.

Donaldson, L., & Scannell, E. (1979). *Human response development: The new trainer's guide*. Reading, MA: Addison-Wesley.

Edwards, J. B., & Lenz, C. L. (1990). The influence of gender on communication for nurse leaders. *Nursing Administration Quarterly, 15*(1), 49–55.

Ehninger, D., Gronbeck, B. E., McKerrow, R. E., & Monroe, A. H. (1986). *Principles and types of speech communications*, 10th ed. Glenview, IL: Scott, Foresman.

Farley, M. J. (1989). Assessing communication in organizations. *Journal of Nursing Administration, 19*(12), 27–31.

Filley, A. C. (1975). *Interpersonal conflict resolution*. Glenview, IL: Scott, Foresman.

Filley, A. C., House, R. J., & Kerr, S. (1976). *Managerial process and organizational behavior*. Madison, WI: A. C. Filley, University of Wisconsin.

Fine, M. G., Johnson, F. L., & Foss, K. A. (1991). Student perceptions of gender in managerial communication. *Women's Studies in Communication, 14*(1), 24–48.

Fulk, J., & Boyd, B. (1991). Emerging theories of communication in organizations. *Journal of Management, 17*(2), 407–446.

Gavett, J. W., Drucker, W. R., McCrum, M. S., & Dickenson, J. C. (1985). *A study of high cost inpatients in Strong Memorial Hospital*. Rochester, NY: Rochester Area Hospital Corporation and University of Rochester.

Gray, J. (1992). *Men are from Mars, women are from Venus*. New York: HarperCollins.

Ingram, C. A., & Siantz, M. L. (1991). How can we become more aware of culturally specific body language and use this awareness therapeutically? *Journal of Psychosocial Nursing Mental Health Services, 29*(11), 38–41.

Jurma & Powell (1994). Perceived gender roles of managers and effective conflict management. *Psychological Reports, 74*(1), 104–106.

Kennedy, C. W., Camden, C. T., & Timmerman, G. M. (1990). Relationships among perceived supervisor communication, nurse morale, and sociocultural variables. *Nursing Administration Quarterly, 14*(4), 38–46.

Kenton, S. (1989). Speaker credibility in persuasive business communication: A model which explains gender differences. *Journal of Business Communication, 26*(2), 143–157.

Kiernan, J. A. (1992). *Conflict management and organizational climate: Head nurse styles and staff nurse perceptions*. Unpublished doctoral dissertation. University of Utah.

Knaus, W. A., Draper, E. A., Wagner, D. P., & Zimmerman, J. E. (1986). An evaluation of outcome from intensive care in major medical centers. *Annals of Internal Medicine, 104*, 410–418.

Leet-Pellegrini, H. (1980). Conversational dominance as a function of gender and expertise. In H. Giles, W. Robinson, & P. Smith (Eds.), *Language: Social psychological perspective* (pp. 97–104). New York: Pergamon.

Levenstein, A. (1984). Negotiation vs. confrontation. *Nursing Management, 15*(1), 52–53.

McElhaney, R. (1996). Conflict management in nursing administration. *Nursing Management, 27*(3), 49–50.

Nations, K. H. (1990a). Coping with difficult people. Part 1. *Medical Laboratory Observer, 22*(9), 22–25.

Nations, K. H. (1990b). Coping with difficult people. Part 2: Dealing with know-it-alls even if you are one yourself. *Medical Laboratory Observer, 22*(10) 29–30, 32.

Nations, K. H. (1990c). Coping with difficult people. Part 3: Effective ways to deflect hostility. *Medical Laboratory Observer, 22*(11), 40–42.

Ribiero, V. E., & Blakely, J. A. (1998). The proactive management of rumor and gossip. In E. C. Hein (Ed.), *Contemporary leadership behaviors: Selected readings,* 5th ed. Philadelphia: Lippincott.

Smith, M. (1975). *When I say no, I feel guilty.* New York: Bantam.

Spitzer, R. B. (1988). Meeting consumer expectations. *Nursing Administration Quarterly, 12*(3), 31–39.

Thomas, K. W. (1992). Conflict and conflict management: Reflections and update. *Journal of Organizational Behavior, 13*(3), 265–274.

Umiker, W. (1990). How to generate power in meetings. *Health Care Supervisor, 9*(1), 33–38.

U. S. Bureau of the Census. (1993). *Statistical abstract of the United States: 1993,* 113th ed. Washington, D.C.: Government Printing Office.

Wheatley, M. J. (1992). *Leadership and the new science: Learning about organizations from an orderly universe.* San Francisco: Berrett-Koehler.

CHAPTER 12

Using Management Information Systems

Information Systems

Management Information Systems
Hospital Information Systems
Nursing Information Systems
Benefits of Using Information
Systems
Obstacles Associated with
Information Systems

Computer Applications in Nursing

Patient Care Applications
Nursing Management Systems
Communication Systems
Educational Applications
Research Applications

Software Selection and System Implementation

Selecting a System: The Decision-
Making Process
Ethical and Social Considerations
The Nurse Informatics Specialist

Future Trends in Informatics

Looking Ahead

Over the past few decades, our society has moved into an age of technologic wizardry. These rapid advances have altered approaches to health care. The applications are endless: Computers can monitor and care for patients, store vast amounts of information, teach and research, and even provide a means for people from around the world to communicate. This chapter provides an introduction to the various systems of information technology that are used within the health care environment.

Objectives

After reading this chapter, you will be able to:

- Describe the contribution of information technology to the efficiency and effectiveness of nursing.
- Discuss considerations used in selecting software and system implementation.
- Discuss the social and ethical considerations related to information technology.

To achieve its goals and maintain efficiency and effectiveness, the organization uses a variety of tools to collect information, analyze data, and make predictions about outcomes. The advent of the personal computer at the end of the 1970s revolutionized this process, and, today, information technology is an important element of health care. This chapter provides an overview of the technology currently available and describes information systems used in nursing.

Information Systems

Information systems are complex automated systems that are integrated through networked computers to process data in order to answer questions, solve problems or make decisions. Common information systems in health care are management information systems, hospital information systems and nursing information systems. A newcomer, the **expert system**, contains a knowledge base that captures the wisdom of experts in the field and makes decisions using an inference engine (Fonteyn & Grobe, 1994). Expert systems also provide complex data processing and reasoning.

Management Information Systems

A **management information system** (MIS) is a defined set of techniques to capture and collect data, analytical tools, operating policies and procedures, and reporting and communications protocols that support management decision making. Management information systems generally provide data about an organization's operations, services, employees, and clients.

Hospital Information Systems

A **hospital information system** (HIS) is an integrated system used in health care settings to manage patient information. Originally, the HIS was an add-on to the hospital accounting system; now, the HIS is primarily a centralized patient record of demographics, health, and financial information. Typical types of information tracked in an HIS are appointments, admissions, transfers, and discharges; order entry and reporting of results; medication profiles; care planning or critical pathways; and patient acuities. Today, this type of information is shared not only among a number of different departments within a hospital but also with clinics and other health care providers through vast networks. One such system is the Colorado Medical

---

Information Network (COMIN), which links hospitals, physicians, pharmacies, and laboratories (Brunner, 1993). (See Figure 12-1.)

Nursing Information Systems

The nursing information system also is an integrated system used to manage patient information. Early systems supported standardized care plans, charting, and integration with hospital information systems for order entries and charges (Manning & McConnell, 1997). As nursing systems have become more sophisticated, automated entry of physiologic parameters is possible, as well as computerization of the patient record, collection of outcome data, and calculation of acuity.

Benefits of Using Information Systems

The complexity of computer systems varies from the relatively simple personal computer to an automated system. Automated information systems linking several departments that access and use a common database within the system form an integrated network; hospital information systems and management information systems are examples. Automated systems offer nursing several benefits (Cox, Harsanyi, & Dean, 1987; Gross, Hoehn, & Rooks, 1993; Zielstorff, McHugh, & Clinton, 1988). These include:

- Efficient organization, management, storage, and retrieval of information
- Logical, consistent, orderly entry of data that enhances accuracy, speed, productivity, and efficiency

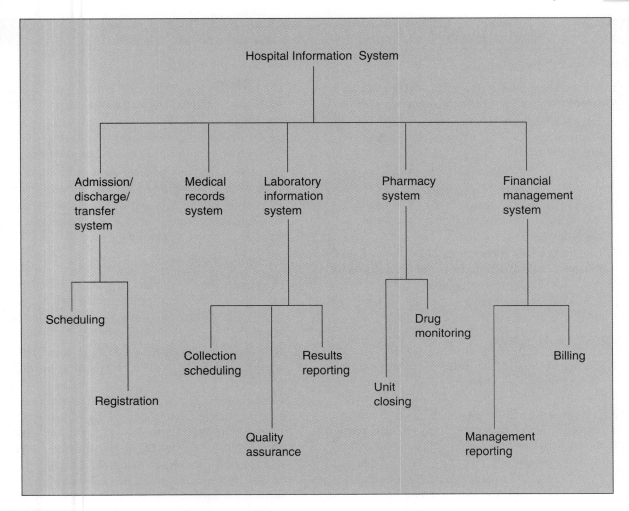

Figure 12-1   **Hospital information system divided into subsystems and functional components, illustrating the types of information tracked.** *Note:* **From
Medical informatics: Computer applications in health care by E. H. Shortliffe
and L. A. Perrault, 1990, Addison-Wesley Publishing Company, Inc. p. 166.**

- Increased access to information and enhanced communication abilities
- Cost containment
- Improved quality of care
- A tool for calculating the cost of nursing care
- Improved nursing satisfaction and retention

Obstacles Associated with Information Systems

Although information systems offer many benefits to nursing, there are also a number of obstacles. One is user resistance. Loss of control over practice, depersonalization of care, previous negative experiences, resistance to change, and fear of losing one's job have all been cited as reasons for user resistance (Zielstorff et al., 1988).

Another concern is the highly structured entry of data. Some propose that the richness of the content entered in progress notes is lost. However, many computer programs allow narrative charting.

Cost also can be prohibitive. Although hardware costs are declining, software is still expensive. In addition, utility costs and the costs of training personnel must be considered.

Until recently, another obstacle to using information systems in nursing was the scarcity of nurses who had the knowledge and expertise to design and evaluate programs specific to nursing. Now, however, graduate programs are preparing nurse informatics

Box 12-1   Criteria for Nursing Information Systems

System Capabilities

1. The system should accommodate the data elements associated with the nursing process.
2. The system should be integrated with or designed to interface with other elements of the patient's automated record.
3. The system should eliminate the need for redundant data entry.
4. The system should be designed to permit nursing data to be transported electronically to other systems.
5. The applications software should be housed in a system specifically designed to facilitate information retrieval and manipulation.
6. To the extent possible, each data item should be defined as a key for retrieval.

User-Machine Interface

1. The system should be flexible enough to permit users to tailor the system to reflect the conceptual framework and vocabulary in use at that site.
2. The system should be flexible enough to permit customization of data entry formats and screens, and of both on-screen and paper-copy data output formats at each user site.
3. The system should permit more efficient data entry and retrieval than preexisting manual systems.
4. The data entry system should be based primarily on structured data entry formats but must also allow limited free text entries.
5. Users should be able to query the database without the assistance of programmers or system analysts.

Hardware Requirements

1. The hardware should provide sufficient processing power to handle the calculated workload.
2. The system should provide a response time of no greater than two seconds during peak usage for data entry and retrieval in client care settings.
3. The system must provide sufficient on line and off-line memory for long-term and short-term storage.
4. The system should be designed to provide enough data entry ports conveniently placed to permit rapid accessibility to all users.

Data Security and Integrity

1. The system should provide software and hardware facilities to protect the security of the data.
2. At least two levels of password security should be required to gain access to the system.
3. The system should be designed to preserve the safety and integrity of the legal record of nursing care.
4. The power to purge a record from the database should be restricted to the database administrator or another person responsible for saving discharged client records onto tape or other permanent storage.
5. The system should permit care plans to be updated as necessary without destroying the outdated information.
6. Backup plans and equipment should be readily available to permit users to function in the event of system failure or recovery from a disastrous event.
7. The system should self-diagnose data transmission and storage problems and notify users and the system operator as soon as difficulties are detected.

Note: Adapted from *Computer design criteria* by R. D. Zielstorff, M. L. McHugh, and J. Clinton, 1988, Kansas City, MO: American Nurses Association, pp. 10–11.

specialists, and criteria have been suggested for developing information systems that support nursing practice. These criteria are listed in Box 12-1.

Computer Applications in Nursing

Computers are used in all businesses, nursing and health care included. Just as health care has changed over the years, so has the demand for information and technology. Computers are used to assess patient status,

provide direct care, communicate with others, manage personnel, teach, conduct research, and analyze data.

Patient Care Applications

Computers have so inundated our world that we are often unaware we are using a computer. Computers are no longer just terminals and keyboards that sit on a desk or are housed in a special room; many pieces of equipment used in health care settings are miniature computers (e.g., blood pressure machines, electronic thermometers). There are three main types of patient care applications: documentation, monitoring, and management systems.

Patient Care Documentation Patient care modules of the HIS are used to distribute necessary information to the appropriate area of responsibility. This component of the HIS allows information to be gathered in such a way that it can be manipulated for an infinite number of purposes, such as billing, inventory control, research, scheduling, and planning. The system allows health care providers to have valuable information that is difficult to collect manually in a timely manner. Nurses use the patient care module to (a) assess patient acuity and condition, (b) prepare an appropriate plan of care or critical path, (c) specify interventions for the patient, (d) document care, and (e) track outcomes and quality control.

The patient care module is a great time saver and efficient tool. For example, if gentamicin is ordered for a neonate in the nursery, the order automatically and instantaneously notifies the pharmacy to send the drug, places the medication on the automated medicine record and schedules the time for administration, notifies the laboratory to expect the blood samples as scheduled, notifies the nurse of the need to draw blood on the neonate at specified times, and sends the appropriate charges for pharmacy, laboratory, and nursing services to the accounting department. Such a system is not only efficient but also more accurate than any other method that uses multiple entry points.

As health care providers merged into larger networks, a need for a unified language became apparent. Until a unified language is developed, the American Nurses Association endorses the use of the North American Nursing Diagnosis Association (NANDA) list of diagnoses, the Nursing Interventions Classification, the Omaha System, and the Home Health Care Classification nomenclatures. (Averill et al., 1998).

Monitoring Patients Monitoring systems provide surveillance, freeing the nurse from routine, repetitive tasks while providing precise measurements. In addition, monitoring systems alert the nurse to abnormal values. Because of these characteristics, monitoring systems are used for surveillance, diagnosis, and treatment. Examples of monitoring systems include cardiopulmonary monitors, pulse oximeters, and fetal monitors.

Patient Management Systems Several types of management systems are used for integrated decision making and monitoring. Electrocardiographic interpretive

KEY TERMS

Point-of-care devices Portable decision-making, monitoring, and management system devices attached to the local area network via radio frequency.

Local area network (LAN) A type of network scheme that joins a group of personal computers and other devices within a particular location or group that is connected to a central file server.

systems are one example. The computer analyzes wave forms according to established criteria and provides a temporary diagnosis.

Documentation, monitoring, and management systems can vary from stationary terminals located at the nursing station or bedside to portable **point-of-care devices**. Point-of-care devices are attached to the local area network via radio-frequency signals. These portable devices provide mobility, minimize the number of devices needed, and can be used in a variety of settings, including the home, clinics, and skilled nursing care facilities.

Nursing Management Systems

Nursing management systems are another component of the HIS. Nursing management systems include applications for fiscal management, employee and patient data management, staffing and scheduling, and quality improvement and utilization review. A number of the different packages are available. In addition, spreadsheet packages such as Lotus 1-2-3 or Microsoft Excel may be used for financial management.

Communication Systems

The initiation of computers has revolutionized communications. No longer does one have to "play phone tag" or "kill trees"; now, communication can occur around the world in a matter of seconds. Communication is made possible by linking groups of computers through a specialized wiring scheme known as a network. There are two types of network schemes. The **local area network (LAN)** is a group of personal computers and other devices (printers, modems, and faxes) within a particular location, group, or department. This group is connected to one or more central

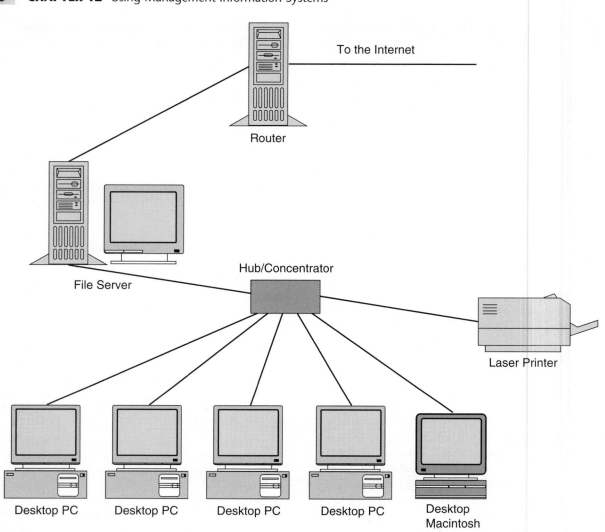

To the Internet

Router

File Server

Hub/Concentrator

Laser Printer

Desktop PC   Desktop PC   Desktop PC   Desktop PC   Desktop Macintosh

Figure 12-2 **Local area network.**

file servers and controlled by networking software (e.g., Novell, Banyan Vines, 3COM) (Figure 12-2). The file server usually contains a number of application programs. To access the network, the user logs in and provides a password, which ensures security and maintains confidentiality of records. **Wide area networks (WANs)** consist of local area networks and other devices, including large-scale computers, connected by specialized hardware and communications protocols. Hardware devices connect these networks and translate and route electronic signals from different types of systems. This type of technology supports the **Internet**, the information superhighway. Access to the World Wide Web is available through browser interface programs (e.g., MOSAIC and Netscape) on the Internet. The Internet provides the means to send an electronic message to an individual in the next office,

across town, or around the world. Services of interest to nurses are the *On-Line Journal of Knowledge Synthesis for Nursing* at Sigma Theta Tau International and the *AJN Network*. Through the Internet, nurses can also communicate with libraries and medical centers around the world.

Health care providers also are taking advantage of the new communication tools. **Telehealth** is the use of telecommunications technology by health care providers to enhance access to quality, affordable health care (ANA, 1997). Telehealth practices include telemedicine, telenursing, and teleradiology that use mechanisms of communication including telephones, cellular and video phones, facsimiles, computers, teleconferencing, video conferencing, and interactive television (NCSBN, 1996). The Texas Tech Telemedicine Project, for example, uses video conferencing to provide referrals to remote sites. Nurses in Kansas are making electronic house calls to the elderly via a two-way cable television line (NCSBN, 1996). Other uses include teleradiology, a technology that digitizes radiographic images and transmits them from one site to another, and home monitoring of ECG, sleep, and uterine contractions (Brunner, 1993).

A new use of the communication networks is development of **community health information networks (CHIN)**. CHINs are wide area networks that provide a population-based index, registry, or directory in a community-based data repository. The Colorado network, mentioned earlier, is an example of a CHIN. Other CHINs are operating in Wisconsin and Ohio (Simpson, 1994).

Educational Applications

Using computers for education is the fastest growing method of distance education (Potempa, Stanley, Davis, Miller, Hassett, & Pepicello, 2000). Distance education used to mean the instructor traveled to an off-campus location, often miles away, to teach a class. Now distance education includes video conferencing, teleconferencing, interactive television, and, more recently, **online instruction** offered by colleges and universities via the Internet. With online courses, instructors provide lectures, case studies, and sometimes clinical slides, graphics, or video, monitor discussion, and answer questions. Students can register for classes, order textbooks and supplementary material, use the library, submit assignments, and take tests, all from a location far from campus. Adult, working students, such as those enrolled in baccalaureate programs for registered nurses and masters degree programs for nurse practitioners, are among those targeted for online instruction.

In addition, other forms of computer-assisted technology can be used to teach nurses, students, patients, or their families essential information about their conditions, treatments, and their care. This technology uses CD-ROMs, the Internet, or Web-based kiosks and typically involves tutorials or simulations, allowing individuals to interact with the system at their own pace. Other applications useful in education are graphics packages that allow the use of clip, live, or graphic art to develop figures; and presentation packages, such as Power Point, to develop slides and overheads.

Research Applications

Whether you are conducting a literature search or an experimental study, computer applications make the work easier and faster. As previously mentioned, a number of library databases are available (e.g., CINAHL, MEDLINE). However, the HIS or community health information networks (CHIN) also can be used as a source of data for research studies. A number of statistical packages, available in both large-scale and desktop versions (e.g., SAS, SPSS), can be used to analyze data. Programs to analyze qualitative data also are available (e.g., NUDIST, ETHNO-GRAPH). Interfaces, spreadsheet packages and statistical programs facilitate data entry and analysis.

Software Selection and System Implementation

Selecting a System: The Decision-Making Process

The process of installing new systems or upgrading existing systems is complex and charged with issues of politics and protocol. Those going through this process are pioneers, who are creating the next generation of medical information systems. The goal of these efforts is to create the first truly electronic patient record that different people or groups of people can access for different purposes, at the same time, and in some cases from different sites. It will eliminate the need to ask, "Who has the patient's chart?" by presenting the patient's history in a way that is clear and understandable without requiring a person to delve into pages of narrative records. Patient information can be presented in various ways; for example, in one way for physicians and in another for nurses. Additional ways of presenting data can be developed for other care team members, such as physical therapists, occupational therapists, and dietitians.

Professionals in a hospital or clinical setting who work to develop these systems must recognize the administrative and cultural issues involved in such an undertaking. Some system interactions are less convenient for some users and better for other users. The goal is to select a system that provides the greatest good for the greatest number of people, that is, an optimal solution. The nurse manager is an integral member of the team involved in developing a new HIS for the organization; including a nurse informatics specialist is also helpful.

When decisions about information technology are made, the following key points should be considered (Adaskin, Hughes, McMullan, McLean, & McMorris, 1994; Jenkins, 1988; Mills & Staggers, 1994):

1. *Involve those who will be using the system and those affected by changes in the system.* It is essential to include representative unit clerks and staff nurses who will use the system in the planning process. If there are differences between nursing subspecialties, make sure to involve representatives from all appropriate areas.
2. *Read the literature.* There is a great deal of current literature in nursing journals, PC magazines, and specialized health care and information technology journals. Information is also available on the Internet and through seminars and forums held by vendors and health care professionals. Make use of these resources.
3. *Network with other users.* Networking with colleagues at other institutions and examining some of the systems at other places can provide invaluable information about not only how to do things but also how not to do things. An easy way to network is to attend vendor-user group meetings on a regular basis.

4. *Select easy-to-use software and systems.* Many questions should be answered: Should a mouse or a trackball be used? Is a light pen more appropriate? What size and type of monitor should I buy? At what height should the bedside terminals be mounted on the wall? An analysis of the setting, the physical and physiological impacts of the system, and other operational considerations is required to decide what types of devices to use, how screens should be designed, and how the system will be implemented. Generally, high-density screens are preferred in clinical settings, as are high-resolution monitors with dark, nonglare glass.
5. *Develop a realistic plan for implementation.* Consider the best time for implementing parts of a new system, for example, at times of the year when patient census is low. Become familiar with the system before implementation; visit other organizations that have the system already in operation. Consider also the method of implementation. Should a phased approach, where one or more pilot units are brought online with one or more functions, be used? Or might the "big bang" approach, which brings all units online at once, be more appropriate? Make reasonable attempts to stick with the plan. Assess progress along the way, and make adjustments to the schedule as necessary. Such efforts will meet with a more positive reception from all involved.
6. *Inform and train users.* It is extremely important that users of a new system know what the system is meant to accomplish. A knowledgeable staff will be more cooperative and more understanding of the need for changes. Make certain to provide user training at times convenient for those who will be required to use a new system. Other considerations, such as training facilities, reference materials, and training staff, all need to be considered when planning implementation and training programs. Current literature provides a wealth of information on training techniques.

Selecting Software One of the first decisions is whether to purchase limited-purpose or customized software. When selecting software, you have a number of factors to take into account (Menzel & McNamara, 1994): What is the market doing? What are other people buying? Does this product have a good reputation for reliability? Does this vendor have a good reputation? What is the financial stability of the

---

Box 12-2 | Common Problems in Selecting Systems and Software

Assessment
Inadequate cost investigation
Expecting computerization to solve all problems
Not involving users, especially nurses, in assessing the system needed

Planning
Trying to automate too much
Not planning an integrated system
Failing to include long-range plans, which results in extensive reprogramming
Ignoring the change process
Not considering confidentiality problems
Appointing committees that are too large
Trying to maintain all reports, forms, etc., exactly as they are in a manual system
Not considering the ergonomics of computerization

Implementation
Trying to implement too fast
Not providing role models
Failing to remember that errors show up faster
Inadequate training in breadth, depth, and time

Evaluation
Failure to plan for evaluation at the beginning
Not establishing base-line data prior to computerization that can be used for a compare–contrast evaluation
Failure to provide for continuous evaluation
Inadequate attention to qualitative evaluation in addition to quantitative evaluation

Note: From *Computers and nursing: Application to practice, education, and research* by H. C. Cox, B. Harsanyi, and L. C. Dean, 1987, Norwalk, CT: Appleton & Lange, p. 181.

---

vendor? What user support will the vendor have available? Who are some of the larger organizations using this software? Will this product easily do what we want it to do? Is it easy to learn? Is it easy to use? Is it compatible with other software and/or systems that we currently have? Does it have a reasonable life span? What continuing costs are involved? Remember that the cost of the hardware and software is only part of such an investment. Training, implementation, and even organizational stress are other, somewhat less readily quantifiable, costs to consider in the decision.

After investigating the companies and available software, solicit demonstrations. As with system selection, representative users should be involved in the selection of software packages. Common implementation problems are noted in Box 12-2.

Ethical and Social Considerations

Malicious intruders such as viruses, Trojan horse programs, and logic or time bombs are threats to the automation and integration of patient records into wide area networks. These threats have provoked a number of concerns: How can integrity of the data be maintained? What about confidentiality? Can more than

one individual access the record at the same time? Who maintains ownership of the record? Who is responsible for information in transit? Many of these questions have yet to be answered; however, a secure system should have the following characteristics (Brunner, 1993; Patrikas, 1993):

- Authorization of users
- Limited access based on the need to know
- Security at each access point

In addition, staff need to be trained not to give out passwords or leave unattended a computer that has been logged on. Many organizations require their employees to sign a statement of confidentiality regarding computer usage, such as the one shown in Figure 12-3.

The Nurse Informatics Specialist

Advances in both medicine and technology have created the need for nurses to become knowledgeable in informatics. Nursing informatics is concerned with the nature of information, its access, and the decisions involved in solving information-related problems. Several specialty graduate-level programs have been developed in nursing informatics.

System User
Confidentiality Statement

1. My computer password is my own individual, personal code for gaining access into the hospital computer system.

2. My computer password allows me to access only the information which I have been authorized to use to perform my hospital responsibilities.

3. My computer password legally acts as my personal signature when performing all computer activities and is legally binding.

4. The information I access through the independence system is confidential and is to be used only in the performance of job-related activities.

5. I am responsible for notifying my immediate supervisor in the event that my password is lost or its confidentiality has been breached, so that my supervisor may take appropriate action.

6. I am responsible for notifying my immediate supervisor should I undergo a name change so that my password can be kept accurate.

I have read the above and understand if I share my code, use someone else's code, or fail to comply with the hospital policies, I will be committing a breach of hospital policy. I understand that I must not disclose confidential information, except as such disclosure is part of the performance of duties. I further understand that such disclosure or breach of hospital policy will result in disciplinary action; possible termination of employment, as per Civil Service Act #75-2949F.

_____   _____
Date   Signature

_____   _____
Department   Witness

Figure 12-3 **Sample statement of confidentiality.** *Note:* **Provided by University of Kansas Medical Center.**

Future Trends in Informatics

Computers will continue to get smaller and more powerful, and their ability to improve patient care, manage data, assist in communication and decision making, and offer instruction—among other uses—will increase. In addition, speech-input interfaces, which will enhance mobility and time management, are being refined (Dillon, McDowell, Norcio, & De-Haemer, 1994). Computers are all around us now, and they will become more and more a part of our lives and practice in the future.

Summary

- In nursing, computers are used to care for patients, manage resources, teach, perform research, and communicate.
- Patient applications include documentation in the patient record, monitoring, and management systems.
- Nursing management systems include applications for fiscal management, employee and patient data management, staffing and scheduling, and quality improvement and utilization review.
- Selecting systems and software packages involves identifying organizational goals, evaluating the product and vendor, considering the benefits and costs, and providing for adequate training and support.
- Confidentiality, integrity, and security are major concerns associated with automated patient records. The nurse is integral to maintaining integrity of the system and patient confidentiality.
- Computer applications will continue to expand in the future, assisting nurses and nurse managers in their work.

■ LEADERSHIP AND MANAGEMENT
in Action

1. How can information technology enhance communication? Time management?
2. What types of computer technology have you used?
3. Describe the social, ethical, and legal concerns associated with computerized patient records.

References

Adaskin, E. J., Hughes, L., McMullan, P., McLean, M., & McMorris, D. (1994). The impact of computerization on nursing: An interview study of users and facilitators. *Computers in Nursing, 12*(3), 141–148.

American Nurses Association (ANA) (1997). *Telehealth— Issues for nursing.* Washington, DC: Author.

Averill, C. G., Marek, K. D., Zielstorff, R., Kneedler, J., Delaney, C., & Milholland, D. K. (1998). ANA standards for nursing data sets in information systems. *Computers in Nursing, 16*(3), 157–161.

Brunner, B. K. (1993). Health care-oriented telecommunications: The wave of the future. *Topics in Health Information Management, 14*(1), 54–61.

Cox, H. C., Harsanyi, B., & Dean, L. C. (1987). *Computers and nursing: Application to practice, education and research.* Norwalk, CT: Appleton & Lange.

Dillon, T. W., McDowell, D., Norcio, A. F., & DeHaemer, M. J. (1994). Nursing acceptance of a speech-input interface: A preliminary investigation. *Computers in Nursing, 12*(6), 264–271.

Fonteyn, M. E., & Grobe, S. J. (1994). Expert system development in nursing: Implications for critical care nursing practice. *Heart & Lung, 23,* 80–87.

Gross, M. S., Hoehn, B. J., & Rooks, C. S. (1993). Clinical information systems: Why now. *Topics in Health Information Management, 14*(1), 1–11.

Jenkins, S. (1988). Nurses' responsibilities in implementation of information systems. In M. J. Ball, K. J. Hannah, U. G. Jelger, & H. Peterson (Eds.), *Nursing informatics: Where caring and technology meet.* New York: Springer-Verlag.

Manning, J., & McConnell, E. A. (1997). Technology assessment: A framework for generating questions useful in evaluating nursing information systems. *Computers in Nursing, 15*(3), 141–146.

Menzel, N. N., & McNamara, J. K. (1994). Occupational health software: Selecting the right program. *AAOHN Journal, 24*(2), 76–81.

Mills, M. E., & Staggers, N. (1994). Nurse-computer performance: Considerations for the nurse administrator. *Journal of Nursing Administration, 24*(11), 30–35.

National Council of State Boards of Nursing [NCSBN] (1996). Telenursing: The regulatory implications for multistate regulation. *Issues, 17*(3), 1–4.

Patrikas, E. O. (1993). Electronic databases and privacy protection: Issues for a free society. *Topics in Health Information Management, 14*(1), 62–68.

Potempa, K., Stanley, J., Davis, B., Miller, K. L., Hasset, M. R., & Pepicello, S. (2001). Survey of distance technology utilization in AACN member schools. *Journal of Professional Nursing, 17*(1), 7–15.

Simpson, R. L. (1994). Taking the future on the CHIN. *Nursing Management, 25*(12), 32.

Thede, L. Q., Taft, S., & Coeling, H. (1994). Computer-assisted instruction: A learner's viewpoint. *Journal of Nursing Education, 33,* 299–305.

Werley, H. H., Devine, E. C., & Zorn, C. R. (1988). The nursing minimum data set: Effort to standardize collection of essential nursing data. In M. J. Ball, K. J. Hannah, U. G. Jelger, & H. Peterson (Eds.), *Nursing informatics: Where caring and technology meet.* New York: Springer-Verlag.

Zielstorff, R. D., McHugh, M. L., & Clinton, J. (1988). *Computer design criteria.* Kansas City, MO: American Nurses Association.

 Additional on-line resources for this chapter can be found on the World Wide Web at http://www.prenhall.com/sullivan_decker. Select Chapter 12 from the drop-down menu.

Stress and Time Management

The Nature of Stress

Causes of Stress
Role Conflict and Role Ambiguity
Consequences of Stress

Managing Stress

Personal Methods
Organizational Methods

Time Management

Goal Setting
Delegation
Time Analysis
Setting Priorities
Daily Planning and Scheduling
Grouping Activities and
    Minimizing Routine Work
Implementation
Personal Organization and
    Self-Discipline
Controlling Interruptions
Paperwork
Respecting Time

Looking Ahead

Do you ever feel as if there aren't enough hours in a day for the work you need to do? We all know how it feels to be stressed and not have enough time to get things done. How do we deal with the constant demands of our environment? Learning to cope with stress and manage time wisely is important to becoming an effective leader and manager. This chapter contains proven strategies to help you identify and manage stress so you can plan and accomplish the endless number of tasks and goals you want to accomplish.

Objectives

After reading this chapter, you will be able to:

- Delineate factors that cause stress.
- Describe the consequences of stress.
- Identify both personal and organizational methods for managing stress.
- Discuss the importance of identifying goals and setting priorities.
- Identify time wasters and describe how to minimize them.

Consider the following scenario. Sue is a medical nurse with 10 years of experience. She is married and has two children under the age of six who attend preschool while Sue is at work. As a nurse manager, Sue has 24-hour responsibility for supervision of two 30-bed medical units. She frequently receives calls from the unit nurses during the evenings and nights, and approximately once a week she has to return to the unit to intervene in a situation or to replace nurses who are absent. Sue is responsible for scheduling all nurses on her unit and has no approval to use agency nurses, in spite of a 20% vacancy rate. In addition, Sue serves on four departmental committees and the hospital task force on consumer relations. She consistently takes work home, including performance appraisals, quality assessment reports, and professional journals. Although provided with an office, Sue has little opportunity to use it because of constant interruptions from nurses, physicians, other departmental leaders, and her clinical director. Recently, Sue saw her family physician, complaining of persistent headaches, weight loss, and a feeling of constant fatigue. After a complete diagnostic workup, Sue was found to have a slightly elevated blood pressure, with a resting pulse of 100. Her physician prescribed an exercise program, and she was advised to lighten her workload, take a vacation, and reduce her stress level.

Steers (1984) defines **stress** as the nonspecific reaction that people have to demands that pose a threat from the environment. Stress results when two or more incompatible demands on the body cause a conflict. Selye (1978), recognized as the pioneer of stress research, suggests that the body's wear and tear results from its response to normal stressors. The rate and intensity of damage increase when an organism experiences greater stress than it is capable of accommodating.

Selye maintains that the physiological response to stress is the same whether the stressor is positive, *enstress*, or negative, *distress*. It is easy to see how negative events, such as job loss, can cause stress. However, positive events also may cause stress. For example, John was the director of nursing for critical care in a 400-bed hospital. He was offered the opportunity to develop a hyperbaric unit. In assuming the additional responsibility, John began putting in long hours and working weekends. As the project progressed, John became unable to sleep and gained 10 pounds. After the unit opened, John's sleep pattern and weight returned to normal. Clearly, John displayed emotional and physical signs of stress although he was experiencing a "positive" promotion and career opportunity.

A certain amount of stress is essential to sustain life, and moderate amounts serve as stimuli to performance, but overpowering stress can cause a person to respond in a maladaptive physiological or psychological manner.

This chapter describes the causes and consequences of stress and proposes several techniques for managing stress. In addition, the chapter provides guidelines to help you use time effectively.

The Nature of Stress

There must be a balance between stress and the capability to handle it. When the degree of stress is equal to the degree of ability to accommodate it, the organism is in a state of equilibrium. Normal wear and tear occur, but sustained damage does not. When the degree of stress is greater than the available coping mechanism, the individual experiences negative aspects of stress. The situation is often described metaphorically through such statements as "carrying a load on one's shoulders" or "bearing a heavy burden." This often leads to physiological and psychological problems for the person and poor performance for the organization. When the degree of stress is not stimulating enough, lack of interest, apathy, boredom, low motivation, and even poor performance can result.

The experience of stress is subjective and individualized. One person's stressful event is another's challenge. One individual can experience an event, positive or negative, that would prove overwhelming for someone else. Even a minor change in organizational policy may cause some individuals to experience stress, whereas others welcome it. Some nurses seem to thrive on the demands of work, family, school, and community involvement, whereas others find even minimal changes in their expectations a source of great discomfort. In the current health care environment, where constant change is the norm, some nurse managers may choose a less demanding position because they find the stress level too high in their current position.

For nurses, stress in the workplace can develop from several sources and may be due to organizational, interpersonal, or individual (intrapersonal) factors.

Causes of Stress

Organizational Factors   Stress can result from job-related factors, such as task overload, conflicting tasks, inability to do the tasks assigned because of lack of preparation or experience, and unclear or insufficient information regarding the assignment. Nurses' jobs are often performed in life-or-death situations; emergencies may cause periods of extreme overload.

The physical environment may also be stressful. Consider the intensive care unit with its constant alarms, beeps, and other noises. Besides noise levels, lighting and other comfort factors may increase stress within the environment. Tight quarters, poorly organized work environments, and lack of equipment also augment stress levels.

The manager's behavior also can be a factor in stress. Authoritarian or punitive supervisory behavior is closely related to stress levels. Participative management, in contrast, reduces job stress (Porter-O'Grady, 1986).

Other organizational factors that can lead to stress include organizational norms and expectations that conflict with an individual's needs. Understaffing and high vacancy levels have historically been seen as stress-producing; more recently, job insecurity due to organizational restructuring has added substantially to the stress of both managers and staff. Managers trying to do more with less, staff working with unlicensed assistive personnel, and more acutely ill patients can lead to an organizational environment that by its very nature is stressful.

Managed care, cost containment, the creation of integrated organizations, and downsizing are creating dramatic changes in health care that are contributing to stress in nursing. New technology, increased expectations from patients and their families, liability concerns, and competition among health care providers (and the increased pressures for efficiency that are associated with it) have made the role of nurses more difficult, conflicting, and stressful.

Interpersonal Factors   To add to the pressures created by organizational changes, nurses must contend with strained interpersonal relationships within the nursing profession and between nursing and other professions (e.g., medicine, administration). Relationships are strained even further as pressures mount. Shorter lengths of stay for patients, supervision of assistive personnel, job redesign, and case management challenge relationships among nursing care providers.

Interdisciplinary difficulties may precipitate tension. For example, in one rehabilitation setting, therapists expect the patients to be bathed, to have eaten breakfast, and to be dressed and ready to start therapy by 8:30 A.M. This expectation places undue stress on rehabilitation nurses, who must motivate patients who complain that they have had far too little sleep. Another example of stress due to interdisciplinary conflict is: A radiology technician responds to a 9:00 P.M. page for a chest x-ray examination and informs the registered nurse that the patient will have to be brought back down because the radiology department is understaffed.

Interactions between physicians and nurses often are not characterized by open communication. Most nurses have experienced an irate response from a physician who is awakened during the night for something the physician thinks should have been handled earlier or might have waited until morning. In one small community hospital, an internist was well known for his outbursts during middle-of-the-night calls. One experienced nurse dealt with necessary calls to him by directly stating when he answered the phone, "This is Jane Jones from St. Matthew's. I have two important things to tell you about Mrs. Smith. . . ." This helped the internist focus on the problem at hand and reduced his outbursts.

The need to fulfill multiple roles is another source of stress. A **role** is a set of expectations about behavior ascribed to a specific position in society (e.g., nurse, mother, husband). Nurses perform a number of roles that often include spouse and parent. Conflict between family roles and professional ones results in stress. Adding to stress is the shift and weekend work required in most nursing jobs. Inpatient organizations must be staffed 24 hours a day, 7 days a week. Nurses who work on evening or night shifts may experience family problems if their spouse and children are on different schedules, especially if the nurse rotates shifts. Studies have demonstrated that it takes several weeks to adjust physiologically to a change in shifts (Levi, 1981); however, most rotation patterns require nurses to change shifts several times a month. Managers can reduce the physiological pressure through ensuring that nurses receive adequate rest and work breaks, rotating staff only between two shifts, and never scheduling "double backs" (working 8 hours, off 8 hours, working 8 hours).

> ### KEY TERMS
>
> *Role*   A set of expectations about behavior ascribed to a specific position.

Instructions: Listed below are various kinds of problems that may—or may not—arise in your work. Indicate to what extent you find each of them to be a problem or concern.

Factor	Responses				
This factor is a problem	Never	Seldom	Sometimes	Usually	Always
Physical environment					
1. Feeling you are too hot or too cold.	1	2	3	4	5
2. Thinking there is a good chance of being seriously injured on the job.	1	2	3	4	5
3. Thinking there is a real possibility of getting some disease from this job.	1	2	3	4	5
Role conflict					
4. Feeling you must do things you personally feel to be unethical.	1	2	3	4	5
5. Having a boss who keeps assigning different tasks with too little time to complete them.	1	2	3	4	5
6. Receiving too many incompatible pressures from too many people.	1	2	3	4	5
Role ambiguity					
7. Not knowing what the people you work with expect you to accomplish.	1	2	3	4	5
8. Being unclear about how you are to perform the tasks in your job.	1	2	3	4	5
9. Not knowing how your manager evaluates your performance.	1	2	3	4	5

Figure 13-1 Stress diagnostic survey. *Note:* From *Management,* 5th ed., by D. Hellreigel and J. W. Slocum, 1989, Reading, MA: Addison-Wesley.

Individual Factors　　Stress can result from personal factors as well. One of these factors is the rate of life change. Changes throughout life, such as marriage, pregnancy, or purchasing a new home, generate stress. Each individual responds to stress differently, but the cumulative effects of stress often lead to the onset of disease or illness (Holmes & Rahe, 1967). The questionnaire in Figure 13-1 can be used to evaluate personal sources of stress.

The ways people interpret events ultimately determine whether the person sees the event as stressful or as a positive challenge.

Deficiency focusing is the habit of focusing on the negatives at the expense of the positives. There is a tendency to exaggerate weaknesses and disregard strengths. Deficiency focusing can lead to an increased sense of threat and a diminished sense of optimism, immobilizing individuals and limiting their ability to solve problems. They become so overwhelmed with what might go wrong that they don't look at options and opportunities that also are present. As resources in health care continue to shrink, nurses are being asked or told to assume responsibility for tasks that had been performed by other departments (i.e., phlebotomy, electrocardiography, respiratory therapy). Nurses can see these responsibilities as an overwhelming amount of work that can't possibly be accomplished given the existing number of staff, or as work that is not appropriate for nurses to do. But if nurses approach the task as a means to improve continuity of care or deliver patient-focused care, they can focus energy on skills in which nurses excel: managing patient care.

Necessitating is the belief that it is imperative or necessary that a particular task be done by a specific person; it is a belief structure that limits choice. Tasks become inflexible demands that must be met. Nurses are especially prone to this type of thinking. Many nurse managers continue to believe that it is necessary to be as clinically competent as their staff. There are many tasks that nursing staff believe only nurses can do. Then, as patient care loads become heavier, their stress level increases. Nurse managers must begin to question old ways of thinking and to evaluate what tasks should belong to the nursing profession in the future. Core competencies for nurse managers include a different set of managerial skills (e.g., facilitation, negotiation, team-building), not excelling at clinical skills. By continually questioning whether the usual activity continues to be appropriate, both the manager and members of the staff can reduce stress.

Low skill recognition is perhaps the least stress-producing of the three habits but may be the one that needs the most attention in an unstable and unpredictable environment. Low skill recognition is a tendency not to recognize the role one's own ability has played in producing one's successes; it affects both managers and staff nurses when they face something unfamiliar. For example, new graduates often do not recognize that they have demonstrated a definitive set of skills and knowledge in having passed all the requirements to become a registered nurse. The stress they experience when changing from the student role to the professional practitioner role has been labeled **reality shock**. It is the surprise and disequilibrium experienced when moving from the familiar school culture to the work culture, where values, rewards, and sanctions are different and often seem illogical. Moving from a staff nurse position to a management position also creates surprise and disequilibrium. The reward structure is totally different for managers. New managers often experience a sense of isolation from the peer group of staff nurses who previously provided support. In each of these cases, the individual often questions her or his abilities to make the transition to the new role. Therefore, low skill recognition is not to be overlooked as a key element in developing stress resiliency.

Stress can also result from incongruence between one's expectations for performance and one's perception of the resulting performance (**intrarole conflict**). Similarly, conflict between the roles of nurse manager and nurse can be a source of stress (**interrole conflict**). Doing a job and directing others to do the job are different. Directing others is stressful, and a person may be tempted to believe that it will be faster to complete a task by doing it herself or himself.

Past experience in coping with stress provides insight into an individual's ability for successful coping in current experiences. People tend to repeat coping behaviors in similar situations, regardless of whether the initial behavior reduced stress.

One's self-esteem also affects coping. Individuals with low self-esteem often have difficulty coping with role conflict and role ambiguity. **Role ambiguity** results from unclear expectations for one's performance. Individuals with high tolerances for ambiguity can deal better with the strains that come from uncertainties and, therefore, are likely to be able to cope with role ambiguity.

Certain personality traits either positively or negatively influence one's responses to stress. Individuals who believe that their life is controlled largely by events external to themselves often perceive less stress and are less likely to react negatively to surrounding events. However, those who perceive factors as being internal react more negatively to situations that are beyond their control. They are more likely to be proactive to situations within their control and engage in positive coping behaviors to change the environment and reduce stresses on themselves (Lazarus & Folkman, 1984).

Role Conflict and Role Ambiguity

Role conflicts occur when an individual has two competing roles, such as when a nurse manager both assumes a patient care assignment and needs to attend a leadership meeting. Another example is the conflict between nurses' personal roles as parents or spouses versus their roles as professional nurses.

Individual role conflict is the result of incompatibility between the individual's perception of the role and its actual requirements. Novice nurse managers experience this type of conflict when they find that administration expects primary loyalty to the organization and its goals, whereas the staff expects the nurse manager's first loyalty to be to their needs.

Role conflict within the profession places nursing at a distinct disadvantage in its relationship with other health care workers. Strife within the profession, differences in educational preparation, the structure of

KEY TERMS

Reality shock   The stress, surprise, and disequilibrium experienced when shifting from a familiar culture into one whose values, rewards, and sanctions are different (e.g., from school culture to work culture).

Intrarole conflict   Conflict resulting from incongruence between one's expectations for performance and one's perception of the resulting performance.

Interrole conflict   Conflict resulting from incongruence between the different roles an individual might play, such as doing a job and directing others to do the job.

Role ambiguity   The frustrations that result from unclear expectations for one's performance.

Burnout   The perception that an individual has used up all available energy to perform the job and feels that he or she doesn't have enough energy to complete the task.

practice settings, and the role of labor and professional organizations contribute to the environment in which nurses must function. This conflict has its roots in a perceived poor regard for nurses. The felt lack of worth is complicated by divisiveness within the profession and the image nursing presents to others.

Role underload and *underutilization* can also occur. Being underutilized or not having much responsibility may be seen as stressful by a person who is a high achiever or who has high self-esteem.

Consequences of Stress

What happens to a person when stress overload occurs? Both physiological and psychological responses can cause structural or functional changes or both. Warning signs of too much stress are (a) undue, prolonged anxiety, phobias, or a persistent state of fear or free-floating anxiety that seems to have many alternating causes; (b) depression, which causes people to withdraw from family and friends, to be unable to experience emotions, and to feel helpless to change the situation; (c) abrupt changes in mood and behavior, which may be exhibited as erratic behavior; (d) perfectionism, which is the setting of unreasonably high standards for oneself and thereby being under

constant stress; and (e) physical illnesses, such as a peptic ulcer, arthritis, colitis, hypertension, myocardial infarction, and migraine headaches.

Ineffective coping methods for reducing stress include excessive use of alcohol and other mood-altering substances, which can result in substance abuse or dependence. Some people become workaholics in an attempt to cope with real or imagined demands. The term **burnout** refers to the perception that an individual has used up all available energy to perform the job and feels that he or she doesn't have enough energy to complete the task. Burnout is a combination of physical fatigue, emotional exhaustion and cognitive weariness, (Kushnir, Rabin, & Azulai, 1997). As a result, the individual may reduce hours worked or change to another profession. One director of nursing at a 120-bed nursing home stated that she could no longer handle the overwhelming needs of the patients; the ever-present shortage of qualified, caring nurses; and consistently dwindling resources. When a for-profit chain purchased the home and further reduced economic resources, the director of nursing left and went back to college to become a court reporter.

The results of employee stress are increased absenteeism and turnover. Although there are various causes of absenteeism (see Chapter 21) and turnover (see Chapter 18), both may result when the individual attempts to withdraw from a stressful situation.

Job performance suffers during times of high stress, so much energy and attention are needed to manage the stress that little energy is available for performance. Such a situation is financially costly in industry but even more costly in human health and well-being.

Managing Stress

There will always be factors in our lives that create stress. To manage those factors effectively and keep stress at levels that enhance one's performance rather than deplete energy, the key is to develop some resiliency. To accomplish this requires a comprehensive approach to managing stress, which involves planning, time, and energy.

Personal Methods

One of the first steps in managing stress is to recognize stressors in the environment and control them. Nurses tend to think they can be "all things to all people." Therefore, it is important to improve one's self-awareness regarding stressors.

Caring for yourself physically (e.g., eating a well-balanced diet, exercising regularly, getting adequate sleep) and developing effective mental habits are also important for coping with stress. These effective habits include role redefinition, improved time-management techniques, and relaxation. Development of interpersonal skills and identifying and nurturing social supports can also facilitate stress management (Kivisto & Couture, 1997).

Role redefinition involves clarifying roles and attempting to integrate or tie together the various roles individuals play. If there is role conflict or ambiguity, it is important to confront others by pointing out conflicting messages. Role redefinition may also involve renegotiation of roles in an attempt to lessen overload.

Much of the stress nurse managers experience results from the perception that staff, patient, and work-group needs must be met immediately and simultaneously. A common feeling is the need to slow down or "get off the train." A notable method of coping with and reducing the stress of time is through time management. We determine how, where, and when our time is used. In the words of Benjamin Franklin (Bliss, 1976), "Time is the stuff of which life is made." Time is the essence of living, and it is the scarcest resource. Because the nurse manager has a limited amount of time, it is essential that time be used expeditiously. One lost hour a day every day for a year results in 260 hours of waste, or 6.5 weeks of missed opportunity, annually. (Time management is discussed later in the chapter.)

It also is important to use positive self-talk and to learn how to relax. This is not easy, especially for an individual with a high-stress job. Some relaxation methods are listening to music, reading, and socializing with friends. Developing outside interests, such as hobbies and recreational activities, can provide diversion and enjoyment and also can be a source of relaxation. Taking regular vacations, regardless of job pressures, is important for renewal and revitalization.

Palliative coping methods, such as overeating, smoking, and drinking alcohol, are ineffective and should be replaced by effective methods (Kivisto & Couture, 1997).

Organizational Methods

Nurse managers are often in the position of helping others identify their level of stress and stressors. If staff appear to be under a great deal of stress, the manager must help identify the source(s) and decide

> **KEY TERMS**
>
> *Role redefinition*   The clarification of roles and an attempt to integrate or tie together the various roles individuals play.
>
> *Time waster*   Something that prevents a person from accomplishing a job or achieving a goal.
>
> *Goals*   Specific statements of achievement that provide direction; in an organization, goals follow the mission and vision.

how these can be reduced or eliminated. In addition to suggesting the techniques previously delineated, the manager should explore work-related sources of stress. The manager must ask, Is role ambiguity or conflict creating the stress? Can the manager help clarify individual staff members' roles, thereby reducing the conflict or ambiguity? Is the manager using an appropriate leadership style? (See Chapter 4.) Does the manager need to clarify a staff member's goals and eliminate barriers that are interfering with goal attainment? Involving staff in decision making is one way to identify and reduce such stress. Is the stress due to feelings of low self-worth? Would additional training or education help reduce the stress? Can the staff person be positively reinforced? Can other sources of support, such as the work group, help the individual deal with stress? Are counseling services available in the organization?

When stress is job-related, several strategies can be used. First, proper matching of the job with the applicant during the selection and hiring process is an important step in reducing stress. (See Chapter 17.) Skills training also reduces stress and promotes better performance and less turnover. (See Chapter 20.) Developing a program of job enrichment matched to the individual's goals and desires often increases autonomy and participation. In turn, greater participation in decisions increases job commitment and reduces stress.

Communication and social support are additional factors in reducing stress. Both upward and downward communication channels should be open. Keeping personnel informed about what is going on in an organization helps reduce suspicion and rumor. Team building encourages staff to build a network of support with each other.

Policies that reduce the stress of shift work also are important. The number of hours in the night shift,

---

Box 13-1   Potential Constraints on the Ability to Manage Time Effectively

- We do what we like to do before we do what we don't like to do.
- We do things we know how to do faster than things we do not know how to do.
- We do things that are easiest before things that are difficult.
- We do things that require a little time before things that require a lot of time.
- We do things for which resources are available.
- We do things that are scheduled (for example, meetings) before nonscheduled things.
- We sometimes do things that are planned before things that are unplanned.
- We respond to demands from others before demands from ourselves.
- We do things that are urgent before things that are important.

- We readily respond to crises and emergencies.
- We do interesting things before uninteresting things.
- We do things that advance our personal objectives or that are politically expedient.
- We wait until a deadline approaches before we really get moving.
- We do things that provide the most immediate closure.
- We respond on the basis of who wants it.
- We respond on the basis of the consequences to us of doing or not doing something.
- We tackle small jobs before large jobs.
- We work on things in the order of their arrival.
- We work on the basis of the squeaky-wheel principle (the squeaky wheel gets the grease).
- We work on the basis of consequences to the group.

---

weekend, and holiday work assignments also can reduce stress. Providing adequate opportunities for breaks and meals is an important function of the organization. (See Chapter 21 for more about how to help employees with stress-related problems.)

Time Management

Time management is a misnomer. No one manages time: What is managed is how time is used. Box 13-1 shows some of the constraints on an individual's ability to manage time effectively. These patterns of behavior must be understood and dealt with to achieve effective time management.

In addition to these patterns of behavior, certain time wasters prevent the nurse manager from effectively managing time. A **time waster** is something that prevents a person from accomplishing the job or achieving the goal. Common time wasters include:

1. Interruptions, such as telephone calls and drop-in visitors
2. Meetings, both scheduled and unscheduled
3. Lack of clear-cut goals, objectives, and priorities
4. Lack of daily and/or weekly plans
5. Lack of personal organization and self-discipline
6. Lack of knowledge about how one spends one's time

7. Failure to delegate, working on routine tasks
8. Ineffective communication
9. Waiting for others, not using transition time effectively
10. Inability to say no

Techniques to deal with these time-management constraints and time wasters are discussed in detail later in the chapter. The basic principles of time management are summarized in Table 13-1.

Goal Setting

Nurses are accustomed to setting both long- and short-range **goals**, although typically such goals are stated in terms of what patients will accomplish rather than what the nurse will achieve. A critical component of time management is establishing one's own goals and time frames. Goals provide direction and vision for actions as well as a timeline in which activities will be accomplished. Defining goals and time frames helps reduce stress by preventing the panic people often feel when confronted with multiple demands. Although time frames may not be as fast as the nurse manager would like (the tendency is to expect change yesterday), necessary actions have been identified.

Individual or organizational goals encourage thinking about the future and what might happen.

Table 13-1	Principles of Time Management

Principle	Discussion/Illustration
Goal setting	Annual determination of unit, department, and organizational goals. The nurse manager also sets long- and short-range personal goals.
Time analysis	Conducting a survey of the way the nurse manager spends the day, in 30- to 60-minute increments. Reviewing the daily schedule and keeping it accurate may demonstrate how time is used. A schedule with no "available" time is as problematic as one in which all time is "available."
Priority determination	Time frames for achievement of goals are identified by the nurse manager. The "to-do" list should be prioritized, by classifying activities as "A" or "1" for urgent, "B" or "2" for nonurgent but important, and "C" or "3" for nonurgent, less important.
Daily planning	To-do lists and scheduling constitute the bulk of daily planning devices.
Delegation	A variety of activities may be delegated by the nurse manager. For example, the nurse manager may delegate responsibility for the quality assurance program.
Interruption control	Identify causes of interruptions and plan to reduce them. The nurse manager might find that consistent interruptions come from a particular physician. To keep this from being an interruption, meeting with the physician could become a planned and scheduled activity, with an alternative time identified for office work.
Evaluation	The nurse manager should make at least a weekly assessment of how effectively time has been used. A good time to complete this review is while identifying priorities for the next week.

Note: Copyright © 1971, by The Regents of the University of California. Reprinted from the *California Management Review,* Vol. 14, No. 2. By permission of The Regents.

Goal setting helps to relate current behavior, activities, or operations to the organization's or individual's long-range goals. Without this future orientation, activities may not lead to the outcomes that will help achieve the goals and meet the ideals of the individual or organization. The focus should be to develop measurable, realistic, and achievable goals. Specific goal setting is discussed more extensively in Chapter 19.

It is useful to think of individual or personal goals in categories, as shown in Table 13-2. This partial listing is a guide to stimulate thinking about goals. In considering individual goals, nurses should think about long-term goals, lifetime goals, and short-term goals. These should be divided into job-related goals and personal goals. Job-related goals may revolve around unit or departmental changes, whereas personal goals may include personal life and community involvement.

Short-term goals should be set for the next 6 to 12 months but need to be related to long-term goals. To manage time effectively, the nurse manager must answer five major questions about these goals:

1. What specific objectives are to be achieved?
2. What specific activities are necessary to achieve these objectives?
3. How much time is required for each activity?

4. Which activities can be planned and scheduled for concurrent action, and which must be planned and scheduled sequentially?
5. Which activities can be delegated to staff?

Delegation

Delegating tasks to others can be an efficient time-management tool. **Delegation** involves assigning tasks, determining expected results, and granting authority to the individual expected to accomplish these tasks. Delegation is perhaps the most difficult leadership skill for nurses to acquire. Today, when more and more assistive personnel are being used to carry out the nurse's work, appropriate delegation and supervisory skills are essential for success. Chapter 14 discusses delegation in detail.

Time Analysis

The first step in time analysis is to identify how time is being used. The second is to determine whether time use is appropriate to the manager's role. Nurse managers find much of their time is taken up doing things that seem to be "busy work" rather than activities that contribute to a particular outcome. In job redesign, there is a stronger emphasis on ensuring that

Table 13-2 Individual Goals

Goal Category	Examples
Department accomplishments	To become involved in one hospital-wide task force by second quarter.
Interpersonal relationships	To develop a solid working relationship with the chief financial officer by third quarter.
Professional growth	To publish one article in a refereed journal by fourth quarter.
Education/personal growth	To complete one continuing education course in human resources by third quarter.
Financial security	To identify financial plan for graduate school by second quarter.
Status	To become a member of the school board of directors by fourth quarter.
Family/personal relations	To remember all birthdays and significant events.
Use of free time	To visit Hawaii by fourth quarter.
Physical well-being	To lose 20 pounds by fourth quarter.
Lifestyle	To work no more than 45 hours a week and no more than one weekend day a month.
Social commitment	To join the Sierra Club by first quarter.
Spiritual growth	To become a member of the church attended by third quarter.

Note: Adapted from *Management: An experimental approach* by H. Knudson, R. Woodworth, and C. Bell, 1973, New York: McGraw-Hill; and *Power and influence* by J. Kotter, 1985, New York: Free Press.

time is spent wisely and that the right individual is correctly assigned the responsibility for tasks.

Time logs, typically kept in intervals of 30 to 60 minutes, are useful in analyzing the actual time spent on various activities. These logs can be reviewed to determine which activities are essential to the nurse manager's job and which activities can be delegated to others or eliminated. Instead of a separate log, the nurse manager's schedule book also may be used to review patterns of time use.

A significant difficulty in moving from a staff nurse position to a leadership position is the need to develop different time-management and organizational skills. In a staff nurse role, the registered nurse has little, if any, free or uncommitted time. Almost every minute

of the shift is assigned to a task. For example, at 6:45 A.M., report is taken; at 7:00 A.M., insulin is administered; at 7:15 A.M., breakfast trays are distributed; from 8:00 A.M. to 10:30 A.M., morning care is administered; and so on. No planning is required, because every minute is taken. In contrast, when the nurse moves to a leadership position, she or he is responsible for defining how time will be spent. Learning to focus on priorities and evaluating time use is an important part of the analysis.

Setting Priorities

Nurse managers should establish priorities, taking into consideration both short- and long-term goals as well as the importance and urgency of each activity. Table 13-3 illustrates examples of five types of activities. Activities can be identified as (a) urgent and important, (b) important but not urgent, (c) urgent but not important, (d) busy work, or (e) wasted time. Activities that are both urgent and important, such as the example described in Table 13-3, must be completed. Activities that are important but not urgent may be those that make the difference between career progression or maintaining the status quo. Urgent but not important activities must be completed immediately but are not considered important or significant. Busy work and wasted time are self-explanatory.

KEY TERMS

Goal setting The relating of current behavior, activities, or operations to the organization's or individual's long-range goals.

Delegation A time-management tool that involves assigning tasks, determining expected results, and transferring responsibility to another individual.

Time logs Journals of activities that are useful in analyzing actual time spent on specific activities.

Table 13-3	Importance-Urgency Chart

Category of Time Use	Examples
Important and urgent	Replacing two call-offs and ensuring sufficient staffing for the upcoming shift.
Important, not urgent	Drafting an educational program for nurses on the changes in Medicare reimbursement.
Urgent, not important	Completing and submitting the "beds available" list for a disaster drill.
Busy work	Compiling new charts for future patient admissions.
Wasted time	Sitting by the phone waiting for return calls.

Daily Planning and Scheduling

Once goals and priorities have been established, the nurse manager can concentrate on scheduling activities. A **to-do list** should be prepared each day, either after work hours the previous day or early before work on the same day. The list is typically planned by workday or work week. Because nurse managers combine many responsibilities, a weekly to-do list may be more effective. Flexibility must be a major consideration in this plan; some time should remain uncommitted to allow the manager to deal with emergencies and crises that are sure to happen. The focus is not on activities and events, but rather on the outcomes that can be achieved in the time available.

A system to keep track of regularly scheduled meetings (staff meetings), regular events (annual or quarterly report due dates), and appointments is also necessary. This system should be used when establishing the to-do list; it should include both a calendar and files. The calendar might include information on the purpose of the meeting, who will be attending, and the time and place. Several commercial planning systems are available, including Franklin Day Planner®, Day Runner®, Day Timer®, and Filofax®. A number of computer software packages for desk-top or hand-held computers (e.g., PalmPilot®) are also available. Any such system includes a daily, weekly, or monthly calendar; a to-do section; a memo or note section; and an address component. An additional consideration is to have a calendar that is small enough to be taken to meetings or home. Files are maintained on the correspondence or reports related to the meeting. These files can be arranged by date so that they are readily retrievable when needed.

Grouping Activities and Minimizing Routine Work

Work items that are similar in nature and require similar environmental surroundings and resources for their accomplishment should be grouped within divisions of the work shift. Set aside blocks of uninterrupted time for the really important tasks, such as preparing the budget. Routine tasks, especially those that are not important or urgent and contribute little to overall objectives, should be minimized. If you insist on doing them, group them together and do them in your least productive time. List a few 5- to 10-minute discretionary tasks. This helps to use the small bits of time that become available.

Much time is spent in transition or waiting. Using time effectively can increase the time available. Commuting time can be used for self-development or planning work activities. We all have to wait sometimes; waiting for a meeting to start or waiting to talk to someone are just two examples. Bring along materials to read or work on in case you are kept waiting. View waiting or transition time as an opportunity.

If you are having difficulty completing important tasks and are highly stressed, doing routine tasks for a while often helps to reduce stress. Pick a task that can be successfully completed and save it for the end of the day. Reaching closure on even a routine task at the end of the day can reduce the sense of overload and stress.

Implementation

Implementation of the daily plan and daily follow-up is essential to time management. In addition, you should repeat your time analysis at least semiannually to see how well you are managing your time, whether the job or the environment has changed, and which requires changes in planning activities. This can help prevent reverting to poor time-management habits.

Personal Organization and Self-Discipline

Some other time wasters are lack of personal organization and self-discipline, including the inability to say no, waiting for others, and excessive or ineffective paperwork. Effective personal organization results from clearly defined priorities based on well-defined, measurable, and achievable objectives. Because the nurse manager does not work alone, priorities and objectives are often related to those of many professionals, as well as to objectives of patients and their families. How time is used is often a matter of resolving conflicts among competing needs. It is easy for the nurse manager to become overloaded with responsibilities and with more to do than should be expected in the time available. This is typical. There is never sufficient time for all the activities, situations, and events in which one might like to become involved. To be effective, the nurse manager must be personally well organized and possess self-discipline. This often includes the ability to say no. Taking on too much work can lead to overload and stress. Being realistic about the amount of work to which you commit is an indication of effective time management. If a superior is overloading you, make sure the person understands the consequences of additional assignments. Be assertive in communicating your own needs to others.

A cluttered desk, working on too many tasks at one time, and failing to set aside blocks of uninterrupted time to do important tasks also indicate a lack of personal self-discipline. Clean your desk, get out the materials you need to complete your highest-priority task, and start working on it immediately. Focus on one task at a time, making sure to start with a high-priority task.

Controlling Interruptions

An interruption occurs any time the nurse manager is stopped in the middle of one activity to give attention to something else. Interruptions can be an essential part of the nurse manager's job, or they can be a time waster. An interruption that is more important and urgent than the activity in which the nurse manager is involved is a positive interruption; it deserves immediate attention. An emergency or crisis, for instance, may cause the nurse manager to interrupt daily rounds.

Some interruptions interfere with achieving the nurse manager's job and are less important and urgent than current activities. As the nurse manager's role expands to a broader span of responsibility, more decision making is placed on the staff nurse. When a manager is interrupted to solve problems within the staff nurse's scope of accountability, the manager should not become responsible for solving the problem. Gently but firmly directing the individual to search for solutions begins to break old patterns of behavior and helps develop individual responsibility. Although time-consuming in the beginning, this practice eventually reduces the number of unnecessary interruptions.

Keeping an **interruption log** on an occasional basis may help. The log should show who interrupted, the nature of the interruption, when it occurred, how long it lasted, what topics were discussed, the importance of the topics, and time-saving actions to be taken. Analysis of these data may identify patterns that the nurse manager can use to plan ways to reduce the frequency and duration of interruptions. These patterns may indicate that certain staff members are the most frequent interrupters and require individual attention to develop problem-solving skills.

Telephone Calls Telephone calls are a major source of interruption, and the interruption log will provide considerable insight for the nurse manager regarding the nature of telephone calls received. Although it is not possible to function today without a telephone, some people do not use the telephone effectively. A ringing telephone is highly compelling; few people can allow it to go unanswered. Nurse managers receive many telephone calls, some of them time wasters. Handling telephone calls effectively is a must:

- Minimize socializing and small talk. If you answer the phone with, "Hello, what can I do for you?" rather than, "Hello, how are you?" the caller is encouraged to get to business first. Be warm, friendly, and courteous, but do not allow others to waste time with inappropriate or extensive small talk. Calls placed and returned just prior to lunchtime, at the end of the day, and on Friday afternoons tend to result in more business and less socializing.
- Plan calls. The manager who plans telephone calls does not waste anyone's time, including that of the person called. Write down topics to be discussed before making the call. This prevents the need for additional calls to inform the other party of an important point or to ask a forgotten question.

- Set a time for calls. The nurse manager may have a number of calls to return as well as calls to initiate. It is best to set aside a time to handle routine phone calls, especially during "downtime." Try not to interrupt what is being done at the moment. If an answer is necessary before a project can be continued, phone immediately; if not, phone for the information at a later time.

- State and ask for preferred call times and the purpose of the call. If a party is not available, state the purpose of the call, and provide several time frames when you will be available for a return call. Have those accepting messages ask for the same information. This makes it easier for the responder to be prepared for the call and helps to prevent "telephone tag" or "trading pink slips" (Mayer, 1990).

Voice mail is an excellent way to send and receive messages when a real-time interaction is not essential. For example, one person or a large group of people can be informed about an upcoming meeting in one voice mail message. They can phone their responses at their convenience, thus obviating the need for continuing to try to reach each other directly. Like other forms of communication, voice mail must be used appropriately. Long messages or sensitive information are better conveyed one-on-one. Also, another person (e.g., unit clerk) may be responsible for taking voice mail messages off the system, so it is important to state the message in a professional manner, omitting personal or confidential information.

E-mail is another tool that enhances time management. E-mail or electronic mail programs (e.g., Microsoft Outlook) minimize time wasted trying to contact individuals and provide a means whereby the urgency of the message can be coded. Tone, however, is difficult to convey by e-mail. Therefore it is advisable to use more personal forms of communication, such as the telephone or in-person contact, for potentially sensitive or troublesome issues.

Drop-in Visitors Although often friendly and seemingly harmless, the typical "got-a-minute?" drop-in visit can last 10 minutes (Mackenzie, 1990). Rather than eliminate drop-in visits, the nurse manager should skillfully direct the visit by identifying the issue or question, arranging an alternative meeting, referring the visitor to someone else, or redirecting the visitor's problem-solving efforts. An additional strategy is to stand up to greet the visitor and remain standing. The gesture appears gracious yet is obvious enough to encourage a short visit.

The nurse manager who is fortunate enough to have an office will find that open doors are open invitations for interruption. Although it is essential that nurse managers be available and accessible, concentration time also is necessary. The manager can obtain concentration time by informing the staff that a specific block of time (a few hours at most) will be available to address issues.

Interruptions also can be controlled by the arrangement of furniture. The nurse manager whose desk is arranged so that immediate eye contact is made with passers-by or drop-in visitors is asking for interruptions. A desk turned 90 or even 180 degrees from the door minimizes potential eye contact.

Encouraging appointments to deal with routine matters also reduces interruptions. Regularly scheduled meetings with those who need to see the nurse manager allow them to hold routine matters for those appointments. Holding such meetings in the other person's office places the nurse manager in charge of keeping the time. It is easier to leave someone's office than to remove an individual from yours.

Paperwork

Health care organizations cannot function effectively without good information systems. In addition to telephone calls and face-to-face conversations, nurse managers spend considerable time writing and reading communications. Increasing government regulations, measures to avoid legal action, new treatments and medications, data processing, work processing, and electronics place pressure on the nurse manager to cope with increasing paperwork (including electronic "paperwork"). Some basic principles can help the nurse manager process information while reducing it as a waster of time.

- Plan and schedule paperwork. Writing and reading reports, forms, e-mail, letters, and memoranda are essential elements of the nurse manager's job. They cannot be ignored. They will, however, become a major source of frustration if their processing is not planned and scheduled as an integral part of the nurse manager's daily activities. Nurse managers should learn the organization's information system and requirements, analyze the paperwork requirements of the position, and make significant progress on that part of the job daily.

- Sort paperwork for effective processing. A system of file folders or trays in which to sort mail can be very helpful. For instance, place all paperwork requiring personal action in a file labeled "A"; it can then be handled according to its relative importance and urgency. Place paperwork that can be delegated in a separate pile, and distribute it appropriately. Place all paperwork that is informational in nature and related to present work in a file labeled "I." Place other reading material, such as professional journals, technical reports, and other items that do not relate directly to the immediate work, in a file labeled "R." The "I" file contains things that must be read immediately, whereas the "R" file materials are not as urgent and can be read later.

  Do not be afraid to throw things away or erase them from the memory of your electronic information system. When they no longer have value, do not let them become clutter. Use trash receptacles in the office and on the electronic system.

- Use the computer, or dictate communications. Handwrite as little as possible. Become proficient in using the computer to construct all letters, memos, and reports. If dictating equipment and secretarial support are available, use them. Dictating is faster than writing, even on the computer.

- Analyze paperwork frequently. Review filing policies and rules regularly, and purge files at least once each year. All standard forms, reports, and memos should be reviewed annually. Each should justify its continued existence and its present format. Do not be afraid to recommend changes and, when possible, initiate those changes.

- Do not be a paper shuffler. "Handle a piece of paper only once," is a common adage, but impossible to follow if taken literally. It really means that each time a piece of paper or e-mail message is handled, some action should be taken to further processing it. Paper shufflers are those who continually move things around on their desks or accumulate unread e-mails. They delay action unreasonably, and the problem mounts. A desktop is a working surface; it is not for files and piles.

Respecting Time

The key to using time-management techniques is to respect one's own time as well as that of others. Nurse managers who respect their time are likely to find others respecting it also. The same values and attitudes indicate respect for one's own time and for that of others. Using the above suggestions regarding time management communicates to those who interact with the nurse manager that respect for time is demanded. The manager, however, must reciprocate by respecting the time needs of others. For example, if the manager needs to talk to someone, it is appropriate to arrange an appointment, particularly for routine matters. One should continually ask, "What is the best use of my time right now?" and should answer in three ways: (a) For myself and my goals, (b) For my staff and their goals, and (c) For the organization and its goals.

Summary

- Stress is a person's reaction to demands from the environment that pose a threat.
- Causes of stress come from job and organizational factors, from interpersonal factors, and from individual factors.
- The consequences of stress are physiological and psychological problems for the individual, poor job performance, low job satisfaction, and high absenteeism.
- Strategies to help individuals, as well as organizations, manage stress include clarifying goals and roles; providing support, including training and education on stress management; using participative management techniques; and practicing personal stress management techniques.
- Nurse managers must use time wisely to accomplish everything that is expected of them; this takes planning.
- The nurse manager's work is subject to many interruptions. An interruption log helps identify patterns that the manager can use to plan ways to reduce unnecessary interruptions.
- Telephone calls are a major source of interruption. They can be controlled by minimizing small talk, planning calls, setting aside time for calls, stating preferred call times, and using voice mail.
- Drop-in visitors are also a source of interruption. One should meet visitors outside the office, keep visits short, encourage appointments, keep staff

informed, and arrange furniture to discourage unscheduled visitors.

- Written communication also can cause interruptions. These can be minimized by planning and scheduling paperwork, sorting, delegating, writing effectively, and using an effective filing system.

- Nurse managers who respect their own time are likely to find others respecting it also.

■ LEADERSHIP AND MANAGEMENT
in Action

1. What are the consequences of stress? Have you experienced any of these consequences? Which ones?

2. Describe personal and organizational methods for managing stress.

3. List four major time wasters. How can each of these be decreased?

References

Adcock, R., & Lee, J. (1971). Time, one more time. *California Management Review, 14*(2), 28–32.

Bliss, E. (1976). *Getting things done.* New York: Bantam.

Holmes, T., & Rahe, R. (1967). The social readjustment rating scale. *Journal of Psychosomatic Research, 11,* 213.

Kivisto, J., & Couture, R. T. (1997). Stress management for nurses: Controlling the whirlwind. *Nursing Forum, 32*(1), 25–33.

Knudson, H., Woodworth, R., & Bell, C. (1973). *Management: An experimental approach.* New York: McGraw-Hill.

Kushnir, T., Rabin, S., & Azulai, S. (1997). A descriptive study of stress management in a group of pediatric oncology nurses. *Cancer Nursing, 20*(6), 414–421.

Lazarus, R., & Folkman, S. (1984). *Stress, appraisal and coping.* New York: Springer.

Levi, L. (1981). *Preventing work stress.* Reading, MA: Addison-Wesley.

Mackenzie, A. (1990). *The time trap.* New York: American Management Association.

Mayer, J. (1990). *If you haven't got the time to do it right, when will you have the time to do it over?* New York: Simon & Schuster.

Porter-O'Grady, T. (1986). *Creative nursing administration: Participative management into the 21st century.* Gaithersburg, MD: Aspen.

Selye, H. (1978). *The stress of life,* 2nd ed. New York: McGraw-Hill.

Steers, R. (1984). *Introduction to organizational behavior,* 2nd ed. Santa Monica, CA: Goodyear.

Effective Delegation

Looking Ahead

Delegation is the act of entrusting and empowering another with responsibility. It is a dynamic process that can often be difficult to learn but is an essential part of the nurse's job. Effective delegation is a tool that benefits both the individual and the organization. Chapter 14 outlines the process of delegation, dealing with both authority and acceptance, and the obstacles faced by those who delegate.

Objectives

After reading this chapter, you will be able to:

- Differentiate delegation from work allocation.
- Discuss the benefits of delegation.
- Describe the delegation process.
- Discuss the difficulties with and obstacles to delegation.

Report is over. Where do you begin? Assessments. Patients to prepare for surgery. Medicines to give. Breakfast trays to deliver and set up. Baths to give. Treatments to do. An admission coming. Charting. Too much to do and so little time. Have you ever felt this way? How can you get it all done, be efficient, provide quality care, and survive the day? Delegate!

It is easy to say delegate, but delegation is a difficult leadership skill for nurses to learn and one that may not have been taught in undergraduate education. With changes in health care delivery, both new graduates and experienced nurses are struggling to develop their delegation skills. Managers also must continually improve their delegation skills to survive. Never before has delegation been as critical a skill for nurses to perfect as it is today, with the emphasis on doing more with less. This chapter describes the delegation process, the benefits and barriers to delegation, and tips on how to avoid ineffective delegation and liability.

Defining Delegation

What is delegation? **Delegation** is the process by which responsibility and authority for performing a task (function, activity, or decision) is transferred to another individual who accepts that authority and responsibility. Although the delegator remains accountable for the task, the delegate is also accountable to the delegator for the responsibilities assumed. Therefore, delegation is a dynamic process that involves responsibility, accountability, and authority. As a process, delegation empowers others and builds trust, enhances communication and leadership skills, and develops teamwork.

Delegation is also a tool. With effective delegation, the delegator can accomplish more tasks, and productivity increases. Delegation can also be a tool to develop skills and abilities of others and to promote harmony in the organization.

To delegate efficiently, the nurse manager must realize delegation is an art and, fortunately, a learnable skill. To perfect this skill, the manager must first appreciate what is and isn't delegation. The place to start is with a clear understanding of the underlying concepts of responsibility, accountability, and authority.

Responsibility and Accountability

Although *responsibility* and *accountability* are often used synonymously, in delegation the two words

> **KEY TERMS**
>
> *Delegation* The process by which responsibility and authority are transferred to another individual.
>
> *Responsibility* An obligation to accomplish a task.
>
> *Accountability* The act of accepting ownership for the results or lack thereof.
>
> *Authority* The right to act or empower.

represent different concepts that go hand in hand. **Responsibility** denotes an obligation to accomplish a task, whereas **accountability** is accepting ownership for the results or lack thereof. In delegation, responsibility is transferred while accountability is shared. The first principle to remember about delegation is *you can delegate only those tasks for which you are responsible*. If you have no *direct* responsibility for the task, then you can't delegate that task. For instance, if a manager is responsible for filling holes in the staffing schedule, the manager can delegate this responsibility to another individual. However, if staffing is the responsibility of a central coordinator, the manager can make suggestions or otherwise assist the staffing coordinator, but cannot delegate the task. Likewise, if an orderly who is responsible for setting up traction is detained and a nurse asks a physical therapist on the unit to assist with traction, this is not delegation, because setting up traction is not the responsibility of the nurse. However, if the orderly (the person responsible for the task) had asked the physical therapist to help, this could be an act of delegation if the other principles of delegation are met. To clearly understand *who* is responsible, it is important to look at practice acts, standards of care, job descriptions, and policy statements. It is also important to realize that an employer cannot decide what to delegate.

The nurse practice acts in each state define the scope of nursing practice. Are responsibilities regarding advanced practice delineated? How does the scope of practice differ between registered and licensed practical/vocational nurses? What is the scope of practice of other health care providers? Is delegation defined? If so, how?

Also, check professional standards. Several organizations have provided position statements regarding delegation. The American Nurses Association (1997) posits that the registered nurse determines what activities may be delegated by considering patient safety

Box 14-1 American Nephrology Nurses' Association Position Statement on Delegation

Criteria for Delegation to Licensed Personnel

Delegation of nursing care activities to LPN/LVNs shall comply with the following criteria:

- The registered nurse must complete an assessment of the patient's nursing care needs prior to delegating any nursing intervention.

- The registered nurse shall be accountable and responsible for all delegated nursing care activities or interventions, and she/he must remain present in the patient-care area for ongoing monitoring and evaluation of the patient's response to the therapy.

- The patient-care activities must be within the scope of practice delineated by the Board of LPN/LVN for the state in which the nurses are practicing and must not require the LPN/LVN to exercise nursing judgment beyond the scope of that practice act.

- The registered nurse shall have either instructed the LPN/LVN in the delegated nursing care activity or verified the individual's competency to perform the activity. Clinical competency of these individuals will be documented and available, and verified at least annually.

Criteria for Delegation to Unlicensed Assistive Personnel

Delegation of nursing care activities to unlicensed assistive personnel shall comply with the following criteria:

- The registered nurse must complete an assessment of the patient's nursing care needs prior to delegating any nursing care activities or interventions.

- The registered nurse shall be accountable and responsible for all delegated nursing care activities or interventions, and she/he must remain present in the patient-care area for the ongoing monitoring and evaluation of the patient's response to the therapy.

- The registered nurse shall have either instructed the unlicensed assistive personnel in the delegated nursing care activity or verified the individual's competency to perform the activity. Clinical competency and knowledge of these individuals will be documented and available, and verified at least annually.

- Since unlicensed assistive personnel practicing in nephrology do not have a recognized scope of practice delineated by an approved state board of occupational regulations, the registered nurse shall be responsible for the ongoing evaluation of the performance of these individuals and supervision of all the nursing care activities performed by them.

- Administration of medication is a nursing responsibility requiring knowledge of the indications, pharmacokinetic action, potential adverse reactions, correct dosage and contraindications, and it is beyond the scope of practice of unlicensed assistive personnel. Administration of medications by unlicensed assistive personnel shall be limited to those medications considered as part of the routine hemodialysis treatment, that is, normal saline and heparin via the extracorporeal circuit and intradermal lidocaine.

- Administration of any blood products and/or intravenous medications by infusion is a nursing responsibility and beyond the scope of practice of unlicensed assistive personnel.

Note: Reprinted with permission from "Delegation of Nursing Tasks to Licensed and Unlicensed Personnel: A Guide for ESRD Facilities" by the American Nephrology Nurses' Association, 1996.

and needs, the education and training of the assistive staff, the extent of supervision required, and staff workload. However, any intervention that requires independent, specialized nursing skill, knowledge, or judgment cannot be delegated; nor can health counseling or teaching. Box 14-1 provides an excerpt from the American Nephrology Nurses' Association statement as an example of a position statement on delegation.

It is also important to be familiar with job descriptions and policy statements at your organization. What may have been allowed at one organization may not be permitted at another.

Authority

The second principle of delegation is that *along with responsibility, you must transfer authority.* **Authority** is the right to act. Therefore, by transferring authority, the delegator is empowering the delegate to accomplish the task. Too often this principle of delegation is neglected. Delegators retain authority, crippling the delegate's abilities to accomplish the task, setting the delegate up for failure, and minimizing efficiency and productivity. This pitfall is discussed later in the chapter.

Differentiating Delegation from Work Allocation

Delegation is often confused with work allocation. As previously discussed, delegation is a mutual transfer of responsibility and authority that occurs on the basis of competence and trust. In **work allocation**, no *transfer* of authority occurs. Instead, assignments are a bureaucratic function that reflect job descriptions and requirements (Manthey, 1990).

Benefits of Delegation

Effective delegation benefits both the individual and the organization. Some of these benefits have been previously mentioned. This section describes the benefits to the delegator, delegate, patient, and organization.

Benefits to the Delegator

Delegation yields a number of personal benefits for the delegator. First, the delegator will be able to devote more time to those tasks that cannot be delegated. With more time available, the delegator can develop new skills and abilities, facilitating the opportunity for career advancement. Having individuals with advanced skills provides continuity in the delegator's absence and offers a ready replacement if the delegator has an opportunity for advancement.

Benefits to the Delegate

The delegate also benefits from delegation. The delegate gains new skills and abilities that can facilitate upward mobility. In addition, delegation can bring trust and support, thereby building self-esteem and confidence. Subsequently, job satisfaction and motivation are enhanced as individuals feel stimulated by new challenges. Morale improves; a sense of pride and belonging develops as well as greater awareness of responsibility. Individuals feel more appreciated and learn to appreciate the roles and responsibilities of others, increasing cooperation and enhancing teamwork.

> **KEY TERMS**
>
> *Work allocation* The assignment of tasks that reflect job descriptions and requirements.

Benefits to the Organization

As teamwork improves, the organization benefits by achieving its goals more efficiently. Overtime and absences decrease. Subsequently, productivity increases, and the organization's financial position may improve.

Benefits to the Patient

As delegation increases efficiency, the quality of care improves. As quality improves, patient satisfaction increases.

The Delegation Process

There are five steps to the delegation process: (a) defining the task, (b) determining to whom to delegate, (c) providing clear communication about expectations regarding the task, (d) reaching mutual agreement about the task at hand, and (e) monitoring and evaluating the results and providing feedback to the individual regarding his or her performance. These steps address the questions what, who, by when, and, in some cases, where and how. Figure 14-1 provides a delegation decision-making tree.

Identifying and Defining the Task and Level of Delegation

Both staff nurses and nurse managers are in positions in which they are not able to do everything that must be done. The first step in delegation is determining what can and should be delegated. Recalling the first principle of delegation, you can delegate only an aspect of your own work for which you have responsibility and authority. These include: (a) routine tasks, (b) tasks for which you do not have time, (c) tasks that have moved down in priority, (d) problem solving, and (e) staff building. In addition, Morrison (1993) suggests you should delegate only what you know best. She contends this is important in providing guidance and feedback. Clearly, lack of expertise in the task hinders the delegator's ability to define the task and associated requirements. Therefore, the third principle of delegation is know well the task to be delegated.

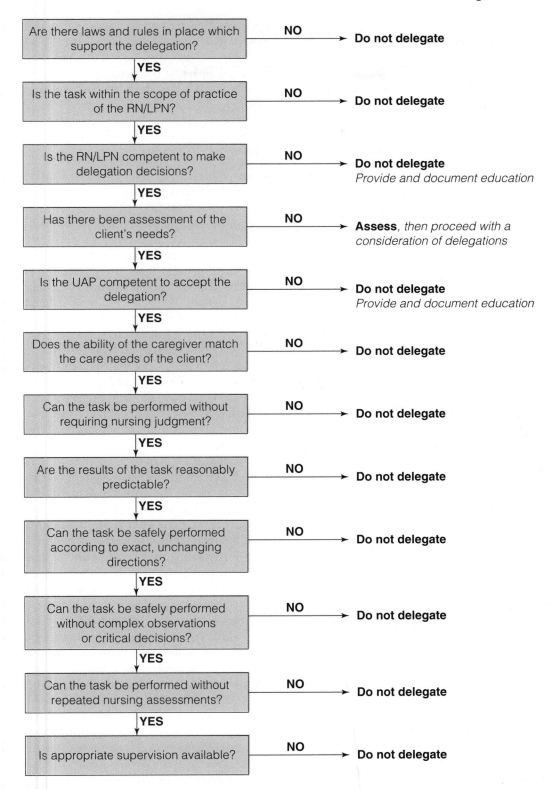

Figure 14-1 Delegation decision-making tree. Authority to delegate varies, so licensed nurses must check the jurisdiction's statutes and regulations. RNs may need to delegate to the LPN the authority to delegate to the UAP. Adapted from the Delegation Decision Tree developed by the Ohio Board of Nursing. *Note:* National Council of State Boards of Nursing (1997). Retrieved August 28, 2000 from the World Wide Web (http://www.ncsbn.org/files/uap/delegationdocs.asp).

Once you have decided what to delegate, the next step is to define the aspects of the task. Ask yourself: Does the task involve technical skills or cognitive abilities? Are specific qualifications necessary? Is performance restricted by practice acts, standards, or job descriptions? How complex is the task? Is training or education required? Are the steps well defined, or are creativity and problem solving required? Would a change in circumstances affect who could perform the task?

While you are trying to define the complexity of the task and its components, it is important not to fall into the trap of thinking no one else is capable of performing this task. Often others can be prepared to perform a task through education and training. The time taken to prepare others can be recouped many times over. An alternative would be to subdivide the task into component parts and delegate the components congruent with the available delegate's capabilities. For example, developing a budget is a managerial responsibility that cannot be delegated, but someone else could explore the types of tympanic thermometers on the market, their costs, advantages, and so on. A committee of staff nurses could evaluate the options and make a recommendation that you could include in the budget justification.

But how do you know what should not be delegated? Before a task is delegated, two questions must be addressed. First, what areas of authority, or what resources, must the person control to achieve the expected results? Second, what are the limits, boundaries, or parameters for each area of authority or resource to be used? A unit manager who is responsible for maintaining adequate supplies needs budget authority. The authority to spend money on supplies, however, may be limited to a specific amount for specific supplies or may be allocated to supplies in general. Uris (1970) suggests certain tasks should never be delegated: (a) total control, (b) discipline, (c) confidential tasks, (d) extremely technical tasks, and (e) controversial topics.

Once the task has been identified and defined, the next step is determining the level of delegation to use (Whetten and Cameron, 1984).

Level 1. Gather information for the delegate so he or she can decide what needs to be done.

Level 2. Determine alternative courses of action from which the delegate may choose.

Level 3. Have the delegate perform one part of the task at a time and obtain approval for each new step.

Level 4. Have the delegate outline an entire course of action for accomplishing the whole task and have it approved before proceeding.

Level 5. Allow the delegate to perform the whole task using any preferred method and report only the results.

Determining Who

Once you have determined what the task entails, what to delegate, and at what level to delegate, the next step is to match the task to the individual. It is important to analyze individuals' skill levels and abilities to evaluate their capability to perform the various tasks; it is also important to determine characteristics that might prevent them from accepting responsibility for the task. A rule of thumb is to delegate to the lowest person in the hierarchy who has the requisite capabilities and who is allowed to do the task legally and by organizational policy.

Education prepares individuals for beginning practice. Experience and individual characteristics, such as initiative, intelligence, and enthusiasm, can expand the individual's capabilities. In general, baccalaureate-prepared nurses are equipped to care for individuals, families, groups, and communities in both structured and unstructured health settings.

Baccalaureate programs provide leadership training and encourage the incorporation of research into practice. Conversely, the associate degree nurse is prepared to care for individuals in a structured health care environment. Research skills are limited to data collection. Usually, associate degree programs do not provide leadership training and community experiences (American Association of Colleges of Nursing and American Organization of Nurse Executives, 1995).

The licensed practical or vocational nurse (LPN/LVN) is prepared to assist in implementing a defined plan of care and perform procedures according to protocol. Assessment skills are directed at differentiating normal from abnormal, and competence is in caring for physiologically stable patients with predictable conditions. The LPN/LVN also has knowledge of asepsis and can perform dressing changes. Knowledge and competence in medication administration varies with the program attended and regulations of the state's nurse practice acts (Wywialowski, 1993).

The scope of practice of unlicensed assistive personnel (UAPs) is the most limited and the most varied. The nursing assistant and other UAPs can assist with a variety of direct patient-care activities, such as bathing, transferring, ambulating, feeding, toileting, and obtaining vital signs and measurements such as height, weight, and intake and output, as well as indirect activities such as housekeeping, transporting, and stocking supplies (Wywialowski, 1993).

The second step in identifying "who" is determining availability. For example, Sue might be the best candidate, but she leaves for vacation tomorrow and won't be back before the project is due.

The final step is considering who would be willing to assume responsibility. This raises the fourth principle of delegation: *Delegation is a contractual agreement that is entered into voluntarily.*

Describing Expectations

The next step in delegation is clearly defining your expectations for the delegate. Communication should be clear and complete. Plan your meeting with the delegate. Attempting to delegate in the middle of a crisis is not delegation; that is directing. Provide for enough time to describe the task and your expectations and to entertain questions. Also, meet in an environment as devoid of distractions as possible. Key behaviors in delegating tasks follow.

1. Describe the task using "I" statements, such as "I would like . . ." and appropriate nonverbal behaviors—open body language, face-to-face positioning, and eye contact. The delegate needs to know what is expected, when the task should be completed and where and how, if that is appropriate. Again, depending on the level of delegation, some delegates can define for themselves the where and how. Decide whether written reports are necessary or if brief oral reports are sufficient. If written reports are required, indicate whether tables, charts, or other graphics are necessary. Be specific about reporting times. Identify critical events or milestones that might be reached and brought to your attention.
2. Provide the delegate with a reason for the task. Describe the importance to the organization, to you, the patient, and the delegate. Provide the delegate with an incentive for accepting both the responsibility and the authority to do the task.
3. Inform the delegate by what standard the task will be evaluated and how often. Clearly describe the expected outcome and the timeline for completion. Establish how closely the assignment will be supervised. Monitoring is important because you remain accountable for the task, but controls should never limit an individual's opportunity to grow.
4. Identify any constraints for completing the task as well as risks. Also identify any situational variables by which authority and responsibility for the task will change. For example, you may ask an assistant to feed a patient for you as long as the patient is coherent and awake, but you would feed the patient if he were confused.
5. Validate understanding of the task and your expectations by eliciting questions and providing feedback.

Reaching Agreement

Once you have outlined your expectations, it is important to seek agreement from the delegate that he or she is accepting responsibility and authority for the task. You need to be prepared to equip the delegate to complete the task successfully. This might mean providing additional information or resources or informing others about the arrangement as needed to empower the delegate. Before meeting with the delegate, anticipate areas of negotiation, and identify what you are prepared and able to provide.

Monitoring Performance and Providing Feedback

Monitoring performance provides a mechanism for feedback and control that ensures that the delegated tasks are carried out as agreed. Give careful thought to monitoring efforts when objectives are established. When defining the task and expectations, clearly establish the where, when, and how. Remain accessible. Support builds confidence and reassures the delegate of your interest in the delegate and negates any concerns about dumping undesirable tasks. Monitoring the delegate too closely, however, conveys distrust. Analyze performance with respect to the established goal. If problem areas are identified, privately investigate and explain the problem(s), provide an opportunity for feedback, and inform the individual how to correct the mistake(s) in the future. Provide additional support as needed. Also, be sure to give the praise and recognition due, and don't be afraid to do so publicly.

Accepting Delegation

When you accept delegation, it is important to understand what is being asked of you. First of all, acknowledge the delegator's confidence in you, but realistically examine whether you have the skills and abilities for the task and the time to do it. If you do not have the requisite skills, it is your responsibility to inform the delegator. However, it does not mean you cannot accept the responsibility. See whether the delegator is willing to train or otherwise equip you to accomplish the task. If not, then you need to refuse the offer. Accepting delegation means you accept full responsibility for the outcome and its benefits or liabilities. Just as the delegator has the option to delegate parts of a task, you also have the option to negotiate for those aspects of a task you feel comfortable with. However, recognize the potential for growth and attempt to capitalize on it, obtaining new skills or resources in the process.

Once you agree on the role and responsibilities you are to assume, make sure you are clear on the time frame, feedback mechanisms, and other expectations. Don't assume anything. As a minimum, repeat to the delegator what you heard said; better yet, outline the task in writing.

Throughout the project, keep the delegator informed. Explore any concerns you have as they come up. Foremost, complete the task as agreed. Successful completion can open more doors in the future.

In the event you are not qualified or do not have the time, do not be afraid to say no. Thank the delegator for the offer and clearly explain why you must decline at this time. Express your interest in working together in the future.

Obstacles to Delegation

Although delegation can yield many benefits, there are potential barriers. Some barriers are environmental; others are the result of the delegator's or delegate's beliefs or inexperience. Table 14-1 summarizes potential obstacles to delegation.

A Nonsupportive Environment

Both environments within and external to the organization may present obstacles to delegation. As described earlier, state practice acts may limit what can be delegated and to whom. Professional standards, job descriptions, and policy statements also may impose limitations. In a study by Thomas & Hume, 1998) new graduates identified support from members of the health care team, especially supervisors, as contributing to successful delegation.

Organizational Culture The culture within the organization may restrict delegation. Hierarchies, management styles, and norms may all preclude delegation. Rigid chains of command and autocratic leadership styles do not facilitate delegation and rarely provide good role models. The norm is to do the work oneself because others are not capable or skilled. An atmosphere of distrust prevails as well as a poor tolerance for mistakes. Additional environmental factors include a norm of crisis management and poorly defined job descriptions or chains of command.

Personal Qualities Poor communication and interpersonal skills can also be a barrier to delegation. Thomas & Hume (1998) note that in addition to good communication skills and respecting and treating staff fairly, a willingness to work with the other, to be open to suggestions, to provide feedback and acknowledgment for work well done is essential. They also note that delegates must be reliable and willing to follow instructions.

Resources Another difficulty frequently encountered is a lack of resources. For example, there may be no one to delegate to. Consider the sole registered nurse in a skilled nursing facility. If practice acts define a task as one that only a registered nurse can perform, there is no one else to whom that nurse can delegate that task.

Another limiting factor may be finances. For instance, there is an expectation that someone from your department must attend the annual conference in your nursing specialty area. However, the organization will only pay the manager's travel and conference expenses, which precludes anyone else from attending.

Educational resources may be another limiting factor. Perhaps others could learn how to do a task if they could practice with the equipment, but the equipment is not available.

Time can also be a limiting factor. For example, it is Friday and the schedule needs to be posted Monday. No one on your staff has experience developing schedules and you need to go out of town for a family emergency, so there is no one else to do the schedule.

An Insecure Delegator

The majority of the barriers to delegation arise from the delegator. Three conflicts have been identified by del Bueno (1993): trust versus control, approval versus affiliation, and the democratic ideal versus the classical hierarchy. Trust is paramount to delegation, but to trust another individual means to give up some

Table 14-1	Potential Obstacles to Delegation

Environmental	Delegator	Delegate
Practice acts	Lack of trust and confidence	Inexperience
Standards	Believe others incapable	Fear of failure and reprisal
Job descriptions	Believe self indispensable	Lack of confidence
Policies	Fear of competition	Overdependence on others
Organizational structure	Fear of criticism	Avoidance of responsibility
Management styles	Fear of liability	
Norms	Fear of blame for others' mistakes	
Resources	Fear of loss of control	
	Fear or overburdening	
	Fear of decreased job satisfaction	
	Insecurity	
	Inexperience in delegation	
	Inadequate organizational skills	

Note: Reprinted with permission from "Delegation: how to deliver care through others," R. Hansten and M. Washburn, 1992, *American Journal of Nursing,* 92(3), 87–88.

control. Everyone has the need for both approval and affiliation, but which is more important—the need to be liked, or the need to belong and be accepted? Which is more valued—teamwork and empowerment, or control and the established hierarchy? These are difficult to address. Hansten and Washburn (1992) have developed a simple quiz, found in Box 14-2, to help identify your readiness to delegate.

Commonly voiced concerns about delegation include (a) "I can do it better," (b) "I can do it faster," (c) "I'd rather do it myself," and (d) "I don't have time to delegate." Often underlying these statements are erroneous beliefs, fears, and inexperience in delegation. As previously indicated, a delegator should delegate those things that the delegator can do well. Therefore, there is a degree of truth in the first three statements; however, one of the roles of a manager is to develop staff. Hence, by failing to delegate, the manager is shirking this responsibility.

Delegation does take time, but failing to delegate is a time waster. Time invested in developing staff today is later repaid many times over.

Additional problems are inherent in the two statements, "I can do it better" and "I can do it faster." These statements suggest a lack of trust and confidence in the staff. The manager also sends the message that the staff is incapable, whereas the manager is indispensable. Both are erroneous. In the process, the staff is demoralized, and the manager loses respect. More often than not, these statements are

smokescreens for the delegator's own fears and weaknesses. Common fears follow.

1. *Fear of competition or criticism.* What if someone else can do the job better or faster than I? Will I lose my job? Be demoted? What will others think? Will I lose respect and control? This fear is unfounded if the delegator has selected the right task and matched it with the right individual. In fact, the delegate's success in the task provides evidence of the delegator's leadership and decision-making abilities.

2. *Fear of liability.* Some individuals are not risk takers and shy away from delegation for this reason. There are risks associated with delegation, but the delegator can minimize these risks by following the steps of delegation, as previously described. More about risks is discussed in the section on liability later in the chapter. A related concern is a fear of being blamed for the delegate's mistakes. If the delegator used prudence in selecting the task and delegate, then the responsibility for any mistakes made are solely those of the delegate; it is not necessary to take on guilt for another's mistakes. To help keep this issue in perspective, it is important to recall the benefits of delegation and balance the rewards with the risks while making the delegation decision.

3. *Fear of loss of control.* Will I be kept informed? Will the job be done right? How can I be sure?

Box 14-2 Delegation Assessment

1. Mr. Jones, a bedridden but stable patient, needs a complete bed bath. You
   a. Assign the task to the nurse assistant.
   b. Work together with the nursing assistant to give the bath.
   c. Do the job yourself because Mr. Jones is a VIP and you know you'll do the best job.

2. You are the charge nurse, and one of your team members is a float nurse who has never worked on the unit before. You
   a. Spend 15 minutes with her assessing her abilities and providing a brief orientation to the unit so that she can take the full assignment.
   b. Give her three of the "easiest patients" and pick up the rest of the assignment yourself.
   c. Call the supervisor and tell her that you have no time to orient someone and the float will be more trouble than she's worth.

3. Another new admission is arriving on your unit. You
   a. Assign the patient to the LPN, recognizing that one of the registered nurses will be overseeing and completing the admission assessment.
   b. Ask the nursing assistant to get the vital signs, and you complete the admission before assigning the patient to another RN.
   c. Take the admission yourself because everyone else seems too busy.

4. You and a nursing assistant are assigned to 10 patients on a medical surgical floor. You
   a. Spend 15 minutes making walking rounds with the nursing assistant, then decide how to distribute patient care tasks.
   b. Assign tasks according to the assignment board from yesterday.

   c. Send the nursing assistant to take vital signs without further information or communication.

5. You are uncertain about a nursing assistant's skill in giving a cleansing enema. You
   a. Review the hospital procedure with the nursing assistant and observe him performing the task so that next time he can do it alone.
   b. Give the enema yourself today, promising that the next time you'll teach the nursing assistant.
   c. You never assign him to give an enema.

6. Your manager tells you that the care delivery system on your unit is changing and you'll need to use assistive personnel. You
   a. Welcome the opportunity to free up some of your time to do more of your professional duties.
   b. Keep an open mind and wait to review the job description of the new assistants.
   c. Take a wait-and-see attitude, but if it doesn't work out in the next two weeks, you'll apply to another hospital in town where you can still be a "real nurse."

If you answered mostly "a"s, congratulations! You have overcome many of the typical barriers to delegation. You can be a mentor to your co-workers who are learning the skill.

If you answered mostly "b"s, you are on the way to overcoming your personal barriers to delegation. Keep an open mind and read on.

If you answered mostly "c"s, oops! You have strong objections to sharing your work load with others. Read on. Learning this skill and applying it will enhance your daily work life.

Note: Reprinted with permission from "Delegation: how to deliver care through others," R. Hansten and M. Washburn, 1992, *American Journal of Nursing, 92*(3), 87–88.

The more one is insecure and inexperienced in delegation, the more this fear is an issue. This is also a predominant concern in individuals who tend toward autocratic styles of leadership and perfectionism. The key to retaining control is to clearly identify the task and expectations and then to monitor progress and provide feedback.

4. *Fear of overburdening others.* They already have so much to do; how can I suggest more? Every-

one has work to do. Such a statement belittles the decisional capabilities of others. Recall that delegation is a voluntary, contractual agreement; acceptance of a delegated task indicates the availability and willingness of the delegate to perform the task. Often, the delegate welcomes the diversion and stimulation, and what the delegator perceives as a burden is actually a blessing. The onus is on the delegator to select the right person for the right reason.

5. *Fear of decreased personal job satisfaction.* Because the type of tasks recommended to delegate are those that are familiar and routine, the delegator's job satisfaction should actually increase with the opportunity to explore new challenges and obtain other skills and abilities.

Additional hindrances to delegation include inadequate organizational skills, such as poor time management, and inexperience in delegation.

An Unwilling Delegate

Inexperience and fear of failure can motivate a potential delegate to refuse to accept a delegated task. Much reassurance and support are needed. In addition, the delegate should be equipped to handle the task. If proper selection criteria are used and the steps of delegation followed, then the delegate should not fail. The delegator can boost the delegate's lack of confidence by building on simple tasks. The delegate needs to be reminded that everyone was inexperienced at one time. Another common concern is how mistakes will be handled. When describing the task, the delegator should provide clear guidelines for handling problems, guidelines that adhere to organizational policies.

Another barrier is the individual who avoids responsibility or is overdependent on others. Success breeds success; therefore, it is important to use an enticing incentive to engage the individual in a simple task that guarantees success.

Ineffective Delegation

When the steps of delegation are not followed or barriers remain unresolved, delegation is often ineffective. Three common forms of inefficient delegation are underdelegation, reverse delegation, and overdelegation.

Underdelegation

Underdelegation occurs when (a) the delegator fails to transfer full authority to the delegate, (b) the delegator takes back responsibility for aspects of the task, or (c) the delegator fails to equip and direct the delegate. As a result, the delegate is unable to complete the task, and the delegator must resume responsibility for its completion.

Reverse Delegation

In **reverse delegation,** someone with a lower rank delegates to someone with more authority. Consider for

> **KEY TERMS**
>
> *Underdelegation*   A common form of ineffective delegation that occurs when full authority is not transferred, responsibility is taken back, or there is a failure to equip and direct the delegate.
>
> *Reverse delegation*   A common form of ineffective delegation that occurs when someone with a lower rank delegates to someone with more authority.
>
> *Overdelegation*   A common form of ineffective delegation that occurs when the delegator loses control over a situation by giving too much authority or responsibility to the delegate.

example, Celina, a staff nurse who says to her nurse manager, "I'm really swamped today. Can you hang Mr. Morino's chemo so I can go to lunch?" Though the manager could assist Celina, this is not an efficient use of her time. Instead, the manager could help Celina organize her own time and efficiently delegate some responsibilities.

Overdelegation

Overdelegation occurs when the delegator loses control over a situation by providing the delegate with too much authority or too much responsibility. This places the delegator in a risky position, increasing the potential for liability.

Liability and Delegation

In delegation, the risk of liability arises from the appropriateness of the assignment and the adequacy of supervision (Barter & Furmidge, 1994). According to the American Nurses Association (ANA) Code for Nurses (1985), the nurse is responsible for exercising informed judgment and basing the decision to delegate on the individual's competencies and qualifications. Failure to do so would constitute negligence. Therefore, it is imperative that the right task be given to the right person at the right time. This means that the delegator must follow the steps of delegation in defining the task and determining who can and should perform the task. In addition, the delegator needs to be delegating for the right reasons; that is, not to gain personal prestige or dump undesirable tasks, but to accomplish the goals of the organization more efficiently.

In addition, the delegator needs to ensure that the task is being completed correctly and that clear guidelines and parameters for the task have been given. If these considerations are included in the steps of delegating, then the risks should be acceptable and liabilities minimal.

Success in the health care environment today necessitates effective delegation strategies. As nurses incorporate delegation into their practice, both professionalism and satisfaction will improve.

Summary

- Delegation is a contractual agreement in which authority and responsibity for a task is transferred by the person accountable for the task to another individual.
- Delegation involves skill in identifying and determining the task and level of responsibility, determining who has the requisite skills and abilities, describing expectations clearly, reaching mutual agreement, equipping the delegate if necessary, and monitoring performance and providing feedback.
- Delegatable tasks are personal, routine tasks that the delegator can perform well, that do not require yielding total control, that do not involve discipline or confidential information, and that are not extremely technical or controversial.
- Delegation benefits the delegator, delegate, organization, and patients.
- Various organizational, delegator, and delegate barriers can prevent effective delegation.
- Ineffective delegation usually results from inadequate or inappropriate transference of authority or responsibility.
- Adhering to the steps of delegation—in particular, prudently selecting a qualified person as delegate and providing appropriate supervision—minimizes the risk of liability.

■ LEADERSHIP AND MANAGEMENT
in Action

1. How does delegation differ from work allocation?
2. List three obstacles to delegation. How can these obstacles be overcome?
3. Describe how delegation can benefit you, the organization, and the patient.

References

American Association of Colleges of Nursing and American Organization of Nurse Executives. (1995). _A model for differentiated practice._ Washington, DC: American Association of Colleges of Nursing.

American Nephrology Nurses' Association. (1996). Delegation of nursing tasks to licensed and unlicensed personnel: A guide for ESRD facilities. _ANNA Journal, 19,_ 337–338.

American Nurses Association (1985). _Code for nurses._ Kansas City: Author.

American Nurses Association (1997). _Registered nurse utilization of unlicensed assistive personnel._ Washington, DC: Author

Barter, M., & Furmidge, M. C. (1994). Unlicensed assistive delegation and supervision. _Journal of Nursing Administration, 24_(4), 36–40.

del Bueno, D. J. (1993). Delegation and the dilemma of the democratic ideal. _Journal of Nursing Administration, 23_(3), 20–21, 25.

Hansten, R., & Washburn, M. (1992). Delegation: How to deliver care through others. _American Journal of Nursing, 92_(3), 87–90.

Manthey, M. (1990). Trust: Essential for delegation. _Nursing Management, 21_(11), 28–30.

Morrison, M. (1993). _Professional skills for leadership: Foundations of a successful career._ St. Louis: Mosby.

National Council of State Boards (1997). Delegation decision-making tree. Retrieved August 28, 2000 from the World Wide Web: http://www.ncsbn.org/files/uap/delegationdocs.asp.

Thomas, S. & Hume, G. (1998). Delegation competencies: Beginning practitioners' reflections. _Nurse Educator, 23_(1), 38–41.

Ward, S., & Westbrich, M. (1990). Delegation and assignment clarification. [Letter]. _AORN, 51,_ 432.

Whetten, D., & Cameron, K. (1984). _Developing management skills._ Glenwood, IL: Scott Foresman.

Wywialowski, E. (1993). _Managing client care._ St. Louis: C. V. Mosby.

Uris, A. (1970). _The executive deskbook._ New York: Van Nostrand Reinhold.

 Additional on-line resources for this chapter can be found on the World Wide Web at http://www.prenhall.com/sullivan_decker. Select Chapter 14 from the drop-down menu.

Building and Managing Teams

Looking Ahead

What distinguishes a group from a team? To understand the concept more clearly, think about an orchestra. The very first day the musicians come together, they are a group of people, each with individual skills and knowledge. The conductor, their leader, gives them a framework: the music. To achieve their goal, creating music, the musicians must learn to cooperate and rely on each other as a team. The orchestra analogy is not unlike nursing, a team-oriented profession with many different types of players. This chapter looks at the different types of groups and group dynamics and offers strategies that nurses and nurse managers can employ to develop teams within the work environment.

Objectives

After reading this chapter, you will be able to:

- Differentiate groups from teams.
- List the phases of group development.
- Describe ways to promote team-building.
- Compare and contrast the different types of groups.
- Discuss ways to manage committees and task forces.

Most often, nursing occurs in a team environment. Work groups that share common objectives function in a harmonious, coordinated, purposeful manner as teams. High-performance teams require expert nurse manager leadership skills. As the health care delivery system becomes more integrated across settings, a team environment becomes increasingly essential. Nurse managers must skillfully orchestrate the activity and interactions of interdisciplinary teams as well as conventional nursing work groups. Understanding the nature of groups and how groups are transformed into teams is essential to the nurse manager's effectiveness.

Unfortunately, research indicates that many managers experience considerable difficulty in transforming work groups into effective teams. Some managers lack the planning and organizing skills needed to facilitate work group performance. The manager may not know how to work with group members to identify goals, tasks, and practical work plans. Managers also may lack skills in conflict management. Although conflict within any work group is inevitable, the manner in which conflict is managed depends on the manager's skill in assisting co-workers to sort out personal differences and to improve their understanding and acceptance of differing views and styles. In addition, some managers have difficulty managing their own interpersonal relationships with group members. They may play favorites, ignore reticent members, give up including the withdrawn individual, or allow animosity to develop with an individual or a subgroup. Achieving balanced relationships with even the most difficult members is part of successful management and is essential to the work group's function. Close teamwork is difficult to achieve when managers lack group planning and organizing skills, do not know how to manage conflict, or cannot maintain healthy interpersonal relationships with group members.

Because staff nurses work in close proximity and frequently depend on each other to perform their work, the quality of group leadership and interaction is vital. A positive climate is one in which there is mutual high regard and in which group members safely may discuss work-related concerns, critique and offer suggestions about clinical practice, and comfortably experiment with new behaviors. Maintaining a positive work group climate and building a team is a complex and demanding leadership task.

Differentiating Groups from Teams

A **group**, quite simply, is an aggregate of individuals who interact and mutually influence each other (Shaw,

KEY TERMS

Group An aggregate of individuals who interact and mutually influence each other.

Formal groups Clusters of individuals designated by an organization to perform specified organizational tasks.

Informal groups Groups that evolve from social interactions that are not defined by an organizational structure.

Real (command) groups Groups that accomplish tasks in an organization and are recognized as legitimate organizational entities.

Task group Several individuals who work together to accomplish specific time-limited assignments.

Committees or task forces Groups that deal with specific issues involving several service areas.

Teams Real groups in which people work cooperatively with each other in order to achieve some goal.

Competing groups Groups in which members compete for resources or recognition.

Ordinary interacting groups Common types of groups; generally have formal leader and are run according to an informal structure with the purpose of solving a problem or making a decision.

1981). Both formal and informal groups exist in organizations. **Formal groups** are clusters of individuals designated temporarily or permanently by an organization to perform specified organizational tasks. Formal groups may be structured laterally, vertically, or diagonally. Task groups, teams, task forces, and committees may be structured in all of these ways, whereas command groups generally are structured vertically. Group membership includes (a) individuals from a single work group or individuals at similar job levels from more than one work group, (b) individuals from different job levels, or (c) individuals from different work groups *and* different job levels in the organization. Groups may be permanent or temporary. Command groups, teams, and committees usually are permanent, whereas task groups and task forces are often temporary.

Informal groups evolve naturally from social interactions. Groups are informal in the sense that they are not defined by an organizational structure. Examples of informal groups include individuals who regularly eat lunch together or who convene spontaneously to discuss a clinical dilemma.

Real (command) groups accomplish tasks in organizations and are recognized as a legitimate organizational entity. Its members are interdependent, share a set of norms, generally differentiate roles and duties among themselves, are organized to achieve ongoing organizational goals, and are collectively held responsible for measurable outcomes. The group's manager has line authority in relation to group members individually and collectively. The group's assignments are usually routine and designed to fulfill the specific mission of the agency or organization. The regularly assigned staff who work together under the direction of a single manager constitute a command group.

A **task group** is composed of several persons who work together, with or without a designated leader, and are charged with accomplishing specific time-limited assignments. A group of nurses selected by their colleagues to plan an orientation program for new staff constitute a task group. Usually, several task groups exist within a service area and may include representatives from several disciplines (e.g., nurse, physician, dietitian, social worker).

Other special groups include **committees** or **task forces** formed to deal with specific issues involving several service areas. A committee responsible for monitoring and improving patient safety or a task force assigned to develop better procedures for specimen collection are examples of special work groups. Health care organizations depend on numerous committees, which nurses participate in and often lead. Some of these committees are mandated by accrediting and regulatory bodies, such as committees for education, standards, disaster, and patient care evaluation. Others are established to meet a specific need (e.g., to formulate a new policy on substance abuse).

Teams are real groups in which individuals must work cooperatively with each other in order to achieve some overarching goal. They demonstrate healthy interdependence. According to Katzenbach and Smith (1993, p. 112), a team is composed of "a small number of people with complementary skills who are committed to a common purpose, set of performance goals, and approach for which they hold themselves mutually accountable." Teams have command or line authority to perform tasks, and membership is based on the specific skills required to accomplish the tasks. Teams may have lateral, vertical, or diagonal member composition; that is, team membership may include (a) individuals from a single work group or individuals at similar job levels from more than one work group,

(b) individuals from different job levels, or (c) individuals from different work groups *and* different job levels in the organization. They may have a short life span or exist indefinitely. Not all work groups are teams. For example, *groups of individuals* who perform their tasks independently of each other are not teams. **Competing groups**, in which members compete with each other for resources to perform their tasks or compete for recognition, also are not teams.

A work group becomes a team when the individuals must apply group process skills to achieve specific results. They must exchange ideas, coordinate work activities, and develop an understanding of other team members' roles in order to perform effectively. Members appreciate the talents and contributions of each individual on the team and find ways to capitalize on them. Most work teams have a leader who maintains the integrity of the team's function and guides the team's activities, performance, and development. Teams may be *self-directed*, that is, led jointly by group members who decide together about work objectives and activities on an ongoing basis.

In a given service area, the entire staff might not function as a team, but a subgroup may. For example, case managers for the inpatient and ambulatory cystic fibrosis population in a children's medical center might be called a team. Individual members of an interdisciplinary team, such as this one, may report formally to different managers, but in delivering care to the cystic fibrosis population there is no designated individual in charge. In meetings, the team members discuss clients' problems and jointly decide on plans of action.

Many different types of groups and teams are used throughout the organization. Examples are ad hoc task groups, quality improvement teams, quality circles, self-directed work teams, councils, and focus groups.

Most groups are considered **ordinary interacting groups**. This type of group usually has a designated formal leader, but it may be leaderless. Most work teams, task groups, and committees are ordinary interacting groups. Discussions usually begin with a statement of the problem by the group leader followed by an open, unstructured conversation. Normally, the final decision is made by consensus (without formal voting; members indicate concurrence with a group agreement that everyone can live with and support publicly). The decision also may be made by the leader or by someone in authority, by majority vote, an average of members' opinions, minority control, or an expert member (Johnson & Johnson, 1994). Interacting groups enhance the cohesiveness and esprit de corps among group members. Participants are able to build strong social ties and will be committed to the solution decided on by the group.

Ordinary interacting groups often are dominated by one or a few members. If the group is highly cohesive, its decision-making ability may be affected by "groupthink." Members may spend excessive time dealing with socioemotional relationships, reducing the time spent on the problem and slowing consensus. Ordinary groups may reach compromise decisions that may not really satisfy any of the participants. Because of these problems, the functioning of ordinary groups is very dependent on the leader's skills. (See Chapter 10 for more about group think.)

Each type of group presents the nurse manager with unique opportunities and challenges. Likert (1961) suggests that an important role of a command group leader, such as a nurse manager, is to link service areas with groups at higher levels in the organization. This link facilitates problem solving, coordination, and communication throughout the organization. Leadership roles in work groups are important and also may be either formal or informal. For example, the nurse manager formally leads the unit or service area staff but may also informally lead a support group of nurse managers.

The leader's influence on group processes, formal or informal, and the ability of the group to work together as a team often determines whether the group accomplishes its goals. Nurse managers may effectively manage work groups and turn them into teams by understanding principles of group processes and applying them to group decision making, team building, and leading committees and task forces.

Group and Team Processes

The modified version of Homans' (1950; 1961) social system conceptual scheme presented in Figure 15-1 provides a framework for understanding group inputs, processes, and outcomes. (See Chapter 8 for more about inputs, processes, and outputs.) The schematic depicts the effects of organizational and individual background factors on group leadership, including dynamics (tasks, activities, interactions, attitudes) and processes (forming, storming, norming, performing, adjourning). Elements of the required group system and processes influence each other and the emergent group system and social structure. This system determines the productivity of the group as well as members' quality of work life (job satisfaction), development, growth, and similarity in thinking. The framework distinguishes required factors that

Forming The initial stage of group development, in which individuals assemble into a well-defined cluster.

Storming The second stage of group development, in which group members develop roles and relationships; competition and conflict generally occur.

Norming The third stage of group development, in which group members define goals and rules of behavior.

Performing The fourth stage of group development, in which group members agree on basic purposes and activities and carry out the work.

Adjourning The final stage of group development in which a group dissolves after achieving its objectives.

Re-forming A stage of group development in which the group reassembles after a major change in the environment or in the goals of the group that requires the group to refocus its activities.

are imposed by the external system from factors that emerge from the internal dynamics of the group.

According to Homans' framework, the three essential elements of a group system are activities, interactions, and attitudes. *Activities* are the observable behaviors of group members. *Interactions* are the verbal or nonverbal exchanges of words or objects among two or more group members. *Attitudes* are the perceptions, feelings, and values held by individual group members, which may be both positive and negative. In order to understand and guide group functioning, a manager should analyze the activities, interactions, and attitudes of work group members.

Phases of Group and Team Development

Homans' framework indicates that background factors, the manager's leadership style, and the organizational system influence the normal development of the group. Groups, whether formal or informal, typically develop in the phases: form, storm, norm, perform, and adjourn or reform. In the initial stage, **forming**, individuals assemble into a well-defined cluster. Group members are cautious in approaching each other as they come together as a group and begin to under-

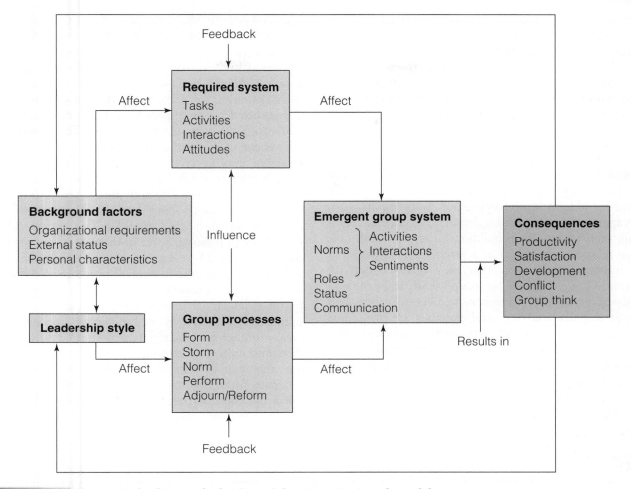

Figure 15-1 Conceptual scheme of a basic social system. *Note:* Adapted from *The human group* by G. Homans, 1950, New York: Harcourt Brace Jovanovich; and *Social behavior: Its elementary forms* by G. Homans, 1961, New York: Harcourt Brace. By permission of Transaction Publishers

stand requirements of group membership. At this stage, the members often depend on a leader to define purpose, tasks, and roles.

As the group begins to develop, **storming** occurs. Members wrestle with roles and relationships. Conflict, dissatisfaction, and competition arise on important issues related to procedures and behavior. During this stage, members often compete for power and status, and informal leadership emerges. During the storming stage, the leader helps the group to acknowledge the conflict and to resolve it in a win–win manner.

In the third stage, **norming**, the group defines its goals and rules of behavior. The group determines what are or are not acceptable behaviors and attitudes. The group structure, roles, and relationships become clearer. Cohesiveness develops. The leader

explains standards of performance and behavior, defines the group's structure, and facilitates relationship building.

In the fourth stage, **performing**, members agree on basic purposes and activities and carry out the work. The group's energy becomes task-oriented. Cooperation improves, and emotional issues subside. Members communicate effectively and interact in a relaxed atmosphere of sharing. The leader provides feedback on the quality and quantity of work, praises achievement, critiques poor work and takes steps to improve it, and reinforces interpersonal relationships within the group.

The fifth stage is either **adjourning** (the group dissolves after achieving its objectives) or **re-forming**, when some major change takes place in the environment or in the composition or goals of the group that requires the group to refocus its activities and recycle through the four stages (Tuckman, 1965; Tuckman & Jensen, 1977). When a group adjourns, the leader must prepare group members for dissolution and facilitate closure through celebration of success and leave-taking. If the group is to refocus its activities, the leader will explain the new direction and provide guidance in the process of re-forming.

Team Building

Team building (or team development) is a popular organizational development technique that can be used to address some work-group dysfunctions, such as aggression, competition, hostility, aloofness, shaming, or blaming. Team building focuses on both task and relationship aspects of a group's functioning and is intended to increase efficiency and productivity (Antai-Otong, 1997). The group's work and problem-solving procedures, member–member relations, and leadership are analyzed, and exercises are prescribed to help members modify their patterns of interaction or processes of decision making. Team building activities may include outside intervention to build team cohesiveness, use internal consultative services, be manager-driven, and/or involve the training and development of the group's members and/or leader.

Most team building, regardless of the facilitator, involves (a) gathering data through individual interviews, questionnaires, and/or group meetings about the team and its functioning; (b) diagnosing the team's strengths and areas in need of development; and (c) holding semistructured retreat sessions, usually directed by an experienced facilitator, aimed at addressing priority team problems. Team building may occur over months during specially arranged retreats or may be confined to "quick fix" activities during regular work time. Most team building involves simulated real-life activities aimed at improving the team's functioning through observing and intervening in the team's actual performance rather than through training. Some of these strategies are depicted in Table 15-1. Retreat sessions ideally are conducted away from the workplace over a period lasting from one day to several days and are insulated from professional or personal interruptions of the participants. Retreat-style team building is intended to create intense prolonged interactions that force conflicts and unhealthy group processes to the surface so that they can be examined and improved under the guidance of an objective, skilled third party. Follow-up in the work setting is often overlooked, but it is an essential final step to ensure application of new

Table 15-1 Strategies for Team Management

Problem	Solution
Member isn't a team player.	• Consider why you want person on team. • Approach person in an assertive manner. • Give person an opportunity to provide feedback on problematic situations. • If person is unable to communicate with other team members, leader might approach for one-to-one dialogue. • Listen actively, using all senses to assess both verbal and nonverbal messages. • Avoid blaming and shaming, which tend to create defensiveness and cause arguments.
Member lacks sense of personal accountability.	• Explain how failure to take responsibility affects team as a whole. (For example, "Mary, last week when you didn't present your part of the report, it set team goals back a week.") • Without blaming or shaming, provide feedback from all team members.
Team lacks clear goals.	• Brainstorm to clarify short-term goals and develop action plan. • Arrive at consensus regarding mission and goals. • Define member responsibilities. • Determine resources needed to accomplish goals, including staff, financial and administrative support, time, and equipment. • Periodically review team progress and goal attainment.
Roles and boundaries are unclear.	• With member input, leader must clarify boundaries. • All team members' roles and responsibilities must be defined, including leader's. • Periodically review team development.

Note: Antai-Otong, D. (1997). Team building in a health care setting. *American Journal of Nursing, 97*(7), 48–51.

collaborative behaviors and ongoing commitments to team development.

The most important initial activities in team building are data gathering and diagnosis. Questions must be asked about the group's context (organizational structure, climate, culture, mission, and goals); characteristics of the group's work, including group members' roles, styles, procedures, job complexity; and the team, its problem-solving style, interpersonal relationships, and relations with other groups.

The following questions may be asked:

1. To what extent do the team's members understand and accept the goals of the organization?
2. What, if any, hidden agendas interfere with the group's performance? **Hidden agendas** are members' individual unspoken objectives that interfere with commitment or enthusiasm.
3. How effective is the group's leadership?
4. To what extent do group members understand and accept their roles?
5. How does the group make decisions?
6. How does the group handle conflict? Are conflicts dealt with through avoidance, forcing, accommodating, compromising, competing, or collaborating?
7. What personal feelings do members have about each other?
8. To what extent do members trust and respect each other?
9. What is the relationship between the team and other units in the organization?

Only after diagnosing the problems of the team can the leader take actions to improve team functioning. A nurse manager may decide to assume personal responsibility for team building when the team is basically functional and simply needs some fine-tuning to deal more effectively with minor interpersonal issues or changing circumstances.

Four qualities are present in successful teams: (a) open and effective communication; (b) involved members who are committed to the team, understand team dynamics, and are emotionally invested in the team; (c) clearly defined goals that identify member roles and responsibilities; and (d) trust and collegiality. (Antai-Otong, 1997) Thoughtful team-building strategies allow group members to acknowledge the developmental process and respond to it in constructive ways. Team-building activities may also be used to facilitate the normal stages of group development (forming, storming, norming, performing, and adjourning or reforming), an important process in managing teams. Team-building techniques also may be used to intervene in traditional work groups that are experiencing problems or in any other type of group, such as a task force or committee. Numerous techniques and commercial resources are available for managers or an intervention specialist to use.

Characteristics of Groups

Norms

Norms are the informal rules of behavior shared and enforced by group members. Norms emerge whenever humans interact. Groups develop norms that members believe must be adhered to for fruitful, stable group functioning. Nursing groups often establish norms related to how members deal with absences that affect the workload of colleagues. Norms may include not calling in sick on Fridays, readily accommodating requests for trading shifts, and returning from breaks in a timely manner. In a team environment, norms are more likely to be linked to each team member's expected contribution to the performance and products of the team's efforts. If an individual agrees to take on a specific assignment on the team's behalf and fails to complete the assignment on time, a group norm has been violated.

Group norms are likely to be enforced if they serve to facilitate group survival, ensure predictability of behavior, help avoid embarrassing interpersonal problems, express the central values of the group, and clarify the group's distinctive identity. Groups go through several stages in enforcing norms with deviant members (Leavitt & Bahrami, 1988). First, members use *rational argument*, or present reasons for adhering to the norms to the deviant individual. Second, if rational argument is not effective, members may use *persuasive* or *manipulative techniques*, reminding the deviant of the value of the group. The third stage is *attack*. Attacks may be verbal or even physical and sometimes include sabotaging the deviant's work. The final stage is *ignoring the deviant*. It becomes increasingly difficult for a deviant to acquiesce to the group as these strategies escalate. Agreeing to rational argument is easy, but agreeing after an attack is very difficult. When the final stage (ignoring) is reached, acquiescence may be impossible because group members refuse to acknowledge the deviant's surrender. A nurse manager has a responsibility to help groups deal with members who violate group norms related to performance, including counseling the employee and preventing destructive conflict.

Roles

Norms apply to all group members, whereas roles are specific to positions in the group. A **role** is a set of expected behaviors that fit together into a unified whole and are characteristic of persons in a given context (Biddle, 1979). Roles commonly seen in groups can be classified as either task roles or socioemotional (nurturing) roles (Bales, 1958). Often, individuals fill several roles. Individuals performing task roles attempt to keep the group focused on its goals. Task roles include the following:

- *Initiator-contributor.* Redefines problems and offers solutions, clarifies objectives, suggests agenda items, and maintains time limits.
- *Information seeker.* Pursues descriptive bases for the group's work.
- *Information giver.* Expands information given by sharing experiences and making inferences.
- *Opinion seeker.* Explores viewpoints that clarify or reflect the values of other members' suggestions.
- *Opinion giver.* Conveys to group members what their pertinent values should be.
- *Elaborator.* Predicts outcomes and provides illustrations or expands suggestions, clarifying how they could work.
- *Coordinator.* Links ideas or suggestions offered by others.
- *Orienter.* Summarizes the group's discussions and actions.
- *Evaluator critic.* Appraises the quantity and quality of the group's accomplishments against set standards.
- *Energizer.* Motivates group to accomplish, qualitatively and quantitatively, the group's goals.

- *Procedural technician.* Supports group activity by arranging the environment (e.g., scheduling meeting room) and providing necessary tools (e.g., ordering visual equipment).
- *Recorder.* Documents the group's actions and achievements.

Nurturing roles facilitate the growth and maintenance of the group. Individuals assuming these roles are concerned with group functioning and interpersonal needs. Nurturing roles include the following:

- *Encourager.* Compliments members for their opinions and contributions to the group.
- *Harmonizer.* Relieves tension and conflict.
- *Compromiser.* Submits own position to maintain group harmony.
- *Gate-keeper.* Encourages all group members to communicate and participate.
- *Group observer.* Takes note of group processes and dynamics and informs group of them.
- *Follower.* Passively attends meetings, listens to discussions, and accepts group's decisions.

Status is the social ranking of individuals relative to others in a group based on the position they occupy. Status comes from factors the group values, such as achievement, personal characteristics, the ability to control rewards, or the ability to control information. Status is usually enjoyed by members who most conform to group norms. Higher-status members often exercise more influence in group decisions than others.

Status incongruence occurs when factors associated with group status are not congruent, such as when a younger, less experienced person becomes the group leader. Status incongruence can have a disruptive impact on a group. For example, *isolates* are members who have high external status and different backgrounds from regular group members. They usually work at acceptable levels but are isolated from the group because they do not fit the group member profile. Sometimes *status incongruence* occurs because the individual does not need the group's approval and makes no effort to obtain it.

The most important role in a group is the leadership role. Leaders are appointed for most formal groups, such as command groups, teams, committees, or task forces. Leaders in informal groups tend to emerge over time and in relation to the task to be performed. Some of the factors contributing to the emergence of leadership in small groups include the ability to accomplish the group's goals, sociability, good communication skills, self-confidence, and a desire for recognition. Guidelines for performing this leadership role are discussed later in this chapter.

Communication in Groups

Groups provide an important channel of communication in organizations. Members of high-performance work teams generally communicate openly, candidly, and clearly with one another about procedures, expectations, and plans. Communication is influenced by the status and roles of the individuals who dominate team discussions. High-status members who are fulfilling key roles in relation to a team's priorities are likely to exercise considerable control over communication in the group by determining topics, setting the tone of the discussion, and influencing how decisions are made.

Effective nurse managers can facilitate communication in groups by maintaining an atmosphere in which group members feel free to discuss concerns, make suggestions, critique ideas, and show respect and trust. An important leadership function related to communication is gate-keeping, that is, keeping communication channels open, refocusing attention on critical issues, identifying and processing conflict, fostering self-esteem, checking for understanding, actively seeking the participation of all group members, and suggesting procedures for discussing group problems.

How Groups Affect Individuals

Group relationships affect individual behavior in many ways. Organizational work groups affect the beliefs, knowledge, attitudes, values, emotions, and social behavior of individuals (Hackman, 1992). Groups profoundly affect the nature and process of communication and interpersonal relationships. On the one hand, they may engender a higher degree of competition and political activity than individual behavior. Group influence is greater than the sum of its parts. A group can bring out the best and the worst in individuals due to the stimulating presence of others. Frequently, this stimulation increases motivation, especially when an individual's potential contribution to the task is fairly clear or easily measured. On the other hand, groups can lead to inordinate conformity among group members. Groups may be tyrannical toward members and ruthless toward nonmembers and thereby contribute to conflict in the organization. Some issues involved in intragroup, intergroup, and intraorganizational conflict are discussed in Chapter 21. The effect of groups on productivity, quality of work life (job satisfaction), and development and growth are discussed below.

Group Productivity and Cohesiveness   Productivity represents how well the work group or team uses the resources available to achieve its goals and produce its services. If patient care is satisfactorily completed at the end of each shift in relation to the levels of staffing, supplies, equipment, and support services used, the group has been productive. Productivity is influenced by work-group dynamics, especially a group's cohesiveness and collaboration.

Cohesiveness is the degree to which the members are attracted to the group and wish to retain membership in it. Cohesiveness includes how much the group members enjoy participating in the group and how much they are willing to contribute. Cohesiveness is also related to homogeneity of interests, values, attitudes, and background factors. Strong group cohesiveness leads to a feeling of "we" as more important than "I" and ensures a higher degree of cooperation and interpersonal support among group members. Group norms may support or subvert organizational objectives, depending on the level of group cohesiveness. High group cohesiveness may foster high or low individual performance, depending on the prevailing group norms for performance. When cohesiveness is low, productivity may vary significantly. Although groups, in general, tend toward lower productivity, nursing education and practice have especially high standards of performance that help to counter this tendency.

Groups are more likely to become cohesive when members: (a) share similar values and beliefs; (b) are motivated by the same goals and tasks; (c) must interact to achieve their goals and tasks; (d) work in proximity to each other, for example, on the same unit and on the same shift; and (e) have specific needs that can be satisfied by involvement in the group. Group cohesiveness is also influenced by the formal reward system. Groups tend to be more cohesive when group members receive comparable treatment and pay and perform similar tasks that require interaction among the members. Similarities in values, education, social class, sex, age, and ethnicity that lead to similar attitudes strengthen group cohesiveness.

Cohesiveness can produce intense social pressure. Highly cohesive groups can demand and enforce adherence to norms regardless of their practicality or effectiveness. In this circumstance, the nurse manager may have a very difficult time influencing individual nurses, especially if the group norms deviate from the manager's values or expectations. For example, operating room nurses may be used to arriving at the time their shift starts and then changing into scrubs. The nurse manager, in contrast, may expect the staff to be changed and ready for work by the time the shift starts. In addition, group dynamics can affect absenteeism and turnover. Groups with high levels of cohesiveness exhibit lower turnover and absenteeism than groups with low levels of cohesiveness.

For most individuals, the work group provides one of the most important social contacts in life; the experience of working on an effective work team contributes significantly to one's professional confidence and to the quality of work life (job satisfaction). Research has indicated that work group relations are an important factor in job satisfaction among staff nurses (Hinshaw, Smeltzer, & Atwood, 1987). For some nurses, the work group provides the primary motivation for returning to the job day after day even though they may be dissatisfied with the employing organization or other working conditions.

Work groups not only perform tasks but also provide the context in which novices learn basic skills and become socialized and experts engage in clinical mentorship, standard setting, quality improvement, and innovation. Work-group relations influence the satisfaction of staff with their jobs, the overall quality of work life, and the quality of the environment for patient care. Managers play key roles in guiding the tasks of work groups and ensuring efficient and effective performance; managers also encourage relationships among members of work teams that will promote coordination and cooperation.

Development and Growth Groups also can provide learning opportunities by increasing individual skills or abilities, the range of resources available, and the ability to function effectively as a group in changed circumstances (Cohen, Fink, Gadon, & Willits, 1988). The group may facilitate socialization of new employees into the organization by "showing them the ropes." The nurse manager must establish an atmosphere that encourages learning new skills and knowledge, creating a group-oriented learning environment by continuously encouraging group members to improve their technical and interpersonal skills and knowledge through training and development. Group cohesiveness and effectiveness improve as staff members take responsibility for teaching each other and jointly seeking new information or techniques.

The Nurse Manager as Team Leader

Influencing group processes toward the attainment of organizational objectives is the direct responsibility of the nurse manager. Leadership is a key factor in developing work-group cohesion, fostering give-and-take, and ensuring involvement in the job (Hansen, 1991). According to Hirschhorn (1991), the manager who wishes to become successful in a team environment must balance empowerment with collaboration. The nurse manager can do a great deal to foster effective individual and group performance by promoting the benefits of group membership and increasing interdependence. By publicizing group accomplishments, creating opportunities for group members to demonstrate new skills, and supporting group social activities, the manager can increase the perceived value of group membership. Indeed, this is one of the manager's primary functions in a nursing organization. Members of groups who have a history of success are attracted to each other more than those who have not been successful.

The manager's communication style also affects group cohesiveness. The nurse manager who maintains a high degree of information power, for instance, controls not only what information is received but also who receives it. Directing information to only a few staff nurses represents a highly centralized communication structure. In a decentralized structure, the nurse manager shares information freely, encouraging a high degree of mutual communication and participative problem solving. In participative groups, each individual has the opportunity, and is encouraged, to seek and share information and to communicate frequently with anyone and everyone in the group.

Managers and staff alike check with each other to ensure that information is clear, to offer suggestions, and to provide feedback.

Group Task

The size of the group can influence its effectiveness, depending on the type of task: additive, disjunctive, divisible, or conjunctive (Steiner, 1972, 1976). The more people who work on an **additive task** (group performance depends on the sum of individual performance), the more inputs are available to produce a favorable result. For example, the game tug-of-war involves the combined effort of the team. For a **disjunctive task** (the group succeeds if one member succeeds), the greater the number of people, the higher the probability that one group member will solve the problem. Consider the Olympics. The more athletes on one team, the greater the opportunity for a gold medal. Regardless of the event, a medalist from the United States team brings recognition to the country, and every citizen is able to share the honor. With a **divisible task** (tasks that can break down into subtasks with division of labor), more people provide a greater opportunity for specialization and interdependence in performing the tasks. For instance, the construction of a car is a complex task. From design of the car to insertion of the last bolt, each individual involved has a specialized task.

On many divisible tasks, the level of interdependance is important. With a **conjunctive task** (the group succeeds only if all members succeed), more people increase the likelihood that one person can slow up the group's performance (e.g., jury trial).

There are three kinds of interdependence: (a) **pooled interdependence**, in which each individual contributes but no one contribution is dependent on any other (e.g., a committee discussion); (b) **sequential interdependence**, in which group members must coordinate their activities with others in some designated order (e.g., an assembly line); and (c) **reciprocal interdependence**, in which members must coordinate their activities with every other individual in the group (e.g., team nursing) (Thompson, 1967).

Group Size and Composition

Groups with five to ten members tend to be optimal for most complex organizational tasks, which require diversity in knowledge, skills, and attitudes and allow full participation (Atwater & Bass, 1994). In larger groups, members tend to contribute less of their individual potential while the leader is called on to take

KEY TERMS

Additive task   A task in which group performance depends on the sum of individual performance.

Disjunctive task   A task in which the group succeeds if one member succeeds.

Divisible task   Tasks that can be broken down into subtasks with division of labor.

Pooled interdependence   A type of interdependence in which each individual contributes to the group but no one contribution is dependent on any other.

Sequential interdependence   A type of interdependence in which members must coordinate their activities with others in some designated order.

Reciprocal interdependence   A type of interdependence in which members must coordinate their activities with every other individual in the group.

Conjunctive task   A task in which the group succeeds only if all members succeed.

Formal committees   Committees in an organization with authority and a specific role.

Informal committees   Committees with no delegated authority that are organized for discussion.

Task forces   Ad hoc committees appointed for a specific purpose and a limited time.

more corrective action, do more role clarification, manage more disruption, and make recognition more explicit. Groups tend to perform better with competent individuals as members. However, coordination of effort and proper utilization of abilities and task strategies must occur as well. Homogeneous groups tend to function more harmoniously, while heterogeneous groups may experience considerable conflict.

Managing Committees and Task Forces

Committees are generally permanent and deal with recurring problems. Membership on committees is usually determined by organizational position and role. **Formal committees** are part of the organization and have authority as well as a specific role. **Informal committees** are primarily for discussion and have no delegated authority. Task forces are ad hoc committees appointed for a specific purpose and a limited time. **Task forces** work on problems or projects that cannot be readily handled by the organization through its normal activities and structures. Task forces often deal with problems crossing departmental boundaries. They tend to generate recommendations and then disband.

Nurse managers often are selected for leadership roles on committees and task forces. In these leadership roles and as unit managers and team leaders, they conduct numerous meetings. The following section provides guidance for leading and conducting meetings.

Guidelines for Conducting Meetings

Although meetings are vital to the conduct of organizational work, they should be held principally for problem solving, decision making, and enhancing working relationships. Other uses of meetings, such as socializing, giving or clarifying information, or soliciting suggestions must be thoroughly justified. Meetings should be conducted efficiently and should result in relevant and meaningful outcomes. Meetings should *not* result in damaged interpersonal relations, frustration, or inconclusiveness.

The first key to a successful meeting is thorough preparation. Preparation includes clearly defining the purpose of the meeting. The nurse manager should prepare an agenda, determine who should attend, make assignments, distribute relevant material, arrange for recording of minutes, and select an appropriate time and place for the meeting. The agenda should be distributed well ahead of time, 7 to 10 days prior to the meeting, and it should include what topics will be covered, who will be responsible for each topic, what prework should be done, what outcomes are expected in relation to each topic, and how much time will be allotted for each topic.

In general, the meeting should include the fewest number of stakeholders who can actively and effectively participate in decision making, who have the skills and knowledge necessary to deal with the agenda, and who adequately can represent the interests of those who will be affected by decisions made. Too few or too many participants may limit the effectiveness of a committee or task force.

Meetings should be held in places where interruptions can be controlled and at a time when there is a natural time limit to the meeting, such as late in the morning or afternoon, when lunch or dinner make natural time barriers. Meetings should be limited to 50 to 90 minutes, except when members are dealing with complex, detailed issues in a one-time session. Meetings that exceed 90 minutes should be planned to include breaks at least every hour. Meetings should start and finish on time. Starting late positively reinforces latecomers, while penalizing those who arrive on time or early. If sanctions for late arrival are indicated, they should be applied respectfully and objectively. If it is the leader who is late, the cost of starting meetings late should be reiterated and an appropriate designee should begin the meeting on time.

The behavior of each member may be positive, negative, or neutral in relation to the group's goals. Members may contribute very little, or they may use the group to meet personal needs. Some members may assume most of the responsibility for the group action, thereby enabling less participative members to avoid contributing. Appropriate behaviors, listed in Box 15-1, facilitate group performance. All attendees should be familiar with behaviors that they may employ to facilitate well-managed meetings. All meeting participants must be helped to understand that they share responsibility for successful meetings.

A leader can increase meeting effectiveness greatly by not permitting one individual to dominate the discussion; separating idea generation from evaluation;

Box 15-1 Guidelines for Group Members

- Come prepared with necessary information.
- Listen to others with an open mind.
- Contribute information, ideas, and opinions.
- Ask other members for ideas and opinions.
- Request clarification of information.

- Recognize opposing points of view.
- Keep remarks on the topic.
- Be willing to state disagreement and give rationale.
- Volunteer to help with the implementation of decisions, when appropriate.

Note: From David P. Gustafson. Used by permission.

Box 15-2 | Guidelines for Leading Group Meetings

- Begin and end on time.
- Create a warm, accepting, and nonthreatening climate.
- Arrange seating to minimize differences in power, maximize involvement, and allow visualization of all meeting activities. (A U-shape is optimal.)
- Use interesting and varied visuals and other aids.
- Clarify all terms and concepts. Avoid jargon.
- Foster cooperation in the group.
- Establish goals and key objectives.
- Keep the group focused.
- Focus the discussion on one topic at a time.

- Facilitate thoughtful problem solving.
- Allocate time for all problem-solving steps.
- Promote involvement.
- Facilitate integration of material and ideas.
- Encourage exploration of implications of ideas.
- Facilitate evaluation of the quality of the discussion.
- Elicit the expression of dissenting opinions.
- Summarize discussion.
- Finalize the plan of action for implementing decisions.
- Arrange for follow-up.

encouraging members to refine and develop the ideas of others (a key to the success of brainstorming); recording problems, ideas, and solutions on a blackboard or flip chart; checking for understanding; periodically summarizing information and the group's progress; encouraging further discussion; and bringing disagreements out into the open and facilitating their reconciliation. The leader is also responsible for drawing out the members' hidden agendas (personal goals or needs). Revealing hidden agendas ensures that these agendas either contribute positively to group performance or are neutralized. Guidelines for leading group meetings are provided in Box 15-2.

Managing Task Forces

There are a few critical differences between task forces and formal committees. For example, members of a task force have less time to build relationships with each other, and, because task forces are temporary, there may be no desire for long-term positive relationships. Formation of a task force may suggest that the organization's usual problem-solving mechanisms have failed. This perception may lead to tensions among task force members and between the task force and other units in the organization. The various members of a task force usually come from different parts of the organization and, therefore, have different values, goals, and viewpoints. The leader will need to take specific action to efficiently familiarize task force members with each other and create bonds in relation to the task.

Preparing for the First Meeting   Prior to the task force's first meeting, the leader must clarify the objectives of the task force in terms of specific measurable outcomes, determine its membership, set a task completion date, plan how often and to whom the task force should report while working on the project, and ascertain the group's scope of authority, including its budget, availability of relevant information, and decision-making power. The task force leader should communicate directly and regularly with the administrator or governing body that commissioned the task force's work so that ongoing clarification of its charge and progress can be tracked and adjusted.

Task force members should be selected on the basis of their knowledge, skills, personal concern for the task, time availability, and organizational credibility. They should also be selected on the basis of their interpersonal skills. Those who relish group activities and can facilitate the group's efforts are especially good members. The group leader also should plan to include one or two individuals who potentially may oppose task force recommendations in order to solicit their input, involve them in the decision-making process, and win their support. By holding personal conversations with task force members before the first meeting, the group leader can explore individual expectations, concerns, and potential contributions. It also provides the leader with an opportunity to identify potential needs and conflicts and to build confidence and trust.

Conducting the First Meeting   The goal of the first meeting is to come to a common understanding of the group's task and to define the group's working procedures and relationships. Task forces must rely on the general norms of the organization to function. The task force leader should legitimize the representative nature of participation on the task force and encourage members to discuss the task force's process with the other members of the organization.

During the first meeting, a standard of total participation should be well established. The leader should remain as neutral as possible and should prevent premature decision making. Working procedures and relationships among the various members, subgroups, and the rest of the organization need to be established. The frequency and nature of full task force meetings and the number of subgroups must be determined. Ground rules for communicating must be established, along with norms for decision making and conflict resolution.

Managing Subsequent Meetings and Subgroups   In running a task force, especially when several subgroups are formed, the leader should hold full task force meetings often enough to keep all members informed of the group's progress. Unless a task force is small, subgroups are essential. The leader must not be aligned too closely with one position or subgroup. A work plan should be developed that includes realistic interim project deadlines. The task force and subgroups should be held to these deadlines. The leader plays a key role in coaching subgroups and the task force to meet its deadlines. The leader also must be sensitive to the conflicting loyalties sometimes created by belonging to a task force. One of the leader's most important roles is to communicate information to both task force members and the rest of the organization in a timely and regular fashion. The leader should solicit feedback from other key organizational representatives during the course of the organization's work.

Completion of the Task Force's Report   In bringing a project to completion, the task force should prepare a written report for the commissioning administrators that summarizes the findings and recommendations. Drafts of this report should be shared with the full task force prior to presentation. To identify any overlooked or sensitive information and reduce defensive reactions, it is especially important that the task force leader personally brief key administrators prior to presenting the report. This gives administrators a chance to read and respond to the report before making recommendations. The leader should consider in-

volving a few task force members in the administrative presentation.

Patient Care Conferences

Patient-related conferences are held for the purpose of addressing the needs of individual patients or patient populations. The purpose of the conference determines the composition of the group. Patient-focused meetings are usually multidisciplinary and used for case management to discuss specific patient care problems. For example, a multidisciplinary team may form to discuss the failure of a rehabilitation regimen to help a home care patient and to develop new plans for intervention. Often nurses also are involved in activities associated with improving the quality of care for various patient groups and their families. For example, a nurse manager might organize meetings with primary care physicians to discuss how to improve discharge planning, to explore strategies to reduce the length of inpatient stays, or to improve the coordination of care for ambulatory patients.

Summary

- A group is an aggregate of individuals who interact and mutually influence each other. Groups may be classified as real or task, formal or informal, permanent or temporary.

- A team is a group of individuals with complementary skills, a common purpose and performance goals, and a set of methods for which they hold themselves accountable.

- Groups develop through five normal stages: forming, storming, norming, performing, and adjourning or re-forming.

- Groups have an impact on cohesiveness and productivity, as well as individual development and growth.

- A group's norms and roles directly influence the productivity and satisfaction of group members and their ability to develop and grow.

- Principles of effective management of meetings include preparing thoroughly, encouraging all members to participate and communicate openly, separating idea generations from evaluations, recording problems, summarizing information and the group's progress, and identifying disagreements and facilitating reconciliation.

■ LEADERSHIP AND MANAGEMENT
in Action

1. What are the differences between groups and teams?
2. Describe how group and leader characteristics differ during each stage of development.
3. What informal groups do you belong to? Formal groups?

References

Antai-Otong, D. (1997). Team building in a health care setting. *American Journal of Nursing, 97*(7), 48–51.

Atwater, D. C., & Bass, B. M. (1994). Transformational leadership in teams. In B. M. Bass & B. J. Avolio (Eds.), *Improving organizational effectiveness through transformational leadership* (pp. 48–83). Thousand Oaks, CA: Sage.

Bales, R. F. (1958). Task roles and social roles in problem-solving groups. In E. E. Maccoby, T. M. Newcomb & E. L. Hartley (Eds.), *Readings in social psychology.* New York: Holt, Rinehart & Winston.

Biddle, B. J. (1979). *Role theory: Expectations, identities, and behavior.* New York: Academic Press.

Cohen, A. R., Fink, S. L., Gadon, H., & Willits, R. D. (1988). *Effective behavior in organizations.* Homewood, IL: Irwin.

Dailey, R., Young, F., & Barr, L. (1991). Empowering middle managers in hospitals with team-based problem solving. *Health Care Management Review, 16*(2), 55–63.

Hackman, J. R. (1992). Group influences on individuals in organizations. In M. D. Dunnette & L. M. Hough (Eds.), *Handbook of industrial and organizational psychology,* vol. 3, 2nd ed. Palo Alto, CA: Consulting Psychologists Press, pp. 199–267.

Hansen, H. E. (1991). Collegiality among staff registered nurses: Test of a conceptual model. (Doctoral dissertation, University of Kansas, 1991). *Dissertation Abstracts International, 53*(11B), 5, 642. University Microfilms No. 92538651.

Hinshaw, A. S., Smeltzer, L. H., & Atwood, J. R. (1987). Innovative retention strategies for nursing staff. *Journal of Nursing Administration, 17*(6), 8–16.

Hirschhorn, L. (1991). *Managing in the new team environment: Skills, tools, and methods.* Reading, MA: Addison-Wesley.

Homans, G. (1950). *The human group.* New York: Harcourt Brace Jovanovich.

Homans, G. (1961). *Social behavior: Its elementary forms.* New York: Harcourt Brace.

Johnson, D., & Johnson, S. (1994). *Joining together: Group theory and group skills,* 5th ed. Boston: Allyn & Bacon.

Katzenbach, J. R., & Smith, D. K. (1993). The discipline of teams. *Harvard Business Review, 71*(2), 111–120.

Lawler, E. E., & Mohrman, S. A. (1988). Quality circles: After the honeymoon. In J. W. Pfeiffer (Ed.), *The 1988 annual: Developing human resources.* San Diego, CA: University Associates.

Leavitt, H. J., & Bahrami, H. (1988). *Managerial psychology,* 5th ed. Chicago: University of Chicago Press.

Likert, R. (1961). *New patterns of management.* New York: McGraw-Hill.

Shaw, M. E. (1981). *Group dynamics,* 3rd ed. New York: McGraw-Hill.

Steiner, I. D. (1972). *Group process and productivity.* New York: Academic Press.

Steiner, I. D. (1976). Task-performing groups. In J. W. Thibaut, J. T. Spence & R. C. Carson (Eds.), *Contemporary topics in social psychology* (pp. 94–108). Morristown, NJ: General Learning Press.

Thompson, J. D. (1967). *Organizations in action.* New York: McGraw-Hill.

Tuckman, B. W. (1965). Developmental sequences in small groups. *Psychological Bulletin, 72,* 384–399.

Tuckman, B. W., & Jensen, M. A. (1977). Stages of small group development revisited. *Group and Organizational Studies, 2,* 419–427.

 Additional on-line resources for this chapter can be found on the World Wide Web at http://www.prenhall.com/sullivan_decker. Select Chapter 15 from the drop-down menu.

Initiating and Managing Change

Nurse as Change Agent

Nurse as Entrepreneur

The Process of Change

Change Theories

Lewin's Force-Field Model
Lippitt's Phases of Change
Havelock's Model
Rogers' Diffusion of Innovations
Using Change Theories in
   Nursing

Planning Change

Assessment
Planning
Implementation
Evaluation

Change Agent Strategies

Power-Coercive Strategies
Empirical-Rational Model
Normative-Reeducative Strategies

Change Agent Skills

Responses to Change

Politics of Change

Looking Ahead

How do you view change? Does it bring up feelings of anxiety and distrust? Or do you see it as a challenge? Today's health care environment is changing rapidly; as we've shown in the opening chapters, it pervades every aspect of our work environment. How can nurses learn to view this transformation as positive and even go so far as to initiate change? This chapter examines the theoretical approach to the process of change and offers insights into planning, implementing, and evaluating change while developing the skills necessary to become an effective change agent.

Objectives

After reading this chapter, you will be able to:

- Describe the change process.
- Compare and contrast change theories.
- Delineate the steps in planned change.
- Compare and contrast change agent strategies.
- Discuss the skills that a change agent needs.
- Describe ways to handle resistance.

The health care system is in the midst of unprecedented change in a climate of uncertainty. Change has become constant, pervasive, and persistent (Hammer & Champy, 1993). Much of this change is economically driven. Federal and state governments, insurance companies, employers, labor unions, and the public are exerting external pressure to control spending and redirect health care from expensive inpatient care to more cost-effective outpatient care. The major payers of health care are pressuring for better management of resource consumption.

Health care organizations must change substantially if they are to weather these pressures. To survive, they must be focused yet flexible (Kanter, 1989). Restructuring is an ongoing activity in health care organizations as outpatient services are expanded and new programs added. New patient care delivery systems are designed to maximize efficiency and quality while controlling cost. These changes require modifications in technology, personnel, and structure. In today's economic environment, organizational change is essential for adaptation; creative change is mandatory for growth.

This climate for change produces new opportunities for nurses. Nurses are rethinking the way health care is organized and delivered. Innovation is in. The participatory approach is popular because status quo management will not work when a whole system is in transition. Transitional times demand new ways of thinking, creative strategies, and fresh opinions.

Change is inevitable, if not always welcome. Change is necessary for growth, although it often produces anxiety and fear. Even when planned, it can be threatening and a source of conflict because **change** is the process of making something different from what it was. There is a sense of loss of the familiar, the status quo. This is particularly true when change is unplanned or beyond human control. Even when change is expected and valued, a grief reaction still may occur. Those who initiate and manage change often encounter resistance from those experiencing unease and, possibly, symptoms of anxiety and grief.

Although nurse managers should understand and anticipate these reactions to change, they need to develop and exude a different approach. They can view change as a challenge and encourage their colleagues to participate. They can become uncomfortable with the status quo and be willing to take risks. Leaders initiate change; followers survive it. Nurse managers must become skilled in implementing organizational change and in initiating change within the organization. Nurse leaders must initiate the changes they

believe are necessary to strengthen nursing practice, provide quality care, and create a better system.

The problem-solving change process described in this chapter synthesizes classical change theory and current nursing, sociological, psychological, and organizational thought.

Nurse as Change Agent

A **change agent** is one who works to bring about a change. The notion of the nurse as change agent is not new. The nurse often acts as an insider, a change agent who is part of the system being altered (managing a unit or team). But nurses can also be outsiders or consultants for change in other systems. There has never been a better time for the nursing profession to take the initiative. As the largest health profession, nurses make the health care system run; they have concrete ideas about how to make it run better. Nurses who can suggest changes to control costs, improve quality, or offer new services will be in great demand.

Changes will continue at a rapid pace with or without nursing's expert guidance. Nurses, like organizations, cannot afford merely to survive changes. If they are to exist as a distinct profession that has expertise in helping individuals respond to actual or potential health problems, they must be proactive in shaping the future. Opportunities exist now for nurses, especially those in management positions, to change the system about which they so often complain.

Nurse as Entrepreneur

Managing patient care with innovative practice and expanding nursing boundaries are demonstrated outcomes of entrepreneurial activity. Many nurses assume the role of entrepreneur when functioning as change agents. The entrepreneurial nurse views change as healthy and seeks to initiate change proactively. Imagination, boldness, ingenuity, leadership, persistence, and determination are key attributes of an entrepreneur (Baumal, 1993). Applying these attributes in nursing has resulted in such innovations as primary nursing, advanced practice roles, case management, critical paths, creative staffing alternatives, professional practice models, and incentive programs for staff. These examples are not exhaustive. Nurses adopting an entrepreneurial role have created and will continue to create numerous changes in the nursing profession.

The Process of Change

Change is a continual unfolding process rather than an either/or event (Conner, 1993). The process begins with the present state, moves through a transition period, and ultimately comes to a desired state. Once the desired state has been reached, however, the process begins again. In today's environment, any permanent state is obsolete. Integrative thinking, skill in applying change theory, and an aptitude for problem solving will help the change agent achieve results during this dynamic and fluid process.

Change Theories

Lewin's Force-Field Model

Lewin (1951) provides a social-psychological view of the change process. He sees behavior as a dynamic balance of forces working in opposing directions within a field (such as an organization). **Driving forces** facilitate change because they push participants in the desired direction. **Restraining forces** impede change because they push participants in the opposite direction. To plan change, one must analyze these forces and shift the balance in the direction of change through a three-step process: *unfreezing, moving,* and *refreezing.* Change occurs by adding a new force, changing the direction of a force, or changing the magnitude of any one force. Basically, strategies for change are aimed at increasing driving forces, decreasing restraining forces, or both.

Lewin's force-field model and an example are diagrammed in Figure 16-1. This scheme shows how a system's driving and restraining forces oppose each other. These forces, which are part of the system's maintenance and adaptive mechanisms, are balanced at the present, or status quo, level. To achieve change, first an imbalance must occur between the driving and restraining forces, which unfreezes the present patterned behavior. Behavior moves to a new level, at

which the opposing forces are brought into a new state of equilibrium. Once participants integrate new patterns of behavior into their personalities and relationships with others, a refreezing takes place. The new level becomes institutionalized into formal and informal behavioral patterns.

Lewin's change strategies fall within this three-step process:

1. Unfreeze the existing equilibrium. Motivate participants by getting them ready for change. Build trust and recognition for the need to change. To thaw attitudes, actively participate in identifying problems and generate alternative solutions.
2. Move the target system to a new level of equilibrium. Get participants to agree that the status quo is not beneficial to them. Encourage participants to view the problem from a new perspective. Stimulate identification by linking group views to those of a respected or powerful leader who supports the change. Help them scan the environment to search for relevant information.
3. Refreeze the system at the new level of equilibrium. Reinforce the new patterns of behavior. Institutionalize them through formal and informal mechanisms (e.g., policies, communications channels).

Lewinian thinking is fundamental to the views of later theorists. Clearly, it is a behavioral approach that nurses find consistent with their theoretical understanding of human behavior. The image of people's attitudes thawing and then refreezing is conceptually useful. This symbolism helps to keep theory and reality in mind simultaneously.

Lippitt's Phases of Change

Lippitt and colleagues (1958) extended Lewin's theory to a seven-step process and focused more on what the change agent must do than on the evolution of change itself. (See Table 16-1 for a comparison of four

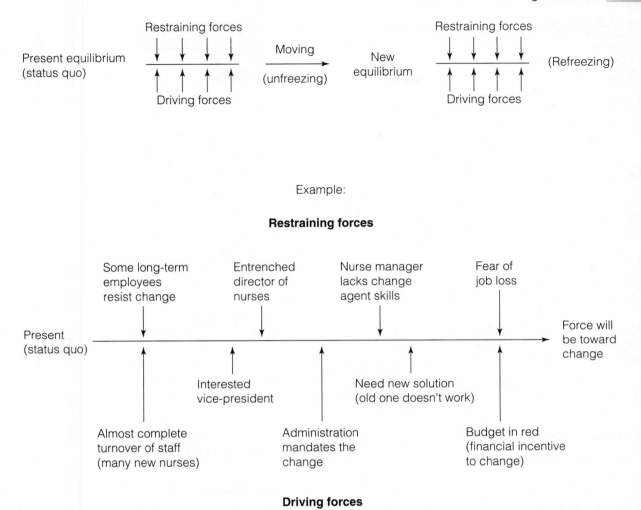

Figure 16-1 Lewin's force-field model of change. *Note: From Field Theory in Social Science* by K. Lewin, 1951, New York: Harper and Row, p. 158.

change theories.) They emphasized participation of key members of the target system throughout the change process, particularly during planning. Communication skills, rapport building, and problem-solving strategies underlie their phases. The seven steps are:

1. Diagnose the problem. Involve key people in data collection and problem solving.
2. Assess the motivation and capacity for change. What are the financial and human resources and constraints? Are the structure and function of the organization conducive to change? What are the possible solutions, and which are preferred?
3. Assess the change agent's motivation and resources. This assessment is important. Consider the change agent's own commitment to change, energy level, future ambitions, and power bases. Starting a change and dropping it midstream can waste valuable personal energy and undermine the confidence of colleagues and subordinates.
4. Select progressive change objects. Develop the action plan, evaluation criteria, and specific strategies.
5. Choose a change agent role. The change agent can act as cheerleader, expert, consultant, or group facilitator. Whichever role is selected, all participants should recognize it so that expectations are clear.
6. Maintain the change. Communication, feedback, revision, and coordination are essential components of this phase.

Table 16-1 Comparison of Change Models

Lewin	Lippitt	Havelock	Rogers
1. Unfreezing	1. Diagnose problem	1. Building a relationship	1. Knowledge
2. Moving	2. Assess motivation	2. Diagnosing the problem	2. Persuasion
3. Refreezing	3. Assess change agent's motivations and resources	3. Acquiring resources	3. Decision
	4. Select progressive change objects	4. Choosing the solution	4. Implementation
	5. Choose change agent role	5. Gaining acceptance	5. Confirmation
	6. Maintain change	6. Stabilization and self-renewal	
	7. Terminate helping relationships		

7. Terminate the helping relationship. The change agent withdraws from the selected role gradually as the change becomes institutionalized.

Havelock's Model

Havelock (1973) described a six-step process, also a modification of Lewin's model (see Table 16-1). Havelock emphasizes the unfreezing or planning stage, which he defines as (a) building a relationship, (b) diagnosing the problem, and (c) acquiring resources. This stage is followed by the moving stage: (d) choosing the solution and (e) gaining acceptance. Refreezing is referred to as (f) stabilization and self-renewal. Havelock describes an active change agent as one who uses a participative approach.

Rogers' Diffusion of Innovations

Rogers (1983) takes a broader approach than Lewin, Lippitt, or Havelock (see Table 16-1). His five-step innovation-decision process details how an individual or decision-making unit passes from first knowledge of an innovation to confirmation of the decision to adopt or reject a new idea. His framework emphasizes the reversible nature of change: Participants may initially adopt a proposal but later discontinue it, or the reverse—they may initially reject it but adopt it at a later time. This is a useful distinction. If the change agent is unsuccessful in achieving full implementation of a proposal, it should not be assumed the issue is dead. It can be resurrected, perhaps in an altered form or at a more opportune time. However, if it is accepted, one also cannot assume permanence.

Rogers' five steps to the diffusion of innovation follow:

1. *Knowledge.* The decision-making unit is introduced to the innovation and begins to understand it.

2. *Persuasion.* A favorable (or unfavorable) attitude toward the innovation forms.
3. *Decision.* Activities lead to a decision to adopt or reject the innovation.
4. *Implementation.* The innovation is put to use, and reinvention or alterations may occur.
5. *Confirmation.* The individual or decision-making unit seeks reinforcement that the decision was correct. If there are conflicting messages or experiences, the original decision may be reversed.

Finally, Rogers stresses two important aspects of successful planned change: Key people and policy makers must be interested in the innovation and committed to making it happen.

Using Change Theories in Nursing

Nurses need to evaluate the plethora of change theories available and select those most appropriate for the situation. The criteria for selecting an appropriate theory to guide change includes the theory's congruence with nursing's world view, significance, clarity, consistency, economy, generality, practicality, and testability. Lutjens and Tiffany (1994) have developed a framework, depicted in Box 16-1, that provides a systematic method of evaluating the change theory for suitability. Thoughtful evaluation and analysis of change theory, selection and application of appropriate theory, and continued research of planned change strengthen nursing's ability to influence change.

Planning Change

A seven-step, eclectic approach comparable to the nursing process can be used by nurses to effect planned change. The nursing process arose in the 1950s, when nurses sought a framework for problem solving in patient care. The process of assessment,

Box 16-1   Evaluation Scale for Planned Change Theory

1. Significance
   - Does the planned change theory address recipients of (targets for) change, wholeness of the social unit, and initiators of planned change?
   - Does the theory allow for unique factors specific to individual social systems?
   - Does the theory have an assessment process that leads the change agent to identification of a problem in social systems, a clear process for planning and implementing the change, and a process for evaluating the change event?
   - Does the theory account for emerging problems and/or goals through the change process?
   - Does the theory prompt nurse change agents to ask if the proposed change is important for nursing?
   - Does the theory advocate for ethical use of power, mutuality, informed decision making, and social justice?

2. Agreement with nursing's world view
   - Does the planned change theory reflect a holistic and dynamic world view?
   - Are the theory's basic assumptions consistent with a world view of change or persistence?

3. Clarity and consistency
   - Is planned change clearly defined?
   - Does the definition of planned change fit with the content of the theory?
   - Are key ideas clearly defined?
   - Do key ideas and relational statements avoid redundancy?
   - Are key ideas and relational statements logically related to one another?
   - Are key ideas used consistently as defined throughout the theory?
   - Are basic assumptions made explicit in the theory?

4. Economy
   - Does the theory focus only on the processes of planned change rather than haphazard, spontaneous, reactive, or developmental change?
   - Do any schematic models offered enhance understanding of planned change and its processes?
   - Does the theory contain only the essential elements of planned change?

5. Generality
   - Is the purpose of the theory to implement planned change in any one of a number of clinical settings, or in one specific setting or area?
   - Can this theory apply to individuals, groups, communities, society, or diverse cultures within and outside the United States?

6. Practicality
   - Does the planned change theory contribute to an understanding of planned change beyond what could be obtained from everyday experience or formal areas of study?
   - Could nurse change agents use this theory to create change in clinical settings, nursing education, and nursing administration, or to conceptualize empirical studies?
   - Does the theory prompt change agents to consider time frames, human resources, staff support resources, financial resources, and organizational support?
   - Does the theory prompt change agents to consider whether the strategies anticipated will agree with expectations of the social unit targeted for change?
   - Does the theory prompt change agents to consider whether they can obtain needed legal and/or political resources for implementing change?
   - Does the theory prompt change agents to consider possible procedural and cultural pitfalls inherent in planned change and suggest ways to address these?
   - Does the theory alert change agents to consider immediate, intermediate, and long-term resistance to change strategies and/or consequences of adoption of proposed innovations (solutions)?

7. Testability
   - Can the theory be tested through research?
   - Can testable hypotheses be derived from the theory?
   - Do empiric indicators exist for key ideas and processes in the theory?

Note: From "Evaluating Planned Change Theories" by L. R. Lutjens and C. R. Tiffany, 1994, *Nursing Management, 25*(3), p. 55.

planning, implementation, and evaluation now structures nurses' thinking and care delivery; it is second nature to the professional nurse. Essentially, managing change follows the same path as the nursing process: assessment, planning, implementation, and evaluation, but the change process includes seven steps. Emphasis is placed on the assessment phase of change for two reasons. First, without thorough data collection and analysis, planned change will not proceed past the "wouldn't it be a good idea if" stage. Second, nurses often are not familiar with the kind of data they need to collect or with the method by which to analyze data to manage and initiate change.

Assessment

Identify the Problem or the Opportunity   Change is often planned to close a discrepancy between the desired and actual state of affairs. Discrepancies may arise because of problems in reaching performance goals or because new goals have been created. Opportunities demand change as much as (or more than) problems do, but they are often overlooked. Be it a problem or an opportunity, it must be identified clearly. If the issue is perceived differently by key individuals, the search for solutions becomes confused. Start by asking the right questions, such as

1. Where are we now? What is unique about us? What should our business be?
2. What can we do that is different from and better than what our competitors do?
3. What is the driving stimulus in our organization? What determines how we make our final decisions?
4. What prevents us from moving in the direction we wish to go?
5. What kind of change is required?

This last question generates integrative thinking on the potential effect of change on the system. Organizational change involves modifications in the system's interacting components: technology, structure, and people. The introduction of new technology may necessitate changes in the structure of the organization. The physical plant will be altered if new services (e.g., open heart surgery) are added. Relationships among the people who work in the system change when the structure is changed. New units open; others close. New rules and regulations, new authority structures, and new budgeting methods may emerge. They, in turn, change staffing needs, requiring people with different skills, knowledge bases, attitudes, and motivations.

Example   Upper management in a medium-sized medical center identified a staffing problem that they wanted to solve by using temporary agency nurses, pulling staff from one floor to float to another, and requesting nurses to remain on duty for an additional 8 hours for overtime pay. However, Marie, a pediatric unit supervisor, saw the problem differently. The problem, in her view, was mismanagement of human resources. Nurses who are experts in the care of children are reluctant to be pulled to units that do not require this expertise or to units that require expertise the child care specialist does not have. During periods of frequent pulling, Marie noticed that these nurses were more likely to call in sick.

With this problem in focus, ideas were generated. The problem was refashioned into an opportunity to create a children's center, a decentralized unit encompassing all pediatric and pediatric intensive care services. The proposal was to staff and manage this unit autonomously, with collaboration between Marie and the pediatric nurses under her jurisdiction. No nurse would float in or out of this unit. Rather, a contingency schedule provided a stable plan for adequate staffing to maintain optimal patient care and, at the same time, promote collegial relationships and accountability. It also lowered overtime costs. Nurses were less likely to call in sick needlessly when they knew their colleagues would be required to cover for them.

Collect Data   Once the problem or opportunity has been clearly defined, the change agent collects data external and internal to the system. This step is crucial to the eventual success of the planned change. All driving and restraining forces are identified so the driving forces can be emphasized and the restraining forces reduced. It is imperative to assess the political pulse. Who will gain from this change? Who will lose? Who has more power and why? Can those power bases be altered? How?

The nurse manager can best assess the political climate by examining the reasons for the present situation. Who is in control who may be benefiting now? Egos, commitment of the involved people, and personality likes and dislikes are as important to assess as the formal organizational structures and processes. The innovator has to gauge the potential for resistance.

The costs and benefits of the proposed change are obvious focal points. The nurse manager also needs to assess resources—especially those the manager can control. A manager who has the respect and support of an excellent nursing staff has access to a powerful resource in today's climate.

To introduce her proposal for a decentralized unit with autonomous staffing prerogatives, Marie had to collect data to support her arguments. Examples of external data included state, regional, and local statistics regarding supply of and demand for general and pediatric nurses; consumer demand for expert pediatric nursing services; staffing policies from competing organizations; and research data regarding motivation of professional employees.

Internal data were derived from different system levels (organizational, group, and personal). At the organization level, the supervisor examined the hospital's philosophy, goals, and marketing plans. She sought evidence that the hospital would benefit from marketing a children's center with a stable staff of specialist nurses. There was no competing focus, which would have been the case if administration had long-range plans to market a different unit. At the group and personal levels, Marie consulted her own staff and discussed the ideas with nurses from other specialized units. If the staff had been organized into a bargaining unit, she would have had to investigate the bargaining unit's negotiated staffing policies and potential support for the idea. The goal was to collect data to support the idea that this change matched the goals, norms, and values of the organization and its members. As a nurse leader, Marie was also interested in demonstrating how this idea reflected the goals and values of the nursing department and the profession.

Quantitative data help document needed change. Historical staffing and turnover data for this unit were compiled. Records were kept demonstrating higher absenteeism during periods of frequent pulling. Incident reports of unit and nonunit members documented the higher quality of care provided by seasoned specialists as opposed to temporary nurses. Finally, Marie estimated the cost savings expected from eliminating the need to hire temporary nurses.

Analyze Data   The kinds, amounts, and sources of data collected are important, but they are useless unless they are analyzed. The change agent should focus more energy on analyzing and summarizing the data than on just collecting it. The point is to flush out resistance, identify potential solutions and strategies, begin to identify areas of consensus, and build a case for whichever option is selected. When possible, a statistical analysis should be made; it is worth the effort, especially when the change agent will need to persuade persons in power. The case should be presented cogently and succinctly using visual aids (e.g., bar graphs and charts) if needed.

Planning

Planning the who, how, and when of the change is a key step. What will be the target system for the change? Members from this system should be active participants in the planning stage. The more involved they are at this point, the less resistance there will be later. Lewin's unfreezing imagery is relevant here. Present attitudes, habits, and ways of thinking have to soften so members of the target system will be ready for new ways of thinking and behaving. Boundaries must melt before the system can shift and restructure.

This is the time to make people uncomfortable with the status quo. Plant the seeds of discontent by introducing information that may make people feel dissatisfied with the present and interested in something new. This information comes from the data collected (e.g., research findings, quantitative data, and surveys of clients or staff). Couch the proposed change in comfortable terms as far as possible, and minimize anxiety about the new change.

Managers need to plan the resources required to make the change and establish feedback mechanisms to evaluate its progress and success. Establish control points with people who will provide the feedback and work with these people to set specific goals with time frames. Develop operational indicators that signal success or failure in terms of performance and satisfaction.

Potential control points and indicators for the children's center proposal might be as follows:

1. Within 6 months, the nurse manager in collaboration with staff nurses will develop a monthly staffing contingency schedule.
2. Within 8 months, there will be a 20% decline in sick leave use.
3. Within 10 months, the staff will meet with upper management to report the effect of the new staffing policy on their professional identity and sense of control.
4. Within 12 months, the nurse manager will submit a recommendation to continue or discontinue the staffing policy based on such evidence as staff turnover, sick time, and use of agency personnel.

Implementation

The plans are put into motion (Lewin's moving stage). Interventions are designed to gain the necessary compliance. The change agent creates a supportive climate, acts as energizer, obtains and provides feedback, and overcomes resistance. Managers are the key change-process actors. Some methods are directed toward changing individuals in an organization, while others are directed toward changing the group.

Methods to Change Individuals   The most common method used to change individuals' perceptions, attitudes, and values is information giving (Katz & Kahn, 1978; Nutt, 1986). External expert consultants or internal staff prepare and disseminate the information, usually in a top-down communication flow. Providing information is prerequisite to change implementation, but it is inadequate unless lack of information is the only obstacle to effecting change. Providing information does not address the motivation to change.

Training is often considered a method to change individuals. Training combines information giving with skill practice. Training typically shows people how they are to perform in a system, not how to change it. Therefore, it is more of a system maintenance mechanism than a change strategy.

Selection and placement of personnel or termination of key people often is used to alter the forces for or against change. When key supporters of the planned change are given the authority and accountability to make the change, their enthusiasm and legitimacy can be effective in leading others to support the change. Conversely, if those opposed to the change are transferred or leave the organization, the change is more likely to succeed.

Methods to Change Groups   Some implementation tactics use groups rather than individuals to attain compliance to change. The power of an organizational group to influence its members depends on its authority to act on an issue and the significance of the issue itself. The greatest influence is achieved when group members discuss issues that are perceived as important and make relevant, binding decisions based on those discussions. Effectiveness in implementing organizational change is most likely when groups are composed of members who occupy closely related positions in the organization.

Individual and group implementation tactics can be combined. Whatever methods are used, participants should feel their input is valued and should be rewarded for their efforts. Some people are not always persuaded before a beneficial change is implemented. Sometimes behavior changes first, and attitudes are modified later to fit the behavior. In this case, the change agent should be aware of participants' conflicts and reward the desired behaviors. It may take some time for attitudes to catch up.

Marie recognized that she was initiating a unit-level change that would have systemwide implications. Both individual and group methods of change were needed. Providing fact sheets to her own unit members heightened their interest and offered a common ground for later discussion. To reduce resistance from other supervisors, she met informally with them one by one. Her tactic was to change attitudes by appealing to their professional values. Group meetings followed, in which she suggested a trial program and requested participation in developing guidelines for contingency scheduling. She began to screen staff nurse applicants as to their desire for autonomy. In addition, she persuaded the chief nurse executive and the nurse recruiter to join her in a visit to another hospital that had already instituted a similar policy in its critical care unit.

Evaluation

Evaluate Effectiveness   At each control point, the operational indicators established are monitored. The change agent determines whether presumed benefits were achieved from a financial as well as a qualitative perspective, explaining the extent of success or failure. Unintended consequences and undesirable outcomes may have occurred.

For example, Marie might discover that the new children's center is successful in attracting patients. However, she would also need to measure staff satisfaction. It is possible the staff resent covering for one another and that conflict is brewing.

Stabilize the Change   The change is extended past the pilot stage, and the target system is refrozen. The change agent terminates the helping relationship by delegating responsibilities to target system members. The energizer role is still needed to reinforce new behaviors through positive feedback. Marie might suggest that the public relations department write an article on the changes in the hospital's in-house magazine, or she might ask some of the nurses in the new unit to speak at a local management meeting. In this way, Marie can recognize the staff's role in the change and promote a progressive image of the hospital at the same time.

Change Agent Strategies

Regardless of the setting or proposed change, the seven-step change process should be followed. However, specific strategies can be used, depending on the amount of resistance anticipated and the degree of power the change agent possesses.

Power-Coercive Strategies

Power-coercive strategies are based on the application of power by legitimate authority, economic sanctions, or political clout. For example, changes are made through law, policy, or financial appropriations. Those in control enforce changes by restricting budgets or creating policies. Those who are not in power may not even be aware of what is happening. Even if they are aware, they have little power to stop it. The change process continues through the seven steps, but there is little, if any, participation by the target system members. Resistance is handled by authority measures: Accept it, or leave.

The federal government's enactment of the prospective payment system for Medicare client's hospitalizations was a power-coercive strategy for changing economic incentives. Health care providers are not paid for a patient's care based on their costs but receive a predetermined fee based on the patient's diagnosis-related group (DRG). Health care organizations thus are motivated to reduce costs.

Power-coercive strategies are useful when a consensus is unlikely despite efforts to stimulate participation by those involved. When much resistance is anticipated, time is short, and the change is critical for organizational survival, power-coercive strategies may be necessary. Marianne, a vice president of nursing, exerted legitimate authority when she appointed Susan as acting nurse manager after the manager was hurt in an auto accident. Although the professional autonomy of the unit's members would be better served if they were given the opportunity to interview and evaluate a candidate, organizational and unit survival needs might supersede this goal for the short run.

Of course, the potential negative consequences of Marianne using this unilateral approach cannot be ignored. If the unit members have been practicing in a decentralized framework and value the accustomed autonomy, they may feel a loss of power. Resistance to Susan as the appointed leader and morale problems might be expected. These strategies should not be used lightly or often if the manager wishes to foster a climate of openness to change.

Empirical-Rational Model

In the **empirical-rational model** of change strategies, the power ingredient is knowledge. The assumption is

that people are rational and will follow their rational self-interest if that self-interest is made clear to them. It is also assumed that the change agent who has knowledge has the expert power to persuade people to accept a rationally justified change that will benefit them. The flow of influence moves from those who know to those who do not know. New ideas are invented and communicated or diffused to all participants. Once enlightened, rational people will either accept or reject the idea based on its merits and consequences.

Because people do not always respond rationally, this strategy should not be used alone (Haffer, 1986). However, empirical-rational strategies are often effective when little resistance to the proposed change is expected and the change is perceived as reasonable. Introduction of new technology that is easy to use, cuts nursing time, and improves quality of care would be accepted readily after inservice education and perhaps a trial use. The change agent can direct the change. There is little need for staff participation in the early steps of the change process, although input is useful for the evaluation and stabilization stages. The benefits of change for the staff and perhaps research findings regarding patient outcomes are the major driving forces. Well-researched, cost-effective technology can be implemented using these strategies.

Normative-Reeducative Strategies

In contrast to the rational-empirical model, **normative-reeducative strategies** of change rest on the assumption that people act in accordance with social norms and values. Information and rational arguments are insufficient strategies to change people's patterns of actions; the change agent must focus on noncognitive determinants of behavior as well. People's roles and relationships, perceptual orientations, attitudes, and feelings will influence their acceptance of change.

In this mode, the power ingredient is not authority or knowledge, but skill in interpersonal relationships. The change agent does not use coercion or nonreciprocal influence, but collaboration. Members of the target system are involved throughout the change process. Value conflicts from all parts of the system are brought into the open and worked through so change can progress.

Normative-reeducative strategies are well suited to the creative problem solving needed in nursing and health care today. With their firm grasp of the behavioral sciences and communication skills, nurses are comfortable with this model. Changing from a traditional nursing system to self-governance or initiating a home follow-up service for hospitalized patients are examples of changes amenable to the normative-reeducative approach. In most cases, the normative-reeducative approach to change will be effective in reducing resistance and stimulating personal and organizational creativity. The obvious drawback is the time required for group participation and conflict resolution throughout the change process. When there is adequate time or when group consensus is fundamental to successful adoption of the change, the manager is well advised to adopt this framework.

Change Agent Skills

Making change is not easy, but it is a mandatory skill for managers. Successful change agents demonstrate certain characteristics that can be cultivated and mastered with practice. Among these are the following:

- The ability to combine ideas from unconnected sources
- The ability to energize others by keeping the interest level up and demonstrating a high personal energy level
- Skill in human relations; well-developed interpersonal communication, group management, and problem-solving skills. Knox and Irving (1997) noted that communication was the most important factor in promoting change.
- Integrative thinking; the ability to retain a big picture focus while dealing with each part of the system
- Sufficient flexibility to modify ideas when modifications will improve the change, but enough

persistence to resist nonproductive tampering with the planned change
- Confidence and the tendency not to be easily discouraged
- Realistic thinking
- Trustworthiness; a track record of integrity and success with other changes
- Ability to articulate a vision through insights and versatile thinking
- Ability to handle resistance

Responses to Change

Response to change varies from ready acceptance to full-blown resistance. Rogers (1983) identified six response typologies: *Innovators* love change and thrive on it. Less radical, *early adopters* are still receptive to change. The *early majority* prefers the status quo, but eventually accept the change; whereas, the *late majority* are resistive, accepting change after most others have. *Laggards* dislike change and are openly antagonistic. *Rejectors* actively oppose and may even sabotage change.

Perlman and Takacs (1990) suggest that the response to change is emotional, leading to a series of defense mechanisms. First, the need for change is *denied*. Next, emotional energies focus on *anger*, *rage*, and *resentment*. Resentment gives way to *bargaining*. Feelings of powerlessness, insecurity and loss of identity develop, resulting in *chaos* and a failure of usual defense mechanisms. This results in *self-pity* and *depression*. Eventually a *resignation* and passive acceptance of change occurs. As change is implemented, an *openness* and *readiness* evolve, leading to a sense of empowerment and a *reemergence* of equilibrium.

Silber (1993) suggests that a person's ability to change depends on flexibility and evaluation of the situation and potential consequences and benefits. Johnston (1998) maintains that confidence in the change agent is a determining factor in the acceptance of change. Whatever the motivation, resistance is to be expected. The change agent should anticipate and look for resistance to change. It will be lurking somewhere, perhaps where least expected. It can be recognized in such statements as:

- We tried that before.
- It won't work.
- No one else does it like that.
- We've always done it this way.
- We can't afford it.
- We don't have the time.
- It will cause too much commotion.

- You'll never get it past the board.
- Let's wait awhile.
- Every new boss wants to do something different.
- Let's start a task force to look at it; put it on the agenda.

Expect resistance and listen carefully to who says what, when, and in what circumstances. Open resisters are easier to deal with than closet resisters. Look for nonverbal signs of resistance, such as poor work habits and lack of interest in the change.

Resistance has positive and negative aspects. On the one hand, resistance forces the change agent to be clear about why the change is needed. The agent must know the change inside and out because she or he must defend it against challengers. The positive part of resistance is the sharper focus and problem solving it encourages. It prevents the unexpected. It forces the change agent to clarify information, keep interest level high, and establish why change is necessary. Resistance is a stimulant as much as it is a force to be overcome. It may even motivate the group to do better what it is doing now, so that it does not have to change.

On the other hand, resistance is not always beneficial, especially if it persists beyond the planning stage and well into the implementation phase. It can wear down supporters and redirect system energy from implementing the change to dealing with resisters. Morale can suffer.

When handling resistance, the change agent must first identify the need to reduce it. Resistance can be used to sharpen decision, for example, and eventually gain consensus. If it is necessary to minimize it, do not personalize the resistance. Remain rational, stick to the problem-solving change process, and proceed with the following guidelines:

1. Communicate with those who oppose the change. Get to the root of their reasons for opposition.
2. Clarify information, and provide accurate feedback.
3. Be open to revisions but clear about what must remain.
4. Present the negative consequences of resistance (e.g., threats to organizational survival, compromised patient care).
5. Emphasize the positive consequences of the change and how the individual or group will benefit. However, do not spend too much energy on rational analysis of why the change is good and why the arguments against it do not hold up. People's resistance frequently flows from feelings that are not rational.
6. Keep resisters involved in face-to-face contact with supporters. Encourage proponents to empathize with opponents, recognize valid objections, and relieve unnecessary fears.
7. Maintain a climate of trust, support, and confidence.
8. Divert attention by creating a different disturbance. Energy can shift to a more important problem inside the system, thereby redirecting resistance. Alternatively, attention can be brought to an external threat to create a bully phenomenon. When members perceive a greater environmental threat (such as competition or restrictive governmental policies), they tend to unify internally.
9. Follow the politics of change.

Politics of Change

Energy is needed to change a system. Power is the main source of that energy. Although few nurses use coercive power sources, they do rely on information, expertise, and possibly positional power to persuade others. They should be politically astute by using these classic political strategies:

1. Analyze the organizational chart. Know the formal lines of authority. Identify informal lines as well.
2. Identify key persons who will be affected by the change. Pay attention to those immediately above and below the point of change.
3. Find out as much as possible about these key people. What are their "tickle points"? What interests them, gets them excited, turns them off? What is on their personal and organizational agendas? Who typically aligns with whom on important decisions?
4. Begin to build a coalition of support before you start the change process. Identify the key people who will most likely support your idea and those who are most likely to be persuaded easily. Talk informally with them to flush out possible objections to your idea and potential opponents. What will the costs and benefits be to them—especially in political terms? Can your idea be modified in ways that retain your objectives but appeals to more key people?

This information helps the change agent develop the most sellable idea or at least pinpoint probable resistance. It is a broad beginning to the data-collection step of the change process and has to be fine-tuned once the idea is better defined.

The politics of change continue through all the steps of the change process. (See Chapter 6.) The astute change agent keeps alert at all times to monitor power struggles. All change agents must follow the cardinal rule: Don't try to change too much too fast. But the savvy change agent develops a sense of exquisite timing by pacing the change process according to the political pulse. For example, the change agent unfreezes the system during a period of coalition building and high interest, while resistance is low or at least unorganized. The change agent may stall the project beyond a pilot stage if resistance solidifies or gains a powerful ally. In this case, the change agent exercises mechanisms to reduce resistance. If resistance continues, two options should be considered: (a) the change is not workable and should be modified to meet the strongest objections (compromise); or (b) the change is fine-tuned sufficiently, but change must proceed now and resistance must be overcome. If the latter option is selected, energy is focused on overcoming resistance. Supporters are mobilized, and constant, consistent pressure is exerted to move ahead.

How the change agent uses the politics of change depends on whether she or he is an insider or outsider. Someone who is part of the system being changed knows that system, has a stake in the outcome, and is familiar with the people, language, and politics. However, being an insider can restrict one's ability to move freely throughout the system. The agent may be locked into certain roles, authority structures, and expectations. Perspective may be limited. However, blinders to insight can be removed. An outsider offers a fresh perspective and is independent of internal policies but is unfamiliar with the system, people's values, and personal agendas. Either agent can accomplish change, but change must be assessed and used differently.

Summary

- In today's health care system, change is rapid, constant, persuasive, and persistent.
- Inevitable conflicts and stresses occur as organizations and individuals learn to grow and adapt to a constant state of transition.
- The change agent has to understand how to move a change plan, how to use and reduce resistance, and how to evaluate outcomes before stabilizing or introducing further change.
- Critical evaluation of planned change theory and selection of theories suitable for nursing provide

guidance and direction for initiating and managing change.

- A seven-step process for implementing change includes identification, data collecting and analysis, strategic planning, implementation, evaluation, and stabilization.
- A change agent needs skills in discovering and handling resistance, understanding the politics of change, and using power appropriately to effect change.

■ LEADERSHIP AND MANAGEMENT *in Action*

1. Identify a needed change in the organization where you practice. Using the change process, outline the steps you would take to initiate change.
2. What types of skills are needed by change agents?
3. How can resistance to change be managed?

References

Baumal, W. J. (1993). *Entrepreneurship, management, and the structure of payoffs.* London: MIT Press.

Conner, D. R. (1993). *Managing at the speed of change.* New York: Villard Books.

Haffer, A. (1986). Facilitating change: Choosing the appropriate strategy. *Journal of Nursing Administration, 16*(4), 18–22.

Hammer, M., & Champy, J. (1993). *Reengineering the corporation: A manifesto for business revolution.* New York: HarperCollins.

Havelock, R. (1973). *The change agent's guide to innovation in education.* Englewood Cliffs, NJ: Educational Technology Publications.

Hickman, C., & Silva, M. (1984). *Creating excellence: Managing corporate culture, strategy and change in the new age.* New York: New American Library.

Johnston, B. (1998). Managing change in health care redesign: A model to assist staff in promoting healthy change. *Nursing Economics, 16*(1), 12–17.

Kanter, R. M. (1989). *When giants learn to dance.* New York: Simon & Schuster.

Katz, D., & Kahn, R. (1978). *The social psychology of organizations,* 2nd ed. New York: Wiley.

Knox, S., & Irving, J. A. (1997). Nurse manager perceptions of healthcare executive behaviors during organizational change. *Journal of Nursing Administration, 27*(11), 33–39.

Lewin, K. (1951). *Field theory in social science.* New York: Harper & Row.

Lippitt, R., Watson, J., & Westley, B. (1958). *The dynamics of planned change.* New York: Harcourt & Brace.

Lutjens, L. R. J., & Tiffany, C. R. (1994). Evaluating planned change theories. *Nursing Management, 25*(3), 54–57.

Nutt, P. (1986). Tactics of implementation. *Academy of Management Journal, 29*(2), 230–261.

Perlman, D., & Takacs, G. J. (1990). The ten stages of change. *Nursing Management, 21*(4), 33–38.

Rogers, E. (1983). *Diffusion of innovations*, 3rd ed. New York: Free Press.

Silber, M. B. (1993). The "Cs" in excellence: Choice and change. *Nursing Management, 24*(9), 60–62.

Tiffany, C. R., Cheatham, A. B., Doornbos, D., Loudermelt, L., & Momadi, G. G. (1994). Planned change theory: A survey of nursing periodical literature. *Nursing Management, 25*(7), 54–59.

Additional on-line resources for this chapter can be found on the World Wide Web at http://www.prenhall.com/sullivan_decker. Select Chapter 16 from the drop-down menu.

P A R T   3

Human Resource Management

Recruiting and Selecting Staff

Looking Ahead

Chapter 17 introduces the human resource management section of this book; the development and management of staff, dealing with problems, and the various obligations and ways of dealing with others that go along with being a manager. This chapter opens the discussion with a focus on the first step, finding quality people who are suitable for a particular job and soliciting their services. This task consists of numerous components, from analyzing the job, developing a diverse recruitment strategy, and conducting interviews to comparing candidates and arriving at a consensual decision. Chapter 17 outlines these issues and helps you develop the human resource skills required of nurse managers.

Objectives

After reading this chapter, you will be able to:

- Describe the recruitment and selection process.
- Explain job analysis.
- Discuss principles for effective interviewing.
- Discriminate appropriate from inappropriate questions to ask during an interview.
- Discuss legal issues involved in hiring.

In service or labor-intensive organizations such as health care organizations, the quality of personnel hired and retained determines whether an organization successfully accomplishes its objectives. The cost of improper selection can be high. The visible cost is in recruiting, selecting, and training an employee who must later be terminated because of unsatisfactory performance. The hidden costs may be even more expensive and include low quality of work performed by the unmotivated employee, disruption of harmonious working relationships, and patients' ill will and dissatisfaction, which may make patients reluctant to return to the particular clinic or hospital. The focus of this chapter is on job analysis, recruitment of applicants, and selection of personnel.

The Recruitment and Selection Process

The purpose of the selection process is to match people to jobs. It includes the following elements: job analysis; methods of recruiting applicants; selection technique(s) that measure applicants' skill, ability, and knowledge; and assurance that the selection techniques developed and used conform to legal requirements.

Responsibility for the selection of nursing personnel in health care organizations is usually shared by the human resources management (HRM) department and nursing management. First-line nursing managers are the most knowledgeable about job requirements and can best describe the job to applicants. HRM performs the initial screening and monitors hiring practices to be sure they adhere to legal stipulations.

Staffing responsibilities and activities can be thought of as a series of steps designed to acquire and retain personnel:

1. Planning the number and types of personnel needed according to patient care delivery systems of the organization.
2. Performing job analyses to define the duties, requirements, tasks, and qualifications of each position.
3. Developing and implementing a recruitment strategy in order to locate and attract enough qualified applicants to provide a pool of potential employees.
4. Interviewing, testing, and selecting needed personnel.
5. Orienting personnel to the job.
6. Enhancing employee performance through staff development and management of job performance.
7. Performance appraisal to provide feedback to the employee.
8. Management of personnel problems.
9. Development and implementation of strategies to retain staff.
10. Career counseling.
11. Developing exit strategies, such as preretirement counseling, exit interviews, and out-placement.

The purpose of recruitment activities is to generate a pool of qualified applicants, whereas the purpose of the selection process is to assess an applicant's ability, skills, and motivation relative to the requirements and rewards of the job so that a matching process can be carried out. To the extent that these matches are made effectively, positive outcomes such as high job satisfaction, low turnover, and high-quality performance can result.

Figure 17-1 shows a flowchart of the recruitment and selection process and suggested responsibilities. As indicated in the chart, this process is a joint effort among the nurse manager, the nursing department, and the HRM department. The recruitment and selection process begins with job analysis, which is a careful determination of job duties and requirements by nursing service, with technical assistance from HRM. Based on the job analysis and subsequent job descriptions, recruiting plans and selection systems are developed and implemented.

Once an applicant makes contact with the organization, HRM reviews the application and may conduct a preliminary interview. If the applicant does not meet the basic needs of the open position or positions, he or she should be so informed. Rejected applicants may be qualified for other positions or may refer friends to the organization and thus should be treated with utmost courtesy.

The next three stages include the selection instruments used: tests, reference checks, and managerial interviews. In most cases, the interview is last, but practices may vary. Even if an applicant does poorly on the selection test or receives poor references, it is prudent to carry out the interview so that the applicant is not aware that the test or reference checking led to the negative decision. In addition, applicants may feel they have a right to "tell their story" and may spontaneously provide information that explains poor references. The nurse manager should participate in the interview process because she or he (a) is generally in the best position to assess applicants' technical competence, potential, and overall suitability and (b) is able to answer applicants' technical, work-related questions more realistically. In some organizations,

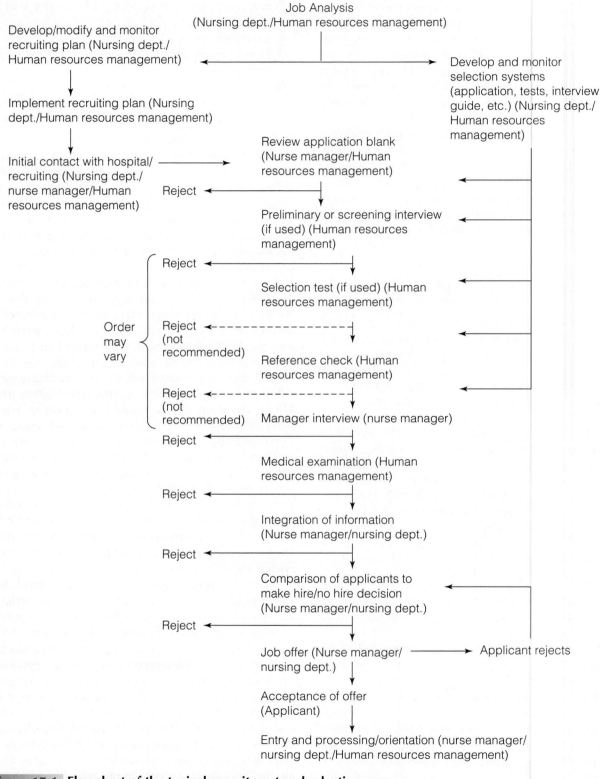

the candidate's future co-workers also participate in the interview process to assess compatibility.

After the managerial interview, the applicant is given a comprehensive medical examination to protect the organization from legal actions. For example, individuals with back problems should not be hired to work on a rehabilitation unit where a great deal of lifting of patients is required. In addition, state boards of health and other regulatory bodies require rubella, tetanus, and tuberculosis testing. The Occupational Safety and Health Administration (OSHA) requires that the hepatitis immune series be offered to health care workers who are not immune to hepatitis.

Once the medical examination has been completed, the nurse manager reviews the information available on each candidate and makes a job offer. The nurse manager must keep others involved in the selection process informed. The nurse manager is usually the first to be aware of potential resignations, requests for transfer, and maternity or family medical leaves that require personnel replacement. The manager also is aware of changes in the work area that might necessitate a redistribution of staff, such as the need for a night nurse instead of a day one. Communicating these needs to HRM promptly and accurately helps ensure effective coordination of the selection process.

Job Analysis

Before recruiting or selecting new staff, those responsible for hiring must be familiar with the job description and the skills, abilities, and knowledge required to perform the job. Duties and requirements are defined through **job analysis**—a process that determines (a) the principal duties and responsibilities involved in a particular job, (b) tasks inherent in those duties, and (c) the personal qualifications (skills, abilities, knowledge, and traits) needed for the job. The outcome of a job analysis is a job description.

If no job descriptions currently exist, then the nurse manager, with the assistance of HRM, should develop one for each job on the unit. All staff members (new or existing) need to have an up-to-date copy of their job description.

An important factor is the job specification, which details the knowledge, skills, and abilities needed, the tasks to be performed, and the behavior required to perform them. Although knowledge, skills, and abilities can be inferred from a description of the tasks to be performed, a description of knowledge, skills, and abilities does not necessarily explain what tasks will

KEY TERMS

Job analysis   A process that determines and defines the duties and requirements involved in a particular job.

be done or what behaviors are expected on the job. Consequently, a job analysis that lists tasks is usually better than one that lists only knowledge, skills, and abilities.

Many tools are available for performing job analysis (Cascio, 1987). They vary substantially in complexity and in applicability to different kinds of jobs. These tools include supervisory conferences, critical incidents, observation (such as work sampling and time and motion studies), interviewing, questionnaires, checklists, and logs.

In a *supervisory conference*, the job analyst brings the supervisors and/or first-line managers together to identify the critical tasks or duties required in a job. Critical incidents require the managers to keep notes on subordinates' behavior that have contributed to particularly successful or unsuccessful job performance. Both methods are time consuming, and critical incident notes do not always give a complete picture of the job because they list only very positive or negative behaviors.

Two commonly used observational techniques for collecting work activity information are work sampling, and time and motion studies (Finkler, Knickman, Hendrickson, Lipkin, & Thompson, 1993). These techniques can be used for jobs that consist of repetitive, short-cycle, manual operations as well as professional positions. In *work sampling*, data are collected at intervals of time, such as twice an hour or at randomly selected times. An inference can be made about overall work activities based on the observed activities. *Time and motion studies* require an observer to record exactly how much time is devoted to each skill, task, or behavior. Observation is done for extended periods. Time and motion studies are labor-intensive and expensive. A drawback to both work sampling and time and motion studies is that employees may change their behavior while being observed.

Interviewing, another common method, relies on staff members providing information about tasks or personal characteristics required for the job. *Questionnaires* and *checklists* also rely on staff members as a source of information on job requirements. Questionnaires may be open-ended, whereas checklists tend to be more structured and may consist of 200 or more items for the individual respondent to check off if performed. These data are analyzed to determine the tasks performed by the majority of persons currently in the job. When a checklist is used as the basis for job analysis, a large number of staff members are needed to supply enough data.

Self-report *logs* may be used by staff members to report their activity at specified times. These logs are considered less reliable than other methods because staff may not record activities in a timely manner and may not be totally honest about what activities they are performing at the designated sampling times (Finkler et al., 1993).

The nurse manager often participates in developing a job analysis, usually through a supervisory conference, by interviewing, or by using questionnaires. Assuming they are free of error and distortion, job descriptions and specifications can be compared to a photograph in that they represent what the job is at the time the analysis is performed. The nurse manager can then use information regarding tasks and duties to develop selection procedures and to construct performance appraisal instruments and training programs.

Recruitment

The purpose of recruitment is to locate and attract enough qualified applicants to provide a pool from which the required number of individuals can be selected. Even though recruiting is primarily carried out by HRM staff and nurse recruiters, nurse managers and nursing staff play an important role in the process. Recruiting is easier when current employees spread the recruiting message, reducing the need for expensive advertising and bounty methods. To a very large extent, proper management can serve as the best recruiting tool. A nurse manager who is able to create a positive work environment through leadership style and clinical expertise will have a positive impact on efforts on recruitment because potential staff members will hear about and be attracted to that area (e.g., hospital unit, home health team). In contrast, an autocratic manager is more likely to have a higher turnover rate and is less likely to attract sufficient numbers of high-quality nurses.

There are essentially four elements in any recruiting strategy: where to look, how to look, when to look, and how to sell the organization to potential recruits. Each of these elements may be affected by market competition, cyclic nursing shortages, reputation, visibility, and location.

Where to Look

For most health care organizations, the best place to look is in their own geographic area. During nursing shortages, however, many organizations conduct national searches. This effort is frequently futile because most nurses look for jobs in their local area. If the agency is in a major metropolitan area, a search may be relatively easy; if it is located in a rural area, however, recruitment may need to be conducted in the nearest city. Organizations tend to recruit where past efforts have been the most successful. Most organizations adopt an incremental strategy whereby they recruit locally first and then expand to larger and larger markets until a sufficient applicant pool is obtained.

During nursing shortages, foreign nurses have been recruited through special legislative initiatives, such as the Immigration Nursing Relief Act of 1989 (INRA). This act and the Professionals Shortage Area Nursing Relief Act of 1997 provided for foreign-educated nurses to meet short-term needs in this country through temporary migration programs (Glaessel-Brown, 1998). However, because proximity to home is a key factor in choosing a job, recruitment efforts should focus on nurses living nearby. The state board of nursing can provide the names of registered nurses by zip code to allow organizations to target recruitment efforts to surrounding areas. Also, personnel officers in large companies or other organizations in the area can be asked to assist in recruiting nurse spouses of newly hired employees.

Students in local schools of nursing are obviously an excellent potential source of employees. One way to recruit them is to serve as a clinical training site and treat students well. Nurses who work with students play a key role in recruitment. Students feel welcomed and valued when their care and contributions are acknowledged. In doing so, the staff conveys a positive impression of the work group.

Employing students as aides may provide another recruitment tool because it allows students to learn first-hand about the organization and what it has to offer. In turn, the organization can evaluate the student as a potential employee post-graduation. Some organizations provide assistance with student loan payments if the student continues to work after graduation. Baccalaureate graduates report, however, that the most critical factor they consider in seeking their first nursing position is the orientation program (Kersten & Johnson, 1992). Graduates look for an orientation that provides successful transition into professional practice. Other top factors they consider are the reputation of the agency, benefits, promotional opportunities, specialty area, and nurse:patient ratio.

How to Look—Recruiting Sources

Employee referrals, advertising in newspapers and professional journals and on the Internet, attendance at professional conventions, job fairs, career days, visits to educational institutions, employment agencies (both private and public), and temporary help agencies are all recruiting sources. Most applicants are drawn to the organization by some form of advertising. During nursing shortages, some organizations offer bonuses to staff members who refer candidates, as well as bonuses to the recruits themselves.

Direct applications and employee referrals are quick and relatively inexpensive ways of recruiting people, but these methods also tend to perpetuate the current racial or social mix of the workforce. It is both legally and ethically necessary to recruit individuals without regard to their race, ethnicity, gender, or disability. In addition, organizations can benefit from the diversity of a staff comprised of persons from a wide variety of social, experiential, and educational backgrounds.

Advertisements may be placed in the classified sections of local newspapers or journals and in the job listings at professional meetings. Advertising can be an effective recruiting tool, but it tends to be expensive. Nevertheless, if the organization intends to add staff, placing display ads in local newspapers reassures currently employed nurses that the organization is serious about its commitment to so so.

Another advertising medium is the Internet. Brooks (2000) noted that an estimated 2.5 million resumes were posted with approximately 29,000 job posting services, and Useem (1999) reported that the Internet is being used significantly for job hunting. Since the Internet is readily accessible, it is an attractive way to explore job opportunities anywhere in the world.

In recruiting, both the medium and the message must be considered. The **medium** is the agent of contact between the organization and the potential applicant. Obviously, it is desirable to find a medium that gives the widest exposure. Unfortunately, these media tend to be inefficient and low in credibility. The more influential media tend to be the more personal ones: present employees and recruiters. Acquaintances or

KEY TERMS

Medium   The agent of contact between the organization and the potential applicant.

4 Ps of marketing   Four strategies included in marketing plans: product, place, price, and promotion.

friends of the recruit have prior credibility and the ability to communicate more subtle aspects of the organization and the job.

Nurses referred by informal methods (e.g., employees) tend to be more productive (Breaugh & Mann, 1984). The reason is that nurses coming from informal sources of referral are likely to have more realistic information about the job and the organization and, therefore, their expectations more closely fit reality. Those who come to the job with unrealistic expectations may experience dissatisfaction as a result. In an open labor market, these individuals may leave the organization, creating high turnover. When nursing jobs are less plentiful, dissatisfied staff members tend to stay in the organization because they need the job, but they are not likely to perform as well as other employees. Consequently, even where applicants are sought may have significant consequences later on.

When to Look

The time lag in recruiting is a concern to nursing, especially when there are severe nursing shortages. Even when there is an excess supply of nurses, there may be spot shortages in certain locations (e.g., rural areas) and specialties (e.g., critical care). Careful planning is necessary to ensure that recruitment begins well in advance of anticipated needs.

How to Sell the Organization

A critical component of any recruiting effort is marketing the organization and available positions to potential employees. The nursing department and/or HRM should develop a comprehensive marketing plan. Generally, four strategies are included in marketing plans and are called the **4 Ps of marketing**: product, place, price, and promotion. The consumer is the key figure around which the four concepts are oriented, and in the recruiting process, the consumer is the potential employee.

Product is the available position(s) within the organization. Consider several aspects of the position and organization, such as professionalism, standards of care, quality, service, and respect. *Place* refers to the physical qualities and location (e.g., accessibility, scheduling, parking), as well as reputation and organizational culture. In recruiting, *price* includes pay and differentials, benefits, sign-on bonuses, and retirement plans. *Promotion* includes advertising, public relations, direct word of mouth, and personal selling (e.g., job fairs, professional meetings). Perry (1989) found that recruitment materials actually may impede hiring because the materials may focus on the organization rather than on the potential employee. Instead, Perry suggests focusing on professional development and why employees at the organization like their jobs.

Developing an effective marketing message is important. Sometimes the tendency is to use a "scatter-gun" approach, sugarcoat the message, or make it very slick. A more balanced message, which includes honest communication and personal contact, is preferable. Overselling the organization creates unrealistic expectations that may lead to later dissatisfaction and turnover. Realistically presenting the job requirements and rewards improves job satisfaction, in that the new recruit learns what the job is actually like. Promising a nurse every other weekend off and only a 25% rotation to nights on a severely understaffed unit and then scheduling the nurse off only every third weekend with 75% night rotations is an example of unrealistic job information. It is important to represent the situation honestly and describe the steps management is taking to improve situations that the applicant might find undesirable. The candidate can then make an informed decision about the job offer.

Cross-Training as a Recruitment Strategy

In today's rapidly changing health care environment, patient census fluctuates rapidly, and staffing requirements must be adjusted appropriately. These conditions may bring about layoffs and daily cancellations and contribute to low morale. Offering cross-training to potential employees may increase the applicant pool. Cross-training has the benefits of increasing morale and job satisfaction, improving efficiency, increasing the flexibility of the staff, and providing a means to manage fluctuations in census. In addition, it gives nurses, such as those in obstetrics and neonatal areas, an opportunity to provide more holistic care. If cross-training is used, care should be taken to provide a didactic knowledge base in addition to

clinical training. How broadly to cross-train is an important decision because training in too many areas may overload the nurse and reduce the quality of care.

Interviewing

The most common selection method, the interview, is an information-seeking mechanism between an individual applying for a position and a member of an organization doing the hiring. After the applicant's initial screening with HRM, the nurse manager usually conducts an interview.

The interview is used to clarify information gathered from the application form, evaluate the applicant's responses to questions, and determine the fit of the applicant to the position, unit, and organization. In addition, the interviewer should provide information about the job and the organization. Finally, the interview should create goodwill toward the employing organization through good customer relations.

Research suggests that decision making is improved if the interviewer postpones reviewing information not needed for the interview, such as test scores, until after the interview. Reviewing such information before the interview may lead to ignoring data that disconfirm this information (Gatewood & Feild, 1990).

An effective interviewer must learn to solicit information efficiently and to gather relevant data. Interviews typically last for 1 or 1½ hours and, as shown in Table 17-1, include an opening, an information-

Table 17-1 **Time Schedule for an Interview**

	1½ Hours	1 Hour
Opening	7 minutes	3
Disclosure of interview procedure	3 minutes	2
Interests	5 minutes	5
Educational history	20 minutes	10
Job history	20 minutes	15
Future plans	10 minutes	5
Information about the organization and position	15 minutes	10
Additional questions and answers	5 minutes	2
Closing	5 minutes	3

Note: Adapted from *Selection interviewing procedures for healthcare managers* by P. J. Decker, copyright 1983, by Phillip J. Decker. Used by permission.

Box 17-1 Staff Nurse Position, Burn Unit: Realistic Preview Information

I. Positive Information
- Lengthy patient stays—lots of patient and family teaching
- Presence of critical as well as recovering patients
- Decision-making opportunities
- Bedside nursing
- Learning environment
- Ability to assist with research
- Small unit, close-knit, dedicated group

- Burns as well as other prior difficulties or concurrent problems to work with
- Children as well as adults

II. Negative Information
- Patients who are sometimes difficult to deal with, that is, young children or elderly—often alcoholics, psychological difficulties
- Emotional stress
- Physical difficulties

Note: Adapted from a form used by Barnes Hospital Service, St. Louis, MO. Used by permission.

gathering and information-giving phase, and a closing. The *opening* is important because it is an attempt to establish rapport with the applicant so she or he will provide relevant information. *Gathering information*, however, is the core of the interview. *Giving information* also is important because it allows the interviewer to create realistic expectations in the applicant and sell the organization if that is needed. However, this portion of the interview should take place after the information has been gathered so that the applicant's answers will be as candid as possible. The interviewer should answer any direct questions the candidate poses. Box 17-1 is an example of realistic information to present to applicants. Finally, the closing is intended to provide information to the candidate on the mechanics of possible employment.

Principles for Effective Interviewing

Preparing for the Interview Most managers do not adequately prepare for the interview, which should be planned just like any business undertaking. All needed materials should be on hand, and the interview site should be quiet and pleasant. If others are scheduled to see the applicant, their schedules should be checked to make sure they are available at the proper time. If coffee or other refreshments are to be offered, advance arrangements need to be made. Lack of advance preparation may lead to insufficient interviewing time, interruptions, or failure to gather important information. Other problems include losing focus in the interview because of a desire to be courteous or because a particularly dominant interviewee is encountered. This typically keeps the interviewer from obtaining the needed information.

In general, when time is limited, it is better to use part of it for planning rather than squander all of it on the interview itself. This is preferable to spending more time later trying to correct the performance of a poor employee. Before the interview, the interviewer should review job requirements, the application and résumé, and note specific questions to be asked. Planning should be done on the morning of the interview or the evening before for an early morning interview. If you are sure that time will be available, planning is best done immediately before an interview or between interviews. Unfortunately, a busy manager may have to deal with unexpected minor crises between interviews and may not be able to use the time to plan the next interview.

A cardinal rule is to review the application or résumé before beginning the interview. (See Companion Website.) If the interviewee arrives with the résumé or application in hand, ask him or her to wait for a few minutes while you review the material. In doing a quick review, consider four things. First, are there clear discrepancies between the applicant's qualifications and the job specifications? If the answer is yes, then only a brief interview may be necessary to explain why the applicant will not be considered. (If a preliminary screening is performed by the HRM, such applicants should not be referred to nurse managers.) Second, look for specific questions to ask the applicant during the interview. Third, look for a rapport builder (something you have in common with the applicant) to break the ice at the beginning of the interview. Fourth, remember that the résumé is prepared by the applicant and is intended to market an applicant's assets to the organization. It does not give a balanced view of strengths and weaknesses. So, examine the résumé critically and make notes about areas where you need more information.

To provide a relaxed, informal atmosphere, the setting is important. Both you and the applicant should be in comfortable chairs, as close as comfortably possible. No table or desk should separate you. If an office is used, arrange chairs so that the applicant is at the side of the desk. There should be complete freedom from distracting phone calls and other interruptions. If the view is distracting, do not seat the applicant so that she or he can look out a window. Box 17-2 provides a set of key behaviors for an effective interview. These should be followed in every interview. These key behaviors also can be typed on a large index card for easy reference during the interview.

Opening the Interview   The interview should start on time. Give a warm, friendly greeting, introduce yourself, and ask the applicant her or his preferred name. Try to minimize status; do not patronize or dominate. The objective is to establish an open atmosphere so applicants reveal as much as possible about themselves. Establish and maintain rapport throughout the interview by talking about yourself, discussing mutual interests such as hobbies or sports, and using nonverbal cues, such as maintaining eye contact. Finally, start the interview by outlining what will be discussed and setting the time limits for the interview.

Be careful not to form hasty first impressions and make equally hasty decisions. Interviewers tend to be influenced by first impressions of a candidate, and such judgments often lead to poor decisions. First impressions may degrade the quality of the interview by coloring the search for information to justify their first impressions, good or bad. If the first impression is negative and you decide not to hire a potentially successful candidate, you have wasted an hour or so and possibly lost a good recruit. If, because of a positive first impression, you hire an unsuccessful candidate, problems may continue for months. Conversely, your personal characteristics may influence the applicant's decisions. You create first impressions by tone of voice, eye contact, personal appearance, grooming, posture, and gestures.

Developing Structured Interview Guides

Unstructured interviews present problems; if interviewers fail to ask the same questions of every candidate, it is often difficult to compare them. With any human skill or trait, no standard or true score exists that can serve as a basis on which to compare applicants. People can only be compared to other people. Consequently, the interview is most effective when the information on the pool of interviewees is as comparable as possible. Comparability is maximized via a structured interview supported by an interview guide. An **interview guide** is a written document containing questions, interviewer directions, and other pertinent information so that the same process is followed and the same basic information is gathered from each

---

Box 17-2   The Effective Interview

- Arrange an appropriate environment and setting.
- Give a warm, friendly welcome.
    a. Relax and smile.
    b. Use the applicant's appropriate name, be consistent, and pronounce it correctly.
- Briefly tell about yourself (e.g., length of employment, role responsibilities) to help the applicant relax.
- Tell applicant the purpose and structure of the interview.
- Use your interview guide. Follow the order and content exactly.
- Take brief notes, and inform the applicant that you intend to do so.

- Probe to get details about negative or unclear information.
- Listen attentively.
- Summarize what you have heard for each main section of the interview.
- Give job preview information that is realistic.
- Give a friendly goodbye.
    a. Outline the next steps in the selection process.
    b. Ask for any additional comments/questions.
    c. Say goodbye, and thank the applicant for coming in.

Note: Adapted from *Selection interviewing procedures for healthcare managers* by P. J. Decker, copyright 1983, by Phillip J. Decker. Used by permission.

applicant. The guide should be specific to the job, or job category, as shown below.

Do job analysis to determine job tasks.

⇓

Use tasks to determine required personal characteristics (skills, abilities, knowledge).

⇓

Write questions and develop behavioral simulations to determine whether the applicant has the required personal characteristics.

⇓

Put these questions and ideas in the interview guide to direct you in the interview.

Figure 17-2 is an interview guide format. This figure can be used to construct your own interview guide, but do not copy the questions verbatim; develop your own questions based on the categories. For example, you may want to add questions on teamwork and collaboration as they relate to your area of responsibility. Box 17-3 is an example of job-related questions for an oncology unit that could be asked in area 6 of the interview guide. As noted earlier, Box 17-1 is an example of the type of information that would be presented in area 8, job preview information.

Interview guides reduce interviewer bias, provide relevant and effective questions, minimize leading

> ### KEY TERMS
>
> *Interview guide*   A written document containing questions, interviewer directions, and other pertinent information so that the same process is followed and the same basic information is gathered from each applicant.

questions, and facilitate comparison among applicants. Space left between the questions on the guide provides room for note-taking, and the guide also provides a written record of the interview.

Using the structured interview guide, take notes, telling the candidate that this is being done to aid recall and that you hope the candidate does not mind. There are various ways of asking questions, but only one question should be asked at a time and, where possible, open-ended questions should be used, such as, "Please tell me about your most rewarding experience as a nurse." Open-ended questions cannot be answered with a single yes, no, or one-word answer and usually elicit more information about the applicant. Closed questions (e.g., what, where, why, when, how many) should only be used to elicit specific information.

Box 17-3 Job-Related Questions for an Oncology Unit

Describe how you would intervene in the following situations:

- A patient whom you admitted with a diagnosis of lymphoma is going to begin chemotherapy, and you are preparing to hang the first dose. When you enter the room she says, "You know, I just can't believe that I have cancer. I know it is what the doctor says, but it just doesn't seem possible to me."

- The wife of a patient overhears some doctors caring for her husband say that the patient has received the incorrect dose of chemotherapy. You are caring for him.

- A young man is diagnosed with acute leukemia and expresses anger and frustration in the presence of his wife. You witness the frequent outbursts and become increasingly aware of the sense of hopelessness on the part of both him and his wife.

- A leukemia patient has been classified as a no-code. On the night shift, the dyspnea develops. The patient becomes uncomfortable and anxious, and screams out periodically. The patient is on 100% oxygen already, but his wife insists that something more be done.

- A physician making rounds notices a discrepancy in your patient's intake and output record. The weights indicate that he has gained 10 pounds, but the intake records do not show how this could have happened.

- You are working nights and caring for an extremely seriously ill man receiving platelets and antibiotic therapy. The patient's blood pressure is continuing to drop. You have talked to the resident on call twice by telephone, and he tells you to continue the present orders. The man's condition continues to decline. What would you do?

Note: Adapted from a form used by Barnes Hospital Nursing Service, St. Louis, MO. Used by permission.

1. Record responses to each question during the interview. Immediately after the interview, indicate your reaction to each answer beneath the response. Use what is appropriate (e.g., education questions may not be necessary for a candidate out of school 10 years with extensive work history).

   Candidate: _____

   Interviewer: _____

   Date: _____   Position sought: _____

   Review of application form: _____

   Items of interest to you on the application: _____

   _____

2. Open the interview and establish rapport.
   ____ Warm friendly greeting.
   ____ Names are important, yours and the applicant's. (Use first and last name correctly.)
   ____ Break the ice—talk about his/her trip to _____, hobbies, weather, and so on, and/or talk briefly about yourself—position, hobbies, and so on.

   Outline topics to be covered in the interview.
   ____ Education
   ____ Work history
   ____ Miscellaneous topics
   ____ Job preview

3. Education

   *1. A. High school name _____

   B. Year graduated _____

   C. Which courses did you like best? _____

   D. Which courses did you like least? _____

   E. Extracurricular activities you enjoyed the most: _____

   _____

   *May skip section if applicant has been out of high school a while.

Figure 17-2 **Interview guide format.** *Note:* Adapted from guides used by Barnes Hospital Nursing Service, St. Louis, MO, and from *Selection interviewing procedures for healthcare managers* by P. J. Decker, copyright 1983, by Phillip J. Decker. Used by permission.

II. A. Nursing school (university or college)

   B. Year graduated _____

   C. Additional college work _____

   D. Additional degrees _____

   E. Which courses did you like best? _____

   F. Which courses did you like least? _____

   G. If you had the opportunity to start your education all over again knowing what you know now, what would you do differently? _____

   H. What were some of the highlights of your years at school?_____

4. Employment history

   A. Tell me about your current job. What are your duties? What kind of decisions do you normally make? _____

   B. What is there about your present position you like most? _____

   C. The least? _____

   D. What aspects of your work is your supervisor especially pleased with? _____

   E. What areas do you feel you could improve on? _____

   F. What is there in your present job that you would change if you could? _____

   G. What things in a job do you consider to be important? _____

   H. What type of supervisor do you prefer working for? _____

   I. Why are you leaving your present job? _____

5. Self-evaluation

   A. What are the most important ways in which you've changed in the past 5–10 years?

   _____

   B. What do you see yourself doing in the next 10 years? _____

   C. What are some of the things you can work on to better your chance of getting where you want to go? _____

Figure 17-2   **(continued)**

D. What do you like to do in your spare time? _____

E. What do you consider to be your strongest asset? _____

F. What are other assets? _____

G. What are 2 or 3 things that you have done in your lifetime of which you are the most proud? _____

H. What is there in your overall background that you feel would enable you to do a good job in this position? _____

6. Job-related situation: Tell me how you would handle this situation . . . (see Box 17-3)

7. Will you work night/weekend rotations? ____ Yes ____ No

8. Job preview information

      A. Unit structure (personnel)
      B. Orientation period
      C. Duties
      D. Available shift
          1. D/E, E, N
          2. 8 hr, 10 hr, 12 hr
      E. Tour of unit—discussion of nursing care in general

9. Closing the interview

      A. Is there anything you would like to add?
      B. Is there anything you would like to know that I haven't covered?

      C. Date available to start _____

      D. Follow-up date _____
      E. Thank you

Figure 17-2 **Interview guide format. (continued)**

Work sample questions are used to determine an applicant's knowledge about work tasks and ability to perform the job. It is easy to ask a nurse whether she or he knows how to care for a patient who has a central intravenous line in place. An answer of yes does not necessarily prove the ability, so you might ask some very specific questions about central lines. Avoid leading questions, in which the answer is implied by the question (e.g., "We have lots of overtime. Do you mind overtime?"). You may also want to summarize what has been said, use silence to elicit more information, reflect back the applicant's feelings to clarify the issue, or indicate acceptance by urging the applicant to continue.

Giving Information Before reaching the information-giving part of the interview, consider whether the candidate is promising enough to warrant spending time in giving detailed job information. Unless the candidate is clearly unacceptable, be careful not to communicate a negative impression, because evaluation of the candidate may change when the entire packet of material is reviewed or more promising candidates decline a job offer. You also must know what information you should give and what is to be provided by others. Detailed benefit or compensation questions are usually answered by HRM. If a promising candidate's questions cannot be answered, arrange for someone to contact the candidate later with the desired information.

In closing the interview, you may want to summarize the applicant's strengths. Make sure to ask the applicant whether she or he has anything to add or questions to ask related to the job and the organization. You may also want to mention the candidate's weaknesses, particularly if they are objective and clearly related to the job, such as lack of experience in a particular field. Mentioning a perception of a subjective weakness, such as poor supervisory skills, may lead to legal problems. Thanking the applicant and completing any notes made during the interview conclude the interview process.

Involving Staff in the Interview Process

Today's trend toward decentralization of decision making may lead to sharing interview responsibilities with staff. Involving staff in interviews helps to strengthen teamwork, improve work group effectiveness, and increase staff involvement in other unit activities (Ott, Esker, Caserza, Anderson, Weeks, & Knapp, 1990). Furthermore, it increases the likelihood

> **KEY TERMS**
>
> *Work sample questions* Used to determine an applicant's knowledge about work tasks and ability to perform the job.
>
> *Intrarater reliability* Agreement between two measures by the same person.
>
> *Interrater reliability* Agreement between two measures by several people.
>
> *Validity* The ability to predict outcomes with some accuracy.

of selecting the best candidate for the position (Secatore & Stengrevics, 1994).

If staff are involved in interviews, several steps must be taken to protect the integrity of the interview process. An organized orientation to interviewing should be given that includes (a) federal, state, and local laws and regulations governing interviewing, as well as any collective bargaining agreements that may affect the process; (b) tips on handling awkward interviewing situations; and (c) time for rehearsing interviewing skills. Just as the manager does, staff should follow a structured interview guide to help standardize the process.

Interview Reliability and Validity

Numerous research studies have been performed on the reliability and validity of employment interviews. In general, agreement between two interviews of the same candidate by the same interviewer (**intrarater reliability**) is fairly high, agreement between two interviews of the same candidate by several interviewers (**interrater reliability**) is rather low, and the ability to predict job performance (**validity**) of the typical interview is very low. Research also has shown that (a) structured interviews are more reliable and valid; (b) interviewers who are under pressure to hire in a short time or meet a recruitment quota are less accurate than other interviewers; (c) interviewers who have detailed information about the job for which they are interviewing exhibit higher interrater reliability and validity; (d) the interviewer's experience does not seem to be related to reliability and validity; (e) there is a decided tendency for interviewers to make quick decisions and therefore be less accurate; (f) interviewers develop stereotypes of ideal applicants against which interviewees are evaluated, and individual interviewers may hold different stereotypes, thus decreasing interrater reliability and validity; and (g) race and gender have been found to influence interviewers' evaluations (Arvey & Faley, 1988).

Possibly the greatest weakness in the selection interview is the tendency for the interviewer to try to assess an applicant's personality characteristics. Although it is difficult to eliminate such subjectivity, evaluations of applicants are often more subjective than they need to be, particularly when interviewers try to assess personality characteristics. Information collected during an interview should answer three fundamental questions: (a) can the applicant perform the job? (b) will the applicant perform the job? and (c) will the candidate fit into the culture of the unit and the organization? The best predictor of the applicant's future behavior in these respects is past performance. Previous work and other experience, previous education and training, and current job performance all should be considered, not personality characteristics, which even psychologists cannot measure very accurately.

Education, Experience, Licensure, and Physical Examinations

Education and experience requirements for nurses have long been important screening factors and bear a close relationship to work sample tests. Educational requirements are a type of job knowledge sample because they tend to ensure that applicants have at least a minimal amount of knowledge necessary for the job. For nurses, educational preparation is particularly important. For example, nurses who are graduates of associate degree and diploma programs are prepared to care for individuals in structured settings and use the nursing process, decision-making process, and management skills in the care of those individuals. Baccalaureate graduates can provide nursing care for individuals, families, groups, and communities using the nursing process and decision-making process. Baccalaureate graduates also are prepared for beginning community health positions and possess the leadership and management skills needed for entry-level management positions.

Making assumptions regarding the type and number of years of experience should be avoided. Factors such as job requirements, patient acuity, autonomy, and degree of specialization vary from organization to organization. Therefore, careful interviewing is needed

to determine the individual applicant's knowledge and skill level.

References and letters of recommendation also are used to assess the applicant's past job experience, but there is little evidence that these have any validity. Because few persons write unfavorable letters of recommendation, such letters do not really predict job performance. Criticisms are likely to be mild and may be reflected by the lack of positive language. Letters with any criticism should be verified with a telephone call, if possible, to avoid overreacting to an unusually honest author. To avoid legal problems, many organizations include in letters of recommendation only employment dates, salary, and whether the applicant is eligible for rehire. Many organizations do not allow supervisors to write letters of recommendation. Negative references may be viewed as potential for slander or other legal recourse. Almost every organization will at least verify position title and dates of employment, which helps to detect the occasional applicant who counterfeits an entire work history. Unfortunately, omission of a position from the work history is more common than including a position not actually held. The only way to detect such omissions is to ask that candidates list year *and month* of all educational and work experiences. Caution is necessary when asking about time between jobs; be careful not to inquire about marital or family status.

In almost every selection situation, an applicant fills out an application form that requests information regarding previous experience, education, and references. Most applications also ask for the applicant's medical history and other personal data. As application forms are reviewed, the critical question to be asked is whether the applicant has distorted responses, either intentionally or unintentionally. Studies indicate that there is usually little distortion, at least not on the easily verifiable information. Applicants may stretch the truth a bit, but rarely are there complete falsehoods. Relative to other predictors, the application form may be one of the more valid predictors in a selection process.

Licensure status can be verified by asking to see the applicant's license at time of employment and by verifying the licensure information with the state board of nursing. The new computerized NCLEX™ examination has changed hiring practices for new graduates. Because rapid notification (7 to 10 days) of licensure examination results are available, state boards no longer issue interim permits to new graduate nurses. Organizations generally wait for new graduates to obtain a license before starting employment.

Preemployment physical examinations can no longer be used to disqualify applicants for a job or benefits. Passage of PL 101-336, the Americans with Disabilities Act of 1990, protects individuals with physical or mental disabilities from discrimination. In fact, reasonable accommodations must be provided for an individual with disabilities. Regardless, disabled employees may be held to the same standards for employment (i.e., they must possess the necessary skills and experience to perform the job) as applicants without disabilities.

Integration of Information

When comparing candidates, first weigh the qualities required for the job in order of importance, placing more emphasis on the most important elements. Second, weigh the qualities desired on the basis of the reliability of the data. The more consistent the observation of behavior from different elements in the selection system, the more weight that dimension should be given. Third, weigh job dimensions by trainability—consider the amount of education, experience, and additional training the applicant can reasonably be expected to receive, and consider the likelihood that the behavior in that dimension can be improved with training. Dimensions most likely to be learned in training (e.g., using new equipment) should be given the least weight so that more weight is placed on dimensions less likely to be learned in training (e.g., being able to care for terminally ill children).

Attempt to compare data across individuals in making a decision. It is more accurate to make decisions based on a comparison of several persons than to make a decision for each individual after each interview. Analysis of the entire applicant pool requires good interview records but lessens the impact of early impressions on the hiring decision because the interviewer must consider each job element across the entire pool.

Legality in Hiring

As a result of Title VII of the Civil Rights Act of 1964, the Equal Pay Act of 1963, the Age Discrimination Act of 1967, and Title I of the Americans with Disabilities Act of 1990, recruitment and selection activities are subject to considerable scrutiny regarding discrimination and equal employment opportunity. Title VII of the Civil Rights Act specifically prohibits discrimination in any **personnel decision** on the basis

KEY TERMS

Personnel decisions   Decisions that affect the terms, conditions, and privileges of employment.

Bona fide occupational qualification (BFOQ) A characteristic that excludes certain groups from consideration for employment.

Business necessity   Discrimination or exclusion that is allowed if it is necessary to ensure the safety of workers or customers.

of race, color, sex, religion, or national origin. "Any personnel decision" includes not only selection but also entrance into training programs, performance appraisal results, termination, promotions, compensation, benefits, and other terms, conditions, and privileges of employment. The act applies to most employers with more than 15 employees, although there are several exemptions—among them, **bona fide occupational qualification** (BFOQ), business necessity, and validity of the procedure used to make the personnel decision (as discussed below). Discrimination is allowed on the basis of national origin (citizenship or immigration status), religion, sex, and age, for instance, if that discrimination can be shown to be a "bona fide occupational qualification reasonably necessary for the normal operation of a business." The classic example of a genuine BFOQ is a sperm donor. More realistic examples are a female part in a play, a Sunday school teacher of a certain religion, or a female correctional counselor at a women's prison. Claims of "customer preference" for female flight attendants or gross gender characteristics such as "women cannot lift over 30 pounds" have not been supported as BFOQs.

A BFOQ allows an organization to exclude members of certain groups (such as all men or all women) if the organization can demonstrate that a selection method is a **business necessity**. Business necessity is likely to withstand legal challenge only in the unusual instances when a selection method that discriminates against a protected group is necessary to ensure the safety of workers or customers. For example, in *Spurlock v. United Airlines*, the court found that a flight time requirement and a college degree requirement were legal in hiring pilot trainees, despite the fact that these requirements discriminated against black applicants. Both requirements were found to be related to flight safety. The fact that hiring members of a particular protected group would lead to an economic loss for the organization is not adequate evidence for business necessity, but customer safety is.

Title VII also is a complaint-oriented law: Any person who feels he or she has been discriminated against may file a complaint with the government against an employer. When a complaint is filed, the Equal Employment Opportunity Commission (EEOC) or the applicable state agency created to enforce the Equal Employment Opportunity (EEO) law sends notice to the employer and initiates an investigation of the complaint. The EEOC has broad investigatory powers and access to all relevant employment records and documents. If it finds there is reasonable cause to believe that illegal discrimination has taken place, it will notify the employer and attempt to settle the complaint through conciliation. If this attempt fails, the EEOC or the individual may file a lawsuit against the company. Any legal action can result in reinstatement and/or back pay of up to 2 years.

When an individual files a complaint of discrimination, initially the person need only prove unequal treatment or that fewer members of minority than of nonminority groups are hired. The latter is known as **adverse impact**. The burden of proof then shifts to the organization, which must justify that its decisions were based on some job-relevant predictor not related to the individual's race, color, sex, religion, national origin, disability status, or other categories that state laws may add. There are two possible methods of justifying this claim: (a) to indicate that the organization did not have the information on race, sex, and so forth in the first place and therefore could not have used it (this is a very difficult claim to make because most applicants are interviewed or are seen in a health

care organization before they are hired) or (b) to prove that the hire/no-hire decision was based on some job-relevant criterion and not on race, sex, color, religion, disability, or national origin.

The EEOC is charged with enforcing and interpreting the Civil Rights Act and has issued Uniform Guidelines on Employee Selection Procedures (43 Federal Register, 1978). The guidelines specify the kinds of methods and information required to justify the job relatedness of selection procedures. These guidelines are not described in detail here; however, the methods of selection discussed in this chapter do follow their specifications. Remember that the law does not say one cannot hire the best person for the job. What it says is that race, color, sex, religion, disability, or national origin must not be used as selection criteria. As long as the decision is not made on the basis of minority status, one is complying with EEO law.

EEO law and succeeding court decisions have had three major impacts on selection procedures. First, organizations are more careful to use predictors and techniques that can be shown not to discriminate against protected classes. Second, organizations are reducing the use of tests, which may be difficult to defend if they screen out a large number of minority applicants. Third, organizations are relying heavily on the interview process as a selection device. Interviews also are subject to EEO and other regulations. Table 17-2 presents questions appropriate to ask in interviews. The basic rule of thumb in interviewing is when in doubt about a question's legality, ask: How is this question related to job performance? If it can be proven that only job-related questions are asked, EEO law will not be violated.

The **Age Discrimination Act** prohibits discrimination against applicants and employees over the age of 40. Questions in recruitment and selection that are appropriate with respect to age are also presented in Table 17-2.

The **Americans with Disabilities Act** took effect in July 1990. The definition of disability in this law is an individual who has a physical or mental impairment that substantially limits one or more of the major life activities, or has a record of such impairment, or is being regarded as having such an impairment. A qualified individual is one who, with or without reasonable accommodation, can perform the essential functions of the position under consideration. Employers with 15 or more employees are required to make accommodations to the known disability of a qualified applicant if it will not impose "undue hardship" on the operation of the business. Reasonable

| Table 17-2 | **Preemployment Questions** |

	Appropriate to Ask	Inappropriate to Ask
Name	Applicant's name. Whether applicant has school or work records under a different name.	Questions about any name or title that indicate race, color, religion, sex, national origin, or ancestry. Questions about father's surname or mother's maiden name.
Address	Questions concerning place and length of current and previous addresses.	Any specific probes into foreign addresses that would indicate national origin.
Age	Requiring proof of age by birth certificate after hiring. Can ask if applicant is over 18.	Requiring birth certificate or baptismal record *before* hiring.
Birthplace or national origin		Any question about place of birth of applicant or place of birth of parents, grandparents, or spouse. Any other question (direct or indirect) about applicant's national origin.
Race or color	Can request *after* employment as affirmative action data.	Any inquiry that would indicate race or color.
Sex		Any question on an application blank that would indicate sex.
Religion		Any questions to indicate applicant's religious denomination or beliefs. A recommendation or reference from the applicant's religious denomination.
Citizenship	Questions about whether the applicant is a U.S. citizen; if not, whether the applicant intends to become one. Questions regarding whether applicant's U.S. residence is legal; requiring proof of citizenship *after* being hired.	Questions of whether the applicant, parents, or spouse are native born or naturalized. Require proof of citizenship *before* hiring.
Photographs	May require after hiring for identification purposes only.	Requesting a photograph *before* hiring.
Education	Questions concerning any academic, professional, or vocational schools attended. Inquiry into language skills, such as reading and writing of foreign languages.	Questions asking specifically the nationality, racial, or religious affiliation of any school attended. Inquiries as to the applicant's mother tongue or how any foreign language ability was acquired (unless it is necessary for the job).
Relatives	Name, relationship, and address of a person to be notified in case of an emergency.	Any unlawful inquiry about a relative or residence mate(s) as specified in this list.
Children		Questions about the number and ages of the applicant's children or information on child-care arrangements.
Transportation		Inquiries about transportation to or from work (unless a car is necessary for the job).
Organization	Questions about organization memberships and any offices that might be held.	Questions about any organization an applicant belongs to that may indicate the race, age, disabilities, color, religion, sex, national origin, or ancestry of its members.

Table 17-2 Continued

	Appropriate to Ask	Inappropriate to Ask
Physical condition/ disabilities	Questions about being able to meet the job requirements, with or without some accommodation.	Questions about general medical condition, state of health, specific diseases, or nature/severity of disability.
Military service	Questions about services rendered in armed forces, the rank attained, and which branch of service. Requiring military discharge certificate *after* being hired.	Questions about military service in any armed forces other than the United States. Request of military service records *before* hiring.
Work schedule	Questions about the applicant's willingness to work the required work schedule.	Questions about applicant's willingness to work any particular religious holiday.
References	General and work references not relating to race, color, religion, sex, national origin or ancestry, age, or disability.	References specifically from clergymen (as specified above) or any other persons who might reflect race, age, disability, color, religion, sex, national origin or ancestry of applicant.
Financial		Questions about banking, credit rating, outstanding loans, bankruptcy, or having wages garnished.
Other qualifications	Any question that has direct reflection on the job to be applied for.	Any non–job-related inquiry that may present information permitting unlawful discrimination. Questions about arrests or convictions (unless necessary for job, such as security clearance).

Note: Adapted from *Americans with Disabilities Act* (EEOC Publication #M-1A), Ohio Civil Rights Commission and United States Equal Employment Opportunities Commission, 1992, Washington, DC: Government Printing Office.

accommodations may include making existing facilities used by employees readily accessible to and usable by individuals with disabilities; job restructuring, part-time or modified work schedules; reassignment to a vacant position; acquiring or modifying equipment or devices; adjusting or modifying examinations, training materials, or policies; and providing qualified readers and interpreters. Interview questions that may be asked of the disabled are also in Table 17-2. The law permits an organization to make an employment offer contingent on the applicant's passing a preemployment physical examination, but only if the examina-tion is required of all applicants in similar jobs and is job-related.

Negligent Hiring

Organizations are liable for the character and actions of the employees they hire. To satisfy this requirement, the employer must check applicants' backgrounds before hiring in regard to licensure, credentials, and references. Failure to do so constitutes **negligent hiring** if that employee harms a patient, visitor, or another employee. Furthermore, an employer is expected to properly train its employees.

KEY TERMS

Negligent hiring Failure of an organization, responsible for the character and actions of all employees, to ascertain the background of an employee.

Summary

- Job analysis, recruitment of applicants, and selection of personnel are important measures to ensure the best fit between employees and the needs of the organizations.

- The selection of staff is a critical function that requires matching people to jobs. Responsibility for hiring is often shared by HRM and nurse managers.
- Job analysis is fundamental to all selection efforts because it defines the job.
- Recruitment is the process of locating and attracting enough qualified applicants to provide a pool from which the required number of new staff members can be chosen. Poor-quality applicants and/or a small pool will result in poorer matches between jobs and applicants.
- Selection processes should be job related and most often include screening application forms, résumés, medical examinations, reference checks, and interviews.
- Interviewing is a complex skill that is intended to obtain information about the applicant and give the applicant information about the organization.
- There are several principles of effective interviewing: plan and structure the interview, respond to the applicant to encourage rapport, elicit information through questioning techniques, give realistic job information, and process the information obtained to make a final placement decision.
- Developing a structured interview guide is a critical element in interviewing because it helps the interviewer "stay on track," provides a mechanism for taking and storing notes that relate the applicant to the job requirements and is legally sound.
- Selection activities are subject to provisions of the Civil Rights Act of 1964, Equal Pay Act of 1963, the Age Discrimination Act of 1967 and the Americans with Disabilities Act of 1990.

■ LEADERSHIP AND MANAGEMENT
in Action

1. How does a job analysis guide the recruitment and selection process?
2. What are the principles for an effective interview?
3. List five questions that would be inappropriate to ask during an interview.

References

Arvey, R. D., & Faley, R. H. (1988). *Fairness in selecting employees.* Reading, MA: Addison-Wesley.

Breaugh, J. A., & Mann, R. B. (1984). Recruiting source effects: A test of two alternative explanations. *Journal of Occupational Psychology, 57,* 261–262.

Brooks, A. M. T. (2000). Journey around the globe [column]. *Journal of Professional Nursing, 16*(3), 130.

Cascio, W. F. (1987). *Applied psychology in personnel management.* Reston, VA: Reston.

Decker, P. J. (1983). *Selection interviewing procedures for healthcare managers.* St. Louis: Author.

Finkler, S. A., Knickman, J. R., Hendrickson, G., Lipkin, M., & Thompson. W. G. (1993). A comparison of work-sampling and time-and-motion techniques for studies in health services research. *Health Services Research, 28,* 577–597.

Gatewood, R. D., & Feild, H. S. (1990). *Human resource selection.* Chicago: Dryden.

Glaessel-Brown, E. E. (1998). Use of immigration policy to manage nursing shortages. *Image: The Journal of Nursing Scholarship, 30*(4), 323–327.

Kersten, J. W., & Johnson, J. S. (1992). Recruitment: What are the new grads looking for? *Nursing Management, 23*(3), 44–48.

Ott, M. J., Esker, S., Caserza, C., Anderson, S., Weeks, M., & Knapp, R. (1990). Peer interviewing: Sharing the hiring. *Nursing Management, 21*(11), 32–33.

Perry, L. (1989). Recruitment materials can impede the hiring of nurses. *Modern Healthcare, 19*(3), 41.

Secatore, J. A., & Stengrevics, S. S. (1994). In search of the perfect match. In R. Spitzer-Lehmann (Ed.), *Nursing management desk reference: Concepts, skills, and strategies* (pp. 159–177). Philadelphia: Saunders.

Spurlock v. United Airlines, 475 F. 2d216 (10th Cir. 1972), pp. 218–219.

United States Equal Employment Opportunities Commission. (1992). *Americans with Disabilities Act.* (EEOC Publication #M-1A). Washington, DC: Government Printing Office.

Useem, J. (1999). For sale online: You. *Fortune, 140*(1), 67–78.

Additional on-line resources for this chapter can be found on the World Wide Web at http://www.prenhall.com/sullivan_decker. Select Chapter 17 from the drop-down menu.

CHAPTER 18

Allocating Staff Resources

Looking Ahead

In the last chapter, we looked at the process of recruiting staff members. The next step is to determine the number of staff needed within the health care organization. There is a fine balance between the number of staff and the quality of patient care delivered. Several questions must be answered: What are the workload patterns? How can staff be distributed in a way that is both efficient and effective? How are the needs of both the staff and the clients balanced? How is staff turnover managed? This chapter will help you find better strategies to face these challenges.

Objectives

After reading this chapter, you will be able to:

- Determine staffing requirements using levels of care, average daily census, and hours of care.
- Compare and contrast different types of patient classification systems.
- Discuss creative ways to staff using a variety of resources.
- Discuss reasons for turnover.
- Identify the consequences of turnover.
- Describe strategies for managing turnover.

Allocating human resources is an important re-sponsibility of the nurse manager. Staffing requires a balance between the quantity of staff available and the numbers needed to provide effective quality nursing care while keeping costs down. This chapter describes guidelines for maintaining that balance. In addition, turnover, a challenge to adequate staffing, is discussed.

Staffing and Scheduling

The goal of **staffing** is to provide the appropriate numbers and mix of nursing staff (nursing care hours) to match actual or projected patient care needs (patient care hours) that will lead to the delivery of effective and efficient nursing care. There is no single or perfect method to achieve efficient and effective staffing and scheduling. There are, however, key elements that contribute to successful and satisfying staffing and scheduling. Because staffing requires continuous fine-tuning, variability in patient census during the year is a big challenge for nursing managers. The unit may experience a steady census during the 7 days of the week or a higher census from Monday to Friday. Its patient days may be distributed evenly during the year, or it may consistently experience peaks in occupancy in certain months (seasonality pattern) such as the months of April, July, and October. For these reasons, staffing is probably the most pressing challenge nurse managers face.

To determine staffing requirements (number of staff), nurse managers must examine workload patterns for the designated unit. This means determining the level of care, average daily census, and hours of care provided 24 hours a day, 7 days a week. The Joint Commission on Accreditation of Healthcare Organizations (JCAHO, 1995) requires that care be based on the patient's specific needs and the severity level of the disease, condition, impairment, or disability. JCAHO does not identify specific levels of nursing care hours for specific patient populations or types of patient care units, or the type of patient classification system to be used.

Patient Classification Systems

Patient classification systems (PCSs), sometimes referred to as *patient acuity systems*, were developed to determine workload requirements and staffing needs objectively. The essential elements of an effective PCS include methods to (a) validate the amount of care given to each category or type of patient on each unit

and shift; (b) predict nursing care requirements for individual patients; (c) evaluate the patterns of care delivered by each unit, shift, and staff level; (d) revalidate, on a periodic basis, the amount of care delivery by patient category; (e) relate nursing care requirements to staff resources allocated on a shift-by-shift and unit-by-unit basis; and (f) monitor the reliability and validity of the PCS over time (DeGroot, 1989). To be most effective, patient classification data are collected midpoint for every shift by the unit nursing staff and analyzed before the next shift to ensure appropriate numbers and mix of nursing staff.

Initially, paper-and-pencil methods based on industrial engineering models that incorporated time and motion study data were used to estimate annual staffing needs and determine the annual personnel budget (Malloch & Conovaloff, 1999). Three methods were commonly used: descriptive, checklist, and time standard. The *descriptive* system is a subjective classification of patient activities by category. Four or five categories are used to describe varying levels of care and dependence. The nurse selects the category that best represents the patient. For example, a new mother ready for discharge would be represented best by the category "feeds self, up ad lib, minimal treatment, PO medications, and routine patient teaching." An elderly patient following a stroke, in contrast, would be considered in the category "needs to be fed, requires enteral/parental feedings, needs passive exercise and frequent turning, incontinent of urine or stool, needs multiple treatments, needs multiple medications." Neither category is an actual representation of the patient's needs or the staff's time. As a result, this type of classification system is rarely used today.

The *checklist* format is another subjective system in which an acuity level is determined by identifying the level of activity within each category for each patient. Points ascribed for each level of activity (eating, bathing, medications, and so on) are totaled and converted to a level of acuity. For example, a new mother following a cesarean section can feed herself (1 point), has a Foley catheter in place (3 points), has an intra-venous catheter (3 points), and needs minimal assistance turning (2 points). Totaled, this patient receives 9 points, which by the hospital's standards converts to an acuity of 2. The checklist format provides a more individualized representation of patients' needs but still may not adequately reflect nursing's time.

In the *time standard* method, work sampling techniques are used to determine time standards associated with various patient care activities. Activities required for patient care are identified; associated time standards are calculated; and, like the checklist method, patient care is totaled and converted to an acuity level. This type of PCS best represents both the patient's needs and nursing's time.

With the advent of computers, patient classification systems became computerized and were used to determine daily staffing needs and predict monthly personnel budgets (Malloch & Conovaloff, 1999). The most common of these are MEDICUS, GRASP, and ARIC.

Medicus   One of the first patient classification systems developed, **Medicus**, was introduced in the late 1960s and continues to be used frequently in the United States. This instrument contains 37 indicators that determine patient dependence on nursing. The result of the applicable indicators is that the patient is placed in one of five levels of care. A patient classified as a 5 requires the greatest intensity of nursing care. Patients are clustered into categories; nursing care requirements are defined in terms of average hours of care per category. A predetermined relative value for the level of care is established by the organization. For example, on a 22-bed acute medical unit with an average patient rating of 3.5, the hours of nursing care required might be 6.8. Total hours of care with this system reflect both direct and indirect care.

GRASP   In 1970, a patient classification system referred to as PETO was introduced. After further study and refinement, **GRASP (Grace Reynolds Application and Study of PETO)** emerged in the mid-1970s (Meyer, 1978). GRASP is probably the most commonly used PCS in the United States. GRASP identifies 40 to 50 direct care activities, as identified by a specific unit, which account for about 85% of the direct care activities. An example is provided in Table 18-1. These direct care activities are determined by the organization; time studies are completed to ensure that the instrument is tailored to the organization. An adjustment factor is added to account for the direct care activities that are unlisted about 15% of the time.

Also, indirect patient care activities are added to determine the total hours of care. In the example provided, the numbers in each column correspond to the total hours of care assigned to that patient care activity. These calculations for every patient are completed every 12 hours and, based on the existing patients, can project nursing interventions and required staff for the next shift. The numbers on the form adjacent to the interventions represent the projected time it takes to complete the activity. The system incorporates interrater reliability testing to verify continued accuracy of the data.

The GRASP system operates as a multidimensional nursing management information system package and includes management reporting, staffing/scheduling, budgeting, cost identification, and quality evaluation. The patient classification portion of the system may be implemented in either a manual pen-and-paper or computerized form.

ARIC   ARIC **(Allocation, Resource, Identification, and Costing)** was developed in the 1970s by the Sisters of Mercy Health Corporation. This system incorporates patient admission, discharge, and transfer information from each patient along with the classification information and recognizes the dependent activities of nurses, physicians' orders and hospital policies, and the independent activities of nurses and their professional judgments. Staffing reports are generated based on the patient classification information entered. The reports identify actual versus needed staffing, the level of productivity, and staff exceeding workload.

Over time, the credibility and usefulness of patient classification systems have been questioned. As patient

Table 18-1   Components of GRASP

Rehabilitation Example

Assessment: (Circle each shift)	Patient A	B	C	D	E	F	G	H	I	J	K	L
Assessment/update assessment	3	3	3	3	3	3	3	3	3	3	3	3
Planning: (circle each shift)												
1. Update/Revise care plan/Problem list	2	2	2	2	2	2	2	2	2	2	2	2
Knowledge deficit: (circle as applicable)												
1. Planned teaching	2	2	2	2	2	2	2	2	2	2	2	2
2. Reinforce teaching	6	6	6	6	6	6	6	6	6	6	6	6
Self-care deficit—feeding: (circle highest applicable)												
1. Feeds self independently	2	2	2	2	2	2	2	2	2	2	2	2
2. Feeds self with assistance by personnel/family	4	4	4	4	4	4	4	4	4	4	4	4
3. Total feed or self-feed with dysphagia training	24	24	24	24	24	24	24	24	24	24	24	24
4. Total feed by staff/feeds self with constant supervision	9	9	9	9	9	9	9	9	9	9	9	9
5. Tube feeding continuous/bolus	6	6	6	6	6	6	6	6	6	6	6	6
Self-care deficit—toileting: (circle highest applicable)												
1. Incontinent care—toilet/bedside commode (BSC) with constant supervision	12	12	12	12	12	12	12	12	12	12	12	12
2. Toilet with assist/BSC/bedpan/urinal	8	8	8	8	8	8	8	8	8	8	8	8
Self-care deficit—bathing/hygiene/grooming: (circle highest applicable)												
1. Total care by staff	6	6	6	6	6	6	6	6	6	6	6	6
2. Moderate care by staff	3	3	3	3	3	3	3	3	3	3	3	3
3. Minimal care by staff	2	2	2	2	2	2	2	2	2	2	2	2
Operation in safety												
1. Restraint	4	4	4	4	4	4	4	4	4	4	4	4
2. Monitor the wandering patient	10	10	10	10	10	10	10	10	10	10	10	10
Other direct: (circle as applicable)												
1. Assistive devices	4	4	4	4	4	4	4	4	4	4	4	4
2. Accucheck	3	3	3	3	3	3	3	3	3	3	3	3
3. Empty Foley/leg bags/drainage collection containers	1	1	1	1	1	1	1	1	1	1	1	1
4. Simple dressing change/remove staples/sutures/steri strips	2	2	2	2	2	2	2	2	2	2	2	2
5. Complex dressing/decubitus care	7	7	7	7	7	7	7	7	7	7	7	7
6. I & O calculation/calorie count	1	1	1	1	1	1	1	1	1	1	1	1
7. Nourishment/supplement feedings/diabetic snacks	1	1	1	1	1	1	1	1	1	1	1	1
Direct care:	10	10	10	10	10	10	10	10	10	10	10	10
Evaluation: (circle each shift)	2	2	2	2	2	2	2	2	2	2	2	2
Unit patient care hour (PCH) Total												
PCH												

Note: Time values on chart have been increased to reflect time for all unlisted activities.

populations and health care needs and delivery systems changed, task-focused classification systems became obsolete (Finnigan, Abel, Dobler, Hudson, & Terry, 1993). Third-generation classification systems are attempting to integrate nursing into hospital information systems in order to predict cost-effective patient outcomes (Diers & Bozzo, 1997; Malloch & Conovaloff, 1999). The new systems still incorporate time and motion data but also incorporate expert nurse judgments. Some include measures of severity, productivity and clinical decision making. One is based on interventions and outcomes from the Iowa Intervention Project (Diers & Bozzo, 1997; Malloch & Conovaloff, 1999). With the increase in technology, fourth-generation classification systems are being envisioned in which caregiver profiles will be matched with patient care needs and caregiver–patient interactions can be tracked and monitored (Malloch & Conovaloff, 1999).

Determining Nursing Care Hours

From the patient classification data, patient workload trends are analyzed for each day of the week (each hour in critical care) or for a specific patient diagnosis to determine staffing needs. For example, if 26 patients with the following acuities required 161 nursing care hours, then an average of 6.19 nursing hours per patient per day (NHPPD) are required. NHPPD are calculated by dividing the total nursing care hours by the total census (number of patients).

Number of Patients	Acuity Level	Associated Hours of Care	Total Hours of Care
3	I	2	6
10	II	6	60
11	III	7	77
2	IV	9	18
Total 26			161

There are no specific standards for nursing care hours (NCHs) for any type of patient or patient care unit. NCHs may vary on the average from 5 to 7 hours of care for patients on medical and/or surgical units, to 10 to 24 hours of care for patients in critical care units, to 24 to 48 hours of care for selected patients, such as new, severely burned patients.

Determining FTEs

Positions are defined in terms of a **full-time equivalent** (**FTE**). One FTE equals 40 hours of work per week

for 52 weeks, or 2080 hours per year. In a 2-week pay period, one FTE would equal 80 hours. One FTE can be filled by one person or any combination of personnel. For example, one nurse may work 24 hours per week, and two other nurses may each work 8 hours per week. Together, the three nurses fill one FTE (24 + 8 + 8 = 40).

Several methods are available for determining the number of FTEs required to staff a unit 24 hours a day, 7 days a week. One technique incorporates information regarding the hours of work for the staff for 2 weeks, average daily census, and hours of care. The average daily census can be determined by dividing the total patient days (obtained from daily census counts for the year) by the number of days in the year.

Example

$$\text{Total patient days} = \frac{9490}{365} = 26 \text{ patients per day}$$

Data

Number of hours worked per FTE in 2 weeks = 80
Number of days of coverage in 2 weeks = 14
Average daily census = 26
Average nursing care hours (from PCS) = 6.15

Formula

$$x = \frac{\substack{\text{average nursing care hours} \times \text{days in} \\ \text{staffing period} \times \text{average patient census}}}{\text{hours of work per FTE in 2 weeks}}$$

$$x = \frac{6.15 \times 14 \times 26}{80} = \frac{2238.6}{80} = 27.98, \text{ or } 28 \text{ FTEs}$$

A second technique uses nursing care hours and annual hours of work provided by one FTE:

Data

Number of hours worked per FTE in 1 year = 2080
Total nursing care hours (from PCS) = 161

Formula

$$x = \frac{\text{Total nursing care hours} \times \text{days in a year}}{\text{Total annual hours per one FTE}}$$

$$x = \frac{161 \times 365}{2080} = \frac{58.765}{2080} = 28.25, \text{ or } 28 \text{ FTEs}$$

As previously delineated, one person working full-time usually works 80 hours (ten 8-hour shifts) in a 2-week period. However, to staff an 8-hour shift takes 1.4 FTEs, one person working ten 8-hour shifts (1.0 FTE) and another person working four 8-hour shifts (0.4 FTE) in order to provide for the full-time person's 2 days off every week. For 12-hour shifts, it takes

Nursing care hours (NCHs) The number of hours of patient care provided per unit of time.

Full-time equivalent (FTE) The percentage of time an employee works that is based on a 40-hour work week.

Staffing mix The type of staff necessary to perform the work of the organization.

2.1 FTEs to staff one 12-hour shift each day, each week; two people each working three 12-hour shifts and one person working one 12-hour shift each week (0.9 FTE = 0.9 FTE = 0.3 FTE = 2.1 FTEs). Therefore, the same number of FTEs is required to staff a unit for 24 hours a day for 2 weeks, regardless of whether the staff are all on 8-hour shifts (1.4 FTEs × 3 shifts = 4.2 FTEs) or 12-hour shifts (2.1 FTEs × 2 shifts = 4.2 FTEs).

Recently the ANA proposed that staffing should focus on the intensity and complexity of care needed rather than on hours spent per patient per day

(Gallagher, Kany, Rowell, & Peterson, 1999). Box 18-1 depicts the ANA's principles for staffing.

Determining Staffing Mix

The same data used to determine FTEs are used to identify **staffing mix**. For example, for patient care needs involving general hygiene care, feeding, transferring, or turning patients, unlicensed assistive personnel (UAPs) can be used. For patient care needs involving frequent assessments, patient education, or discharge planning, RNs will be needed because of the skills required. A high RN-skill mix allows for greater staffing flexibility and has been found to decrease patient length of stay, while introducing various skill levels increase the number of people to manage, educate, and evaluate and increases staffing costs (Melberg, 1997). Again, information on typical or usual patient needs is obtained by using trends from the patient classification system.

Determining Distribution of Staff

For many patient care units, the distribution of staff varies shift to shift and by days of the week. Patient census on a surgical unit will probably fluctuate

Box 18-1 | American Nurses Association's Principles for Nurse Staffing

A. Patient Care Unit Related

1. Appropriate staffing levels for a patient care unit reflect analysis of individual and aggregate patient needs.
2. There is a critical need to either retire or seriously question the usefulness of the concept of nursing hours per patient day (HPPD).
3. Unit functions necessary to support delivery of quality patient care must also be considered in determining staffing levels.

B. Staff Related

1. The specific needs of various patient populations should determine the appropriate clinical competencies required of the nurse practicing in that area.
2. Registered nurses must have nursing management support and representation at both the operational level and the executive level.

3. Clinical support from experienced RNs should be readily available to those RNs with less proficiency.

C. Institution/Organization Related

1. Organizational policy should reflect an organizational climate that values registered nurses and other employees as strategic assets and exhibits a true commitment to filling budgeted positions in a timely manner.
2. All institutions should have documented competencies for nursing staff, including agency or supplemental and traveling RNs, for those activities that they have been authorized to perform.
3. Organizational policies should recognize the myriad needs of both patients and nursing staff.

Note: Gallagher, R. M., Kany, K. A., Rowell, P. A., & Peterson, C. (1999). ANA's nurse staffing principles. *American Journal of Nursing, 99*(4), 50, 52–53.

throughout the week, with a higher census Monday through Thursday and a lower census over the weekend. In addition, some surgical units may have more complex cases earlier in the week and short-stay surgical cases later in the week. Surgical patients may have a shorter length of stay (LOS) than many medical patients. The patient census on a medical unit rarely fluctuates Monday through Friday, but may be less on weekends, when diagnostic tests are not done.

The workload on many units also varies within the 24-hour period. The care demands on a surgical unit will be heaviest early in the morning hours prior to the start of the surgical schedule; midmorning, when the unit receives patients from critical care unit(s); late in the afternoon, when patients return from the postanesthesia recovery unit; and in the evening hours, when same-day surgical patients are discharged. Critical care units may have greater care needs in the mornings when transferring patients to medical or surgical units and in the early afternoon hours when admitting new surgical cases. Medical units usually have the heaviest care needs in the morning hours, when patients' daily care needs are being met and physicians are making rounds. On skilled nursing and rehabilitation units, care needs are greatest before and immediately after mealtimes and in the evening hours; during other times of the day, patients are often away from the unit and involved in various therapeutic activities.

In contrast with the medical, surgical, critical care, and rehabilitation units that have definite patterns of patient care needs, labor-and-delivery and emergency department areas cannot predict when patient care needs will be most intense. Thus, labor-and-delivery and emergency department areas must rely on **block staffing** to ensure that adequate nursing staff are available at all times. Block staffing involves scheduling a

set staff mix for every shift. However, there may be trends in peak workload hours in emergency departments, when additional staff (RN, UAP, or secretary) beyond the block staff are necessary. Examples of peak workload hours within the emergency department may be from 6:00 P.M. to 10:00 P.M. to accommodate patient needs after physicians' offices close or from 12:00 A.M. to 3:00 A.M. to accommodate alcohol-related injuries. All these patterns of care needs must be known when staffing requirements and work schedules are established. Data reflecting peak workload times must be continuously monitored to maintain the appropriate levels and mix of staff.

Table 18-2 presents a staffing template for a 30-bed unit with fluctuating needs. This table illustrates numbers of staff and numbers of FTEs (the latter appear in brackets), as well as the staffing mix required for every shift. The direct care totals include only those nursing personnel providing direct patient care. Leadership and unit clerk positions are excluded from the direct care numbers. The decision to include or exclude these two groups of staff is a very important decision that affects the unit's productivity report. The total number of FTEs involved in direct care is based on the average NHPPD of 6.15 hours and an average patient census of 26 patients (86.7% occupancy). Average occupancy rates are determined by dividing

Table 18-2 Staffing Template*

Shift	Leadership Unit Manager/ Assistant Unit Manager	RNs	LPNs	UAPs	Unit Clerk	Direct Care	Total Nursing Care Hours	All Staff
Day	1 [1.0]	4 [5.6]	2 [2.8]	2 [2.8]	1 [1.4]	8 [11.2]	64	10 [13.6]
Evening	1 [1.0]	4 [5.6]	1 [1.4]	2 [2.8]	1 [1.4]	7 [9.8]	56	9 [12.2]
Night	0 [0.0]	2 [2.8]	2 [2.8]	1 [1.4]	0 [0.0]	5 [7.0]	40	5 [7.0]
Total	2 [2.0]	10 [14.0]	5 [7.0]	5 [7.0]	2 [2.8]	20 [28.0]	160	24 [32.8]

*This is a 30-bed unit, but it is staffed for an average patient census of 26 (86.7% occupancy) and an average number of hours of care of 6.15 (calculated using only direct care staff). In each column (except for "Total Nursing Care Hours"), the number on the left indicates the number of staff; the bracketed number to the right indicates the number of FTEs.

the average patient days (obtained by dividing total annual census by number of beds on unit) by number of days in a year.

Example

Data

Annual census = 9490
Number of beds on unit = 30

Formula

$$\text{Average patient days} = \frac{\text{Annual census}}{\text{Number of beds}}$$

$$\text{Occupancy rate} = \frac{\text{Average patient days}}{\text{Days in a year}}$$

$$\text{Average patient days} = \frac{9490}{30} = 316.33$$

$$\text{Occupancy rate} = \frac{316.33}{365} = 86.7\%$$

Scheduling

Cyclic nurse shortages and current restrictions in salary budgets have made creative and flexible staffing patterns necessary and probably everlasting. Combinations of 4-, 6-, 8-, 10-, and 12-hour shifts and schedules that have nurses working 6 consecutive days of 12-hour shifts with 13 days off, and staffing strategies such as weekend programs and split shifts are common. Table 18-3 presents a 2-week working schedule for RNs based on the master staffing template; four types of shifts and a weekend option are incorporated. Note that the work schedule has fewer RNs on weekends and more RNs Monday through Friday. However, the average nursing care hours would be unchanged; more LPNs and UAPs would be included. A decrease in patient census and intensity of patient care needs on weekends (as identified from trend analysis) justify this alteration. Distribution of all staff is based on the overall data on actual patient care needs.

Flexible staffing patterns, as presented in Table 18-3, can be a major challenge for the nurse manager, and in some cases a mathematical challenge. However, once a schedule is established and agreed to by the nurse manager and the staff, it can become a cyclic schedule for an extended period of time, such as 6 to 12 months. This allows staff members to know their work schedule many months ahead of time.

The use of 8-hour and 12-hour shifts is fairly straightforward. Problems with combined staffing patterns may include (a) the perception that nurses don't work full time when they work several days in a row

and then are off for several days in a row, (b) disruption in continuity of care if split shifts are used (7:00 A.M. to 11:00 A.M.; 11:00 A.M. to 3:00 P.M.; 3:00 P.M. to 7:00 P.M.; 7:00 P.M. to 1:00 A.M.; 1:00 A.M. to 7:00 A.M. shifts), and (c) immense challenges for nurse managers to communicate with all staff in a timely manner. Advantages of using combined staffing patterns are that it (a) better meets patient care needs during peak workload times, (b) improves staff satisfaction, and (c) maximizes the availability of nurses. Ten-hour shifts (not included in Table 18-3) provide greater overlap between shifts to permit extra time for nurses to complete their work; for this reason, 10-hour shifts may increase salary expenditures. There are a few specialty units in which 10-hour shifts would be cost-efficient: postanesthesia recovery areas, operating departments, and emergency departments are examples.

Creative Staffing and Scheduling

Some hospitals have instituted **self-staffing**. With this model, nurse managers and their staff completely manage staffing and schedules. This is an empowerment strategy that allows unit staff the authority to use their backup staffing options if the patient workload increases or if unscheduled staff absences occur. Likewise, staff can and must go home early if the patient workload decreases.

Hospitals can no longer arbitrarily staff patient care units on weekends or at nights with marginal numbers or levels of qualified staff. The acuity of patients in hospitals, including medical and surgical patients, mandates staffing units on the weekends by the same principles used for weekdays. Thorough trend analysis of patient classification data can provide the justification necessary to appropriately decrease the number of RNs, at least for some levels, because of differences in patient care needs throughout the day. Another creative method for staffing includes a weekend program, in which a nurse agrees to work 24 hours every weekend (usually two 12-hour shifts) for full-time benefits and full-time salary or premium salary. Yet other units have tried expert panels to determine staff requirements (Dunn et al., 1995).

Supplemental Staff

When there is a need for additional staff because of scheduled or unscheduled absences, increased workload demands, or existing staff vacancies, the nurse manager or staffing person must find additional staff.

Table 18-3 Sample 2-Week Schedule for RNs on Surgical Unit Using 4-, 6-, 8-, and 12-Hour Shifts and Weekend Option (Average Patient Census of 26)

Name	Position	FTE	Week 1 S	M	T	W	T	F	S	Week 2 S	M	T	W	T	F	S
Taber	Head Nurse (HN)	1.0	-	D	D	D	D	D	-	-	D	D	D	D	D	-
Carson	Assistant HN	1.0	E	E	E	E	E	-	-	-	E	E	E	E	-	E
Lewis	RN	1.0	-	D	D	D	D	-	D	-	D	D	D	D	D	-
Cass	RN	1.0	-	D	D	D	D	D	-	-	-	D	D	D	D	D
Freeze	RN	0.9	A	A	A	-	-	-	-	-	-	-	-	A	A	A
Ritz	RN	0.9	-	-	-	-	A	A	A	A	A	A	-	-	-	-
Jakarti	RN	0.9	-	-	A	A	A	-	-	A	A	-	A	-	-	-
Chow	RN	.55	-	-	D	6	-	D	E	-	-	D	6	-	-	-
Smith	RN	0.4	-	A	-	-	-	-	-	-	-	A	-	D	-	-
Burch	RN	0.4	-	-	-	D	-	-	D	-	D	-	E	-	-	-
Jones	RN	PRN	-	-	-	5	4	-	-	-	-	-	5	-	-	A
Betz	RN	PRN	A	-	-	-	-	-	-	-	-	-	-	A	-	-
Zipp	RN	PRN	-	-	-	-	-	A	-	-	-	-	A	-	-	-
Simon	RN	PRN	-	-	-	-	D	-	-	-	-	-	-	-	A	-
Link	RN	0.9	-	E	E	E	-	E	E	-	E	E	E	E	-	-
White	RN	0.9	-	E	E	P	N	-	-	-	E	E	N	-	-	P
Turner	RN	0.9	P	P	P	-	-	-	-	P	P	P	-	-	-	-
Short	RN	0.9	P	P	P	-	-	-	-	-	P	-	-	P	P	-
Melton	RN	.75	-	-	-	P	-	P	-	-	-	P	P	P	-	-
Graham*	RN	0.6	-	-	-	-	-	P	P	-	-	-	-	-	P	P
Allen	RN	0.5	-	-	-	3	E	E	-	-	-	-	E	4	R	-
Pascheco	RN	0.5	-	E	-	-	E	-	-	-	-	E	-	E	E	-
King	RN	0.4	-	-	3	3	E	-	-	P	-	-	4	-	-	-
Boyer	RN	PRN	-	-	4	4	P	-	-	-	-	-	-	3	-	-
Lui	RN	PRN	-	-	-	-	-	-	N	-	-	-	-	N	-	-
†7 A.M.–3 P.M.			2	4	5	5	5	4	3	2	4	5	5	5	4	3
†3 P.M.–7 P.M.			2	5	5	5	5	4	2	2	5	5	5	5	4	2
†7 P.M.–11 P.M.			2	5	5	5	5	4	2	2	5	5	5	5	4	2
†11 P.M.–7 A.M.			2	2	2	2	2	2	2	2	2	2	2	2	2	2
Daily RN Nursing Care Hours			48	88	96	96	96	80	56	48	88	96	96	96	80	56

Legend: D = 7 A.M.–3 P.M.; E = 3 P.M.–11 P.M.; N = 11 P.M.–7 A.M.; A = 7 A.M.–7 P.M.; P = 7 P.M.–7 A.M.; PRN = as needed; 1 = 7 A.M.–11 A.M.; 2 = 11 A.M.–3 P.M.; 3 = 3 P.M.–7 P.M.; 4 = 7 P.M.–11 P.M.; 5 = 7 A.M.–1 P.M.; 6 = 1 P.M.–7 P.M.

*Weekend option (works 12-hour shifts every Saturday and Sunday "A" *or* Friday and Saturday "P").
†Number of RNs scheduled to work each shift based on average patient acuity and census.

Options include using PRN staff (staff scheduled on an as-needed basis), part-time staff, or float pool staff; allowing overtime for full-time staff; scheduling nurse manager(s) for direct care assignments; using extra nurses from another unit; using outside agency nurses; or asking staff for suggestions or help.

Supplemental staff are needed when workload increases beyond that which the existing staff can manage, staff absences and resignations occur, and staff vacancies exist. Chronic staffing problems need to be addressed in a proactive manner involving the nurse manager, chief nurse executive, and the nursing personnel on the unit having the problem. Strategies for dealing with turnover are given later in this chapter, and strategies for managing absenteeism are discussed in Chapter 21.

Internal Pools Acute staffing problems can be addressed by establishing internal float **pools** using nursing staff and unlicensed assistive personnel (UAPs). Internal float pools of nurses can provide supplemental staffing at a substantially lower cost than using

KEY TERMS

Pools   Internal or external groups of workers that are used as supplemental staff by the organization.

Turnover   The numbers of staff members that vacate a position.

agency nurses. Internal float pools can be centralized or decentralized. A centralized pool is the most efficient. A pool of RNs, LPNs, UAPs, and unit clerks are available for placement anywhere in the institution. However, it may be difficult to place the person with the correct skills for a particular unit at the needed time. In decentralized pools, a staff member usually works only for one nurse manager or on only one unit. The advantages of decentralized pools include better accountability, improved staffing response, and improved continuity of care. Critical care units, operating rooms, maternal–child units, and other highly specialized or technical areas tend to use a decentralized system. Other pools often used include PRN or per diem staff. PRN staff also can be centralized or decentralized. These employees, however, receive premium pay instead of benefits.

External Pools   For some institutions, agency nurses become part of the regular staff contracted to fill vacancies for a specified period of time (e.g., traveling nurses). However, most agency nurses are used as supplemental staff. All agency nurses require orientation to the facility and unit; they must work under the supervision of an experienced in-house nurse. The nurse manager must verify valid licensure, ensure that either the agency or agency nurse has current malpractice insurance, and develop a mechanism to evaluate the agency nurse's performance. Although an agency nurse may meet an urgent staffing need, continuity of care may be compromised and there may be some staff resentment because these nurses may earn two to three times the salary of in-house nurses.

Use of Existing Staff   Nurse managers also must explore opportunities to use nurse extenders, referred to as unlicensed assistive personnel (UAPs). Persons in these roles are nonprofessionals and may or may not provide direct patient care. Sometimes, UAPs complete nonnursing tasks and allow nurses time to assume direct care. Emptying trash, getting supplies, transporting patients, distributing linens, and passing drinking water and food trays are all nonnursing tasks that take nurses away from the patient's professional care. As the demands for nursing care continue, more efficient and effective use of UAPs will remain a strong option, permitting RNs to focus exclusively on direct patient care.

Nurse managers also may provide direct patient care if there are no other solutions to the staffing crisis. This option is the least desirable because it frequently inhibits problem-solving interventions to resolve staffing and patient care issues.

Turnover

One of the most challenging issues in relation to staffing and scheduling of nursing personnel is **turnover** and its cyclic nature. Nursing shortages and high turnover rates alternate with periods of adequate numbers of nurses and low turnover. In the 1980s, the yearly turnover rate in health care institutions averaged between 18% and 25%, according to the Bureau of National Affairs. In 1990, Jones (1990) reported an average turnover rate of 27%.

Marketplace changes in health care are shifting practice to new sites (e.g., clinics) and new models of delivery (e.g., integrated systems). The effect on where nurses practice and what mix of nursing staff is required to adequately care for tomorrow's patients is shifting. It is difficult to estimate the actual dollar cost of nursing turnover. However, given the numerous expenses incurred in hiring a new nurse (e.g., recruiting, selection, orientation, on-the-job training) and temporarily replacing a nurse who quits or is fired (e.g., paying other nurses to work overtime or filling the vacancy with a temporary replacement), the costs are certainly sizable. Jones (1990) estimates the cost of a nurse's resignation at $3,000 or more.

Given its cyclic appearance and its cost, nursing turnover clearly needs to be understood better and controlled more effectively. Turnover has been thought of in simplistic terms and seen as universally negative. Such a primitive view of turnover is not helpful to managers as they attempt to deal with this costly problem. Rather, varieties of turnover need to be differentiated: Did the employee leave of her or his own accord, or was the person asked to leave? Was the departed individual's performance exceptional or mediocre? Did the employee leave for career development (e.g., return to school) or because of dissatisfaction with the organization? Will the departed nurse be easy or difficult to replace? Questions such as these have only recently been asked by health care organizations. Yet until they are answered, it is difficult to establish whether the organization truly has a turnover problem and, if so, what can be done about it.

The discussion in this chapter focuses on voluntary turnover. If an organization finds a significant amount of involuntary turnover (i.e., employees being terminated), then it needs to carefully examine the way it recruits, selects, trains, and motivates employees. These topics are addressed in detail in other chapters in this book.

Measurement Issues

Before a supervisor can hope to manage turnover, its causes must be understood. Traditionally, organizations have attempted to determine the reason(s) for voluntary turnover through two sources: The exiting employee's supervisor is asked why the employee is leaving, and an exit interview with the departing employee is conducted by someone in the human resources department. Although such an approach for determining the cause of voluntary turnover is certainly straightforward, its validity has been questioned. Hinrichs (1975) has shown that the reasons that departing employees give in their exit interviews differ greatly from their responses to surveys completed several months after leaving the organization. Hinrichs argues that because future employers often ask for reference information from prior employers, exiting employees provide safe responses (e.g., "a better opportunity came along") during an exit interview. In summarizing his results, Hinrichs found it was rare that departing employees would say anything negative about an organization they were leaving or about their immediate supervisor.

Although this tendency for departing employees to make safe responses is understandable, it makes it difficult to determine why turnover is occurring. Surveys sent to former employees several weeks after they have resigned may be more useful. Former employees need to be assured that their responses will not influence any future reference information furnished about them, but rather will be used only to help the organization identify the reasons why nurses are leaving. Another way to attempt to discover the cause of nurse turnover is to conduct interviews with the former employee's co-workers, who often know why an employee left.

Turnover is either functional or dysfunctional (Dalton, Krackhardt, & Porter, 1981). Losing a nurse who is an excellent performer is a greater loss than losing a mediocre performer. Similarly, if a nurse can be replaced easily, the loss to the organization is less

than if she or he is hard to replace. Thus, a nurse manager needs to be particularly concerned about turnover when the nurses who are leaving are of high quality and difficult to replace (i.e., dysfunctional turnover). In contrast, if poorly performing nurses who can be easily replaced resign, the organization actually may benefit from the turnover (i.e., functional turnover). Managers need to disregard the myth that all turnover is bad and replace it with an appreciation of the numerous factors that should be involved in determining whether turnover is a problem meriting attention.

Consequences of Turnover

Although turnover obviously involves real costs to the organization, turnover also can have undesirable effects on patients, co-workers, and others. And, as discussed earlier, voluntary turnover is not always undesirable. Anyone with work experience can remember some individual (e.g., a co-worker, a supervisor) whose departure would have improved the organization's functioning significantly. In evaluating the consequences of turnover, a nurse manager (and the organization) must remember that voluntary turnover can have costs and/or benefits. What may be seen as a desirable departure by some (e.g., the nurse manager) may be viewed as a loss by others (e.g., a subset of co-workers).

However, turnover has consequences that go far beyond direct dollar costs. Turnover can have a number of repercussions among other nurses who worked with the departed nurse. Steers and Stone (1982) suggest that turnover can be interpreted by co-workers as a rejection of the job and a recognition that better job opportunities exist elsewhere. For those who remain, ways must be found to reconcile their decision to stay in light of evidence from others that the job may not be good. As a result, those who remain may reevaluate their present position in the organization and develop more negative job attitudes. In addition, nurses who remain may have to work longer hours (overtime) or simply work harder to cover for a departed nurse; this can cause both physical and mental strain and may result in additional departures. Thus, one often finds a turnover spiral (Staw, 1980). If temporary replacements are used, problems still can result as the workflow of the unit is disturbed and communication patterns within the unit are disrupted. Turnover, and the resultant decrease in the number of nurses, also may cause the organization to postpone, cancel, or not pursue potentially profitable new ventures. An organization may delay opening new clinics or services or even close existing units.

There are, as suggested earlier, several desirable consequences of turnover, especially if the departed nurse was a poor performer. Steers and Stone (1982) state that among these are the possibility that performance may improve: Recently trained employees may be more enthusiastic; long-running conflicts between people will be reduced or eliminated through attrition; opportunities for promotion and transfer will increase for those who remain, and innovation and adaptation brought about by the introduction of fresh ideas will be enhanced.

To this list of desirable consequences could be added three additional outcomes: the opportunity for overtime (some nurses desire voluntary overtime as a way to increase wages), the stimulation of needed policy changes (as a result of losing a "star performer," an organization may be stimulated to change a troublesome policy), and the avoidance of layoffs (natural attrition may lessen or eliminate the need for forced reduction of staff during tight labor markets).

Although a detailed discussion of the consequences of turnover is beyond the scope of this chapter, the abbreviated discussion provided should make clear the numerous issues that need to be considered in attempting to determine whether a given turnover rate actually is a "turnover problem." If the nurse manager decides that she or he has a turnover problem,

then action should be initiated. The turnover model introduced in the next section should be a useful vehicle for helping the manager diagnose the cause of voluntary turnover and actively manage it (e.g., attempt to reduce the overall turnover rate, influence who is resigning).

A Model of Employee Turnover

According to the model shown in Figure 18-1, voluntary turnover is a direct function of a nurse's perceptions of both the ease and the desirability of leaving the organization. Perceived ease of movement depends on the nurse's personal characteristics (e.g., education, area of specialization, age, geographic mobility, contacts at other hospitals, and transportation) as well as market forces (e.g., number of job openings at other hospitals, non–health care organizations hiring nurses for nursing or nonnursing positions).

As with ease of movement, perceptions of the desirability of movement can be affected by several factors. Three important ones are the existence of job alternatives within the health care organization, work characteristics, and organizational characteristics. The more a nurse perceives that other work opportunities (positions) exist within the organization, the less voluntary turnover there should be; that is, a nurse may be able to leave her or his current position by means of a lateral transfer, promotion, or demotion. Thus, a

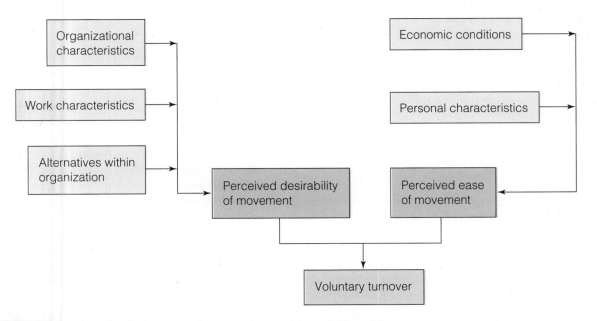

Figure 18-1 Model of voluntary employee turnover. *Note:* Adapted from *Organizations* by J. G. March and H. A. Simon, 1958, New York: Wiley, pp. 90–106. Used by permission.

nurse who is having problems with a co-worker may be able to transfer to a new unit rather than leave the organization. To some degree, a nurse manager may be able to facilitate alternative job opportunities (e.g., helping a nurse transfer) as a way to reduce voluntary turnover. Work characteristics (e.g., autonomy, communication, group cohesion, job stress, job satisfaction, organizational commitment) and organizational characteristics (e.g., unit structure, distributive justice) also can affect perceived desirability of movement. A number of studies have shown that the greater an employee's satisfaction level or level of organizational commitment, the lower the probability of the individual's quitting. Job satisfaction is affected by various facets of the work environment, including relationships with the nurse manager, other staff nurses and unit employees, patients, and physicians, as well as the shift worked (e.g., day versus evening, rotating versus fixed), compensation level, and equal and fair distribution of rewards and punishments.

In dealing with turnover, managers need to be aware of three important considerations. First, voluntary turnover can be caused by several factors, only some of which the nurse manager can influence. Second, the manager needs to assess why nurses are leaving; this may be done in cooperation with the human resource department. Box 18-2 presents a list of several possible causes of turnover. Typically, an organization determines the reasons for turnover by means of exit interviews. However, as noted earlier, the use of exit questionnaires (mailed several weeks after a resignation) and interviews with remaining co-workers often provide more accurate data on turnover causes. Finally, the nurse manager must realize that any action taken to reduce voluntary turnover may have other unintended ramifications. The nurse manager should carefully think through a strategy for dealing with turnover prior to implementing it.

Strategies for Controlling Turnover

The turnover model presented in Figure 18-1 provides a useful organizing framework for deriving strategies to control turnover. The nurse manager's goal should be to reduce dysfunctional voluntary turnover. The manager's first opportunity to reduce turnover is when the decision to hire is made. An individual's length of stay at past employers is an indication of how long the person could be expected to stay on a new job (Breaugh & Dossett, 1989).

In order to retain a valued employee in the organization, the manager can facilitate movement within

the organization. Thus, if a staff nurse is "burned out" from working on an oncology floor, one option is to allow a transfer to another service area in the organization (e.g., home care). Unfortunately, many nurse managers hinder or even prohibit such a transfer (particularly if the potential transferee is an excellent performer), not wanting to lose a good nurse. However, this perspective is shortsighted. If the staff nurse cannot transfer to another area (intraorganizational mobility), she or he may leave the organization entirely (interorganizational mobility).

Work characteristics (e.g., job satisfaction, group cohesion, job stress) and organizational characteristics (e.g., unit structure) also can be influenced by the nurse manager both directly and indirectly by such actions as providing a realistic job preview, enriching or redesigning the staff nurse's job, facilitating upward and downward communication, linking rewards and performance, developing group cohesiveness, helping resolve interpersonal conflicts, and providing training and educational opportunities.

Although the appropriate strategy for addressing nursing turnover will vary depending on the unique circumstances of the work unit, it is important for the nurse manager to be proactive. Landstrom, Biordi, and Gillies (1989, p. 23) found that 88% of RNs who left their jobs reported that "an appropriate managerial intervention early in their leave-taking decision process would have halted their decision to leave."

A Systems Perspective

Employee absenteeism and turnover have been referred to as withdrawal behaviors because they allow an employee to leave the workplace, in one case temporarily and, in the other, permanently. In many cases, these withdrawal behaviors share a common cause: job dissatisfaction. Many effective strategies for reducing absenteeism (e.g., providing child care, improving supervisory behavior, coordinating car pools, offering stress management workshops, creating a cohesive work group) also have a positive effect on turnover.

The nurse manager must avoid the temptation to look for a quick fix in dealing with turnover. In addition, the manager must recognize that what appears to be a simple change (e.g., trying to enrich the job of a high-performing nurse) may not be. For example, providing additional duties to enrich a nurse's job may lead to complaints of favoritism from other nurses or the human resource department may worry about assigning duties that are not included in the job

Box 18-2 Categories of Reason for Turnover

Dissatisfaction

Wages—amount
Wages—equity
Benefits
Hours or shift
Working conditions
Supervision—technical
Supervision—personal
Co-workers
Job security
Job meaningfulness
Use of skills and abilities
Career opportunities
Policies and rules
Communication
Stress
Respect

Living conditions

Housing
Transportation
Child care
Health care facilities
Leisure activities
Physical environment
Social environment
Education opportunities
Other: _____

Personal

Spouse transferred
To be married
Illness or death in family
Personal illness
Personal injury
Pregnancy

Alternatives

Returning to school
Military service
Government service
Starting own business
Similar job: same industry
Similar job: other industry
Different job: other industry
Voluntary early retirement
Voluntary transfer to subsidiary (loss of seniority)
New position
   Organization
   Position
   Location
   Earnings

Organization initiated

Resignation in lieu of dismissal
Violation of rules, policy
Unsatisfactory probation period
Attendance
Performance
Layoff
Layoff: downgrade refused
Layoff: transfer refused
End of temporary employment
Reduction in force

Other

Transfer to: _____
Leave of absence from: _____
On loan to: _____
Retirement
Death

Note: Adapted from *Employee turnover: Causes, consequences, and control* by W. H. Mobley, 1982, Reading, MA: Addison-Wesley, p. 38.

description. Such potential difficulties should not cause a nurse manager to revert back to status quo behavior. Rather, the manager needs to anticipate such potential problems and deal with them (e.g., be able to justify the differential treatment through the use of performance appraisal data, have the affected nurse agree to the additional duties in writing).

An environment that rewards good performance is the goal. Obviously, this calls for careful attention to the performance appraisal process (see Chapter 19).

Such a performance-oriented climate increases the likelihood of functional turnover (i.e., the departure of poorly performing nurses) and decreases the probability of dysfunctional turnover.

Work scheduling (self-scheduling, fixed versus rotating shifts, flexible work hours, job sharing) is a particularly important area not only because of its relationship to voluntary turnover but also because of its frequent linkage to unionization attempts. It should not be surprising that working conditions that lead to turnover also can motivate interest in unionization. Two key causes of turnover-related unionization are staff shortages and rotating work schedules. Innovative work schedules have had positive impacts on both nurse recruitment and retention. Although changing to work schedules that staff nurses see as more advantageous (e.g., fixed shifts, flexible hours, job sharing) obviously involves costs (e.g., coordination time, paperwork), it also provides benefits. Most nurses prefer fixed shifts. If possible, nurses also prefer flexible hours. For many nurses with child care responsibility, job sharing provides a perfect means for remaining in health care and, at the same time, fulfilling parental responsibilities.

Before implementing such innovative work schedules, considerable planning (e.g., cost–benefit analysis) clearly needs to take place. Unfortunately, many health care organizations, even those that are having trouble recruiting and retaining nurses, simply dismiss such schedules. As with a number of the strategies for reducing turnover, a single nurse manager is unlikely to be able to change an organization's policy concerning work schedules. However, if several managers coordinate their efforts, change is more likely to occur. To increase their likelihood of a successful attempt, the group of managers may need to build a persuasive case for the program they are suggesting (e.g., document the success of job sharing at other hospitals, cost out the possible financial gain—often, part-time nurses are paid at a lower rate and do not receive pension benefits).

Sometimes a nurse manager may simply need to adapt to a high turnover rate. Even if this is the case, the manager may be able to lessen potential problems by doing two things. First, the nurse manager may want to "manage" beliefs about why a nurse left. Sometimes, the reason is unclear, and the grapevine often will provide an inaccurate and less attractive reason from the organization's perspective (e.g., "she left for $1.05 more an hour at a competitor institution"). Second, the nurse manager may be able to provide human resources with a preferred list of replacement workers. One health care organization keeps an up-to-date list of former nurses who will fill in on an occasional basis. Such former employees are more familiar with organizational procedures and thus can handle things more efficiently.

A nurse manager wants to do everything possible to lessen the problem of turnover. Sometimes this involves coordinating efforts with other managers to change organizational policy. The strategies outlined in this chapter have been shown to be effective in reducing turnover. However, not all are equally applicable to all situations. As a manager, the nurse must be able to analyze situational factors and determine what is appropriate for the set of circumstances. For example, flexible work hours may be suitable for a clinic but not for an around-the-clock operation. By being creative, nurse managers not only can reduce the overall turnover rate but also can have an influence on which nurses leave by providing incentives for the exceptional nurse to stay and by doing less to retain mediocre nurses.

Summary

- The goal of staffing is to provide an adequate mix of nursing staff to match patient care needs. Expected productivity levels, patient acuity levels, and nursing care hours must be continuously analyzed.

- Patient classification systems provide a mechanism to objectively determine acuity levels of patients, determine nursing hours of care, staffing, and staffing mix. The most commonly used systems are Medicus, GRASP, and ARIC.

- Reduction of salary budgets due to reduced reimbursement for patient services have made flexible and creative staffing and scheduling techniques increasingly necessary. Use of PRN staff, part-time staff, and split shifts provide the most flexible arrangements.

- Although turnover may be functional or dysfunctional, it is costly to the organization. In addition, turnover may lead to negative job attitudes, distorted workflow, and overtime. Positive outcomes may include increased productivity, opportunities for promotion or transfer, and the avoidance of forced staff reductions.

- Turnover can be minimized by using appropriate hiring strategies, facilitating movement within the organization, redesigning jobs, facilitating communication, linking rewards to performance, developing group cohesiveness, resolving interpersonal conflicts, appropriately using power, and providing educational opportunities.

■ LEADERSHIP AND MANAGEMENT
in Action

1. What types of information are used in determining staffing requirements?
2. Describe four different ways to meet temporary staffing needs.
3. Identify and discuss two types of turnover. What are the organizational consequences of each?

References

Breaugh, J. A., & Dosset, D. L. (1989). Rethinking the use of personal history information. *Journal of Business and Psychology, 3,* 371–385.

Bureau of National Affairs (1988). *Bulletin to Management.* Washington, DC: Author.

Dalton, D., Krackhardt, D., & Porter, L. (1981). Functional turnover. *Journal of Applied Psychology, 66,* 716–721.

DeGroot, H. A. (1989). Patient classification system evolution. Part I: Essential system elements. *Journal of Nursing Administration, 19*(6), 30–35.

Diers, D., & Bozzo, J. (1997). Nursing resource definition in DRGs. *Nursing Economics, 15*(3), 124–130, 137.

Dunn, M. G., Norby, R., Cournoyer, P., Hudec, S., O'Donnell, J. & Donaldson-Snider, M. (1995). Expert panel method for nurse staffing and resources management. *Journal of Nursing Administration, 25*(10), 61–67.

Finnigan, S. A., Abel, M., Dobler, T., Hudson, L., & Terry, B. (1993). Automated patient acuity: Linking nursing systems and quality measurement with patient outcomes. *Journal of Nursing Administration, 23*(5), 62–71.

Gallagher, R. M., Kany, K. A., Rowell, P. A., & Peterson, C. (1999). ANA's Nurse staffing principles. *American Journal of Nursing, 99*(4), 50, 52–53.

Hinrichs, J. (1975). Measurement of reasons for resignation of professionals: Questionnaire versus company and consultant interviews. *Journal of Applied Psychology, 60,* 530–532.

Joint Commission on Accreditation of Healthcare Organizations (JCAHO). (1995). *Comprehensive accreditation manual for hospitals.* Chicago: Author.

Jones, C. B. (1990). Staff nurse turnover costs: Measurements and results. *Journal of Nursing Administration, 20,* 27–32.

Landstrom, G. L., Biordi, D. L., & Gillies, D. A. (1989). The emotional and behavioral process of staff nurse turnover. *Journal of Nursing Administration, 19,* 23–28.

Malloch, K., & Conovaloff, A. (1999). Patient classification systems, Part 1: The third generation. *Journal of Nursing Administration, 29*(7/8), 49–56.

Melberg, S. E. (1997). Effects of changing skill mix. *Nursing Management, 28*(11), 47–48.

Meyer, D. (1978). *GRASP: A patient information and workload management system.* Morganton, NC: MCS.

Staw, B. M. (1980). The consequences of turnover. *Journal of Occupational Behavior, 1,* 253–273.

Steers, R., & Stone, T. (1982). Organizational exit. In K. Rowland & G. Ferris (Eds.), *Personnel management.* Boston: Allyn and Bacon.

Performance Appraisal

Looking Ahead

Evaluating job performance by determining the strengths and weaknesses of individual employees within the organization and the motivation of those employees is a vital function of managers. It helps determine and develop the future role of an employee and provides a basis for administrative decisions. This chapter explains the importance of this process and provides methods of evaluation, criteria to take into consideration, and the accuracy and problems of performance appraisal.

Objectives

After reading this chapter, you will be able to:

- Discuss how motivation and ability affect job performance.
- Compare and contrast motivational theories.
- Describe how motivational theories can help a manager.
- Describe criteria used to evaluate employee performance.
- Compare and contrast methods for appraising performance.
- Discuss typical problems in appraising performance.
- List key behaviors for the performance interview.

Acontinual and troublesome question facing nurse managers today is why some employees perform better than others. Making decisions about who performs what tasks in a particular manner without first considering individual behavior can lead to irreversible long-term problems. Each employee is different in many respects. A manager needs to ask how such differences influence the behavior and performance of the job requirements. Ideally, the manager performs this assessment when the new employee is hired. In reality, however, many employees are placed in positions without the manager's having adequate knowledge of their abilities and/or interests. This often results in problems with employee performance, as well as conflict between employees and managers.

Employee performance literature ultimately reveals two major dimensions as determinants of job performance: motivation and ability (Hersey & Blanchard, 1988). This chapter describes a model of job performance and presents techniques for evaluating performance.

A Model of Job Performance

Nurse managers spend considerable time making judgments about the fit among individuals, job tasks, and effectiveness. Such judgments are typically influenced by both the manager's and the employee's characteristics. For example, ability, instinct, and aspiration levels—as well as age, education, and family background—account for why some employees perform well and others poorly. Based on these factors, a model that considers motivation and ability as determinants of job performance is presented in Table 19-1.

This performance model identifies six categories likely to be viewed as important by the nurse manager: daily job performance, attendance, punctuality, adherence to policies and procedures, absence of incidents/errors/accidents, and honesty and trustworthiness. Although there is conceptual overlap in these

categories, separate designation of each helps emphasize their importance.

When using this model, the nurse manager should carefully consider several factors. First, the health care organization should establish and communicate clear descriptions of daily job performance so that deviations from expected behaviors can be easily identified and documented. Second, behaviors considered troublesome in one department may be acceptable in another department. Finally, some behaviors are viewed as serious only when repeated (e.g., being late to work), whereas others are classified as troublesome following only one incident (e.g., a medication error with severe consequences).

Employee Motivation

Motivation describes the factors that initiate and direct behavior. Because individuals bring to the workplace different needs and goals, the type and intensity of motivators vary among employees. Nurse managers prefer motivated employees because they strive to find the best way to perform their jobs. Motivated employees are more likely to be productive than are nonmotivated workers. This is one reason that motivation is an important aspect of enhancing employee performance.

Motivational Theories

Historically, motivational theories were concerned with three things: (a) what mobilizes or energizes human behavior, (b) what directs behavior toward the accomplishment of some objective, and (c) how such

Table 19-1 A Simplified Model of Job Performance

Motivation	and	Ability	=	Employee Performance
Compensation		Responsibilities		Daily job performance
Benefits		Education—basic/advanced		Attendance
Job design		Continuing education		Punctuality
Leadership style		Skills/abilities		Adherence to policies and procedures
Recruitment and selection				Absence of incidents/errors/accidents
Employee needs/goals/abilities				Honesty and trustworthiness

behavior is sustained over time. The usefulness of motivational theories depends on their ability to explain motivation adequately, to predict with some degree of accuracy what people will actually do, and, finally, to suggest practical ways of influencing employees to accomplish organizational objectives. There are some distinct differences among motivational theories that allow them to be classified into at least two different groups: content theories and process theories.

Content Theories In general, **content theories** emphasize individual needs or the rewards that may satisfy those needs. There are two types of content theories: instinct and need. Instinct theorists characterized **instincts** as inherited or innate tendencies that predisposed individuals to behave in certain ways. These theories were attacked for their difficulty in pinpointing the specific motivating behaviors and the acute awareness of the variability in the strengths of instincts across individuals. In addition, the development of need theories supported the concept that motives were learned behaviors. Perhaps the most noted of the need theorists were Abraham Maslow, Clayton Alderfer, and Frederick Herzberg.

Maslow (1943, 1954) identified five hierarchical needs. A lower-level need controls behavior until it is satisfied, and then the next higher need energizes and directs behavior. This hierarchy, from the lowest to the highest level, is as follows: (a) physiological needs, such as hunger and thirst; (b) safety needs, that is, bodily safety; (c) belongingness or social needs, such as friendship, affection, and love; (d) esteem needs, such as recognition, appreciation, and self-respect; and (e) self-actualization, that is, developing one's whole potential (Figure 19-1). Maslow's theory is frequently used in nursing to provide an explanation of human behavior.

Alderfer (1972) suggested three, rather than five, need levels in his existence–relatedness–growth theory: (a) existence needs, which include both physiological and safety needs; (b) relatedness needs (Maslow's belongingness or social needs); and (c) growth needs, which include the needs for self-esteem and self-actualization. This theory is similar to Maslow's in that it assumes that the satisfaction of needs on one level activates a need at the next higher level (Figure 19-1). An example is that staff who have a sense of job security will strive for a means of feeling related or connected to the organization or unit. Today's employees want to have a voice in how things are done; they want to make a difference and feel that they are valued by the organization. Empowerment, self-managing teams, and continuous quality improvement programs are built on recognition of these needs.

Alderfer suggests, however, that frustrated higher-level needs cause a regression to and reemphasis of the next lower-level need in the hierarchy. In addition, Alderfer's model suggests that more than one need may operate at any point in time. Although it is somewhat less rigid than Maslow's hierarchy, it presents little that is new or substantially different from Maslow's.

Herzberg's two-factor theory explains motivation as a function of job satisfaction (Herzberg, 1966; Herzberg, Mausner, & Snyderman, 1959). Herzberg states that job satisfaction and job dissatisfaction are not opposite ends of the same continuum; rather, they are two different phenomena. The factors that lead to no job satisfaction are quite different from those that lead to no job *dis*satisfaction, and the resulting

Maslow	Alderfer	Herzberg
Self-actualization	Growth needs	Motivating factors
Esteem needs		
Belongingness (social needs)	Relatedness needs	Hygiene factors
Safety needs	Existence needs	
Physiological needs		

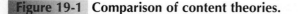 **Figure 19-1** **Comparison of content theories.**

KEY TERMS

Content theories Motivational theories that emphasize individual needs or the rewards that may satisfy those needs, or attempt to explain why a person behaves in a particular manner.

Instincts Inherited or innate tendencies that predispose individuals to behave in certain ways.

Process theories Motivational theories that emphasize how the motivation process works to direct an individual's effort into performance.

Reinforcement theory (behavior modification) The motivational theory that views motivation as learning and proposes behavior is learned through a process called operant conditioning.

Operant conditioning Process by which a behavior becomes associated with a particular consequence.

Punishment A process used to inhibit an undesired behavior by applying a negative reinforcer.

Extinction The technique used to eliminate negative behavior, in which a positive reinforcer is removed and the undesired behavior is extinguished.

behaviors from these two states are also quite different. Based on this concept, Herzberg proposed that hygiene factors and motivating factors, respectively, affect dissatisfaction and satisfaction. Hygiene factors are extrinsic to the job itself; they include pay, supervision, organizational policies, relationships with coworkers, working conditions, personal life, status, and job security. Unsatisfactory hygiene factors lead to dissatisfaction, which, in turn, leads to increased absences, grievances, or resignations. Herzberg likens hygiene factors to a water filtration plant. Not having one will likely result in illness, but drinking purified water will not necessarily keep one from becoming sick.

Satisfaction and motivation then result from factors intrinsic to the job, such as a sense of achievement for performing a task successfully, recognition and praise, responsibility for one's own or another's work, growth, and advancement or changing status through promotion. To the extent that these intrinsic, or motivating, factors are present, an employee is assumed to experience job satisfaction and hence will be highly motivated to perform the job effectively.

Process Theories Whereas content theories attempt to explain why a person behaves in a particular manner, **process theories** emphasize *how* the motivation process works to direct an individual's effort into performance. These theories add another dimension to the manager's understanding of motivation and help to predict employee behavior in certain circumstances. Examples of process theories are reinforcement theory, expectancy theory, equity theory, and goal-setting theory.

Reinforcement theory, also known as behavior modification, views motivation as learning (Skinner, 1953). According to this theory, behavior is learned through a process called **operant conditioning**, in which a behavior becomes associated with a particular consequence. In operant conditioning, the response–consequence connection is strengthened over time—that is, it is learned.

Consequences may be positive, as with praise or recognition, or negative. Positive reinforcers are used for the express purpose of increasing a desired behavior. For example, Kyle, a staff nurse, offered a creative idea to redesign work flow on the unit. His manager supported the idea and helped Kyle implement the new process. In addition, the manager praised Kyle for the extra effort and publicly recognized him for the idea. Kyle was encouraged by the outcome and sought other solutions to work-flow problems.

Negative reinforcers are used to inhibit an undesired behavior. **Punishment** is a common technique. In order to get Rose to chart adequately, the manager required her to come to his office daily with her patient charts until she achieved an acceptable level of charting. Rose found the task laborious and humiliating. As a result, Rose soon was charting appropriately. Because punishment is negative in character, an employee may fail to improve and also may avoid the manager and the job, as well. Research has shown that the effects of punishment are generally temporary. Undesirable behavior will be suppressed only as long as the manager monitors the situation and the threat of punishment is present. Conversely, research has demonstrated that positive reinforcement is the best way to change behavior.

Extinction is another technique used to eliminate negative behavior. By removing a positive reinforcer, undesired behavior is extinguished. Consider the case of Jasmine, a chronic complainer. To curb this behavior, her manager chose to ignore her many complaints and not try to resolve them. Initially Jasmine complained more, but eventually she realized her behavior was not getting the desired response and stopped complaining.

A problem with operant conditioning (behavior modification) is that there is no sure way to elicit the desired behavior so that it can be reinforced. In addition, staff and the manager may view consequences differently. Take Thad, for example. As a new employee, Thad conscientiously completed critical paths for his assigned patients. When the manager recognized Thad for his good work, his peers began to exclude him from the group. Although the manager was attempting positive reinforcement, Thad quit completing critical paths because he felt the manager had alienated him from his co-workers.

Another procedure is **shaping**. Shaping involves selectively reinforcing behaviors that are successively closer approximations to the desired behavior. Consider the case of Betty, who was chronically late to work. Her uniform was always wrinkled and sometimes soiled, her personal hygiene left something to be desired, and her general attitude was quite unpleasant. For Betty, it was not a matter of not knowing what to do; she had been reprimanded and counseled innumerable times on appropriate job behavior. Her problem did not appear to be lack of knowledge, but a simple lack of motivation.

The nurse manager tried for a week to find a single, positive behavior to reinforce. The following week, she found occasion to praise Betty several times. One day, for example, Betty came to work only 10 minutes late, and her relative punctuality was promptly reinforced. Similarly, she seemed to have made at least an attempt to comb her hair, so she was positively reinforced for her improved appearance. On every occasion, however, the manager was met with a low grunt and an occasional icy glare from Betty, who continued about her own business. After a few weeks, however, she seemed to respond more favorably to the praise and increased interest (rewards) of the nurse manager. Her hair appeared fairly well groomed on most days, and although wrinkled, her uniform was relatively clean.

Within a period of approximately 2 months, Betty's performance, although not perfect, was substantially improved, and she had ceased to be an embarrassment to her colleagues and the hospital. Moreover, her disposition had improved, and she had actually begun to develop some friendships with other members of the staff. Her appearance and hygiene were, for the most part, quite acceptable, although her punctuality had improved only slightly. She was clearly no star

performer, but she had come to be regarded as a valuable and necessary member of the staff.

The main point of this story is that behavior modification via the principles of positive reinforcement may take some time, especially when shaping procedures must be implemented. Each successively closer approximation to the desired behavior is reinforced and well established before progressive reinforcement is given to closer approximations of the desired behavior. When people become clearly aware that desirable rewards are contingent on a specific behavior, their behavior will eventually change.

Behavior modification works quite well, provided that rewards can be found that, in fact, employees see as positive reinforcers and provided that supervisory personnel can control such rewards or make them contingent on performance. This does not mean that all rewards work equally well or that the same rewards will continue to function effectively over a long time. If a nursing manager praised someone four or five times a day every day, the praise would soon begin to wear thin; it would cease to be a positive reinforcer. Care must be taken not to overdo a good thing. For this reason, a *continuous schedule* of reinforcement—reinforcement every time a desired behavior occurs—may result in the reinforcer's losing its effectiveness over time (Table 19-2).

Partial schedules of reinforcement, reinforcing behavior with every second or third occurrence, is more effective in changing behavior. This *fixed-ratio schedule* of reinforcement requires very close monitoring to

Table 19-2 Effects of Different Reinforcement Schedules

Arrangement of Reinforcement Contingencies	Schedules of Reinforcement Contingencies	Effect on Behavior When Applied	Effect on Behavior When Removed
Positive reinforcement	Continuous reinforcement	Fastest method to establish a new behavior	Fastest method to extinguish a new behavior
	Partial reinforcement	Slowest method to establish a new behavior	Slowest method to extinguish a new behavior
	Variable partial reinforcement	More consistent response frequencies	Slower extinction rate
	Fixed partial reinforcement	Less consistent response frequencies	Faster extinction rate
Avoidance reinforcement		Increased frequency over preconditioning level	Return to preconditioning level
Punishment extinction		Decreased frequency over preconditioning level	Return to preconditioning level

Note: Adapted from "Present theories and new directions in theories of work effort" by O. Behling, C. Schreisheim, and J. Tolliver, *Journal Supplement Abstract Service* of the American Psychological Corporation.

reinforce every *n*th response and is obviously not very practical. Reinforcing on a fairly regular basis is known as a *variable-ratio schedule* of reinforcement; an example is the distribution of weekly or monthly paychecks.

Some rather interesting research findings have emerged over the years on continuous and partial schedules of reinforcement. On the one hand, for example, we know that a continuous schedule of reinforcement is the fastest method of establishing or learning a new behavior, whereas any kind of partial schedule of reinforcement is much slower. On the other hand, behaviors learned under a continuous schedule also extinguish very quickly once reinforcement stops. Behavior learned on a partial schedule continues for a much longer time without being reinforced. In addition, continuous schedules of reinforcement are probably better when money is used rather than other reinforcers, such as praise.

Like reinforcement theory, **expectancy theory** (Vroom, 1964) emphasizes the role of rewards and their relationship to the performance of desired behaviors. Expectancy theory regards people as reacting consciously and actively to their environment.

Vroom asserts that individuals are motivated by their expectancies (beliefs) about future outcomes (consequences of behavior) and by the value they place on those outcomes. Three components are important in predicting what and how much effort a person will exert. First, **expectancy** is the perceived probability that effort will lead to a specific performance level or behavior, that is, the degree to which people expect they "can do" something. Second, **instrumentality** is the belief that a given performance level or behavior will lead to some outcome (reward or punishment). Third, **valence** is the perceived value (attractiveness or unattractiveness) of an outcome. Thus, a manager must determine an individual's beliefs regarding the expectancy that will achieve the desired result (expectancy), that the achievement will yield rewards (instrumentality), and how the rewards are valued (valence). In an effort to improve the amount of delegation by the nurses on her unit, Andrea approached the situation from an expectancy theory perspective. She identified that the nurses wanted to assign more duties to assistive personnel but were reluctant because of concerns about liability. Once Andrea was able to clarify liability issues, the nurses were eager to delegate nonprofessional tasks in order to be able to devote more time to their professional responsibilities.

The net effect of these three components is the amount of effort an individual will exert. Thus, when any one component is drastically reduced, so is motivation (effort). If staff members do not believe that they are capable of performing a task (expectancy), or if they believe there is little chance of reward for their work (instrumentality), or if the value of the outcome (valence) is low, motivation is reduced.

Expectancy theory also considers multiple outcomes. Consider the possibility of a promotion to nurse manager. Even though a staff nurse believes such a promotion is positive and is a desirable reward for competent performance in patient care, the nurse also realizes that there are possibly some negative outcomes (e.g., working longer hours, losing the close camaraderie enjoyed with other staff members). These multiple outcomes will influence the staff nurse's decision.

Expectancy theory is useful because of its clear managerial implications. First, managers can maximize expectancies by assigning to employees tasks that they are capable of performing or by providing them with the necessary training. In addition, removing obstacles (inadequate resources, lack of information or cooperation from others) increases employees' expectancies. Second, instrumentalities can be maximized by making certain that rewards (and punishment) are made contingent on performance. Finally, rewards must be perceived as desirable enough to make the effort toward high performance worthwhile. Similarly, to act as a successful deterrent to inappropriate job behavior, punishment must be regarded as sufficiently undesirable.

Similarly, **equity theory** suggests that effort and job satisfaction depend on the degree of equity, or perceived fairness, in the work situation (Adams, 1963; 1965). **Equity** simply means that a person perceives that one's contribution to the job is rewarded in the same proportion that another person's contribution is rewarded. Job contributions include such things as ability, education, experience, and effort, whereas rewards include job satisfaction, pay, prestige, and any other outcomes an employee regards as valuable. Thus, equity theory is concerned with the conditions under which employees perceive their contributions to the job and the rewards obtained as fair and equitable. Equity does not in any way imply equality; rather, it suggests that employees who bring more to the job will receive greater rewards. Inequity occurs when an employee's effort and rewards are perceived to be disproportional to that of another person, whether a coworker or a person doing a similar job for a different employer. Inequity, then, motivates a change in behavior that may either increase or decrease actual effort and job performance. However, reducing inequity may or may not change performance.

Employees can try to restore what they perceive as equity in a variety of ways. First, they can increase or decrease effort. Nurses can attempt to increase their status by assuming more patient care assignments, spending more time on charting, or exhibiting other behaviors reflecting additional effort. Second, they

may attempt to persuade the person(s) to whom they are comparing themselves to increase or decrease their inputs—persuading nursing assistants to work less, for instance. Third, they may attempt to persuade the organization to change either their own rewards or those of the comparison persons (e.g., salary changes or perquisites). Fourth, they may psychologically distort the perceived importance and value of their own contributions and rewards ("How could they run this unit without me?"). Fifth, they may distort the perceived importance and value of the comparison persons' contributions or rewards ("What can you expect of assistants?").

Psychologically distorting the perceptions of a comparison person's outcomes or inputs is probably the easiest way to restore equity without actually changing one's effort. Alternatively, the staff member may select a different comparison person, someone who is seen as more relevant for the comparison being made, such as the nurse manager. Finally, the individual may actually leave the organization.

The important point is that perceived fairness of rewards affects the manner in which individuals view their jobs and the organization, and it can affect the amount of effort they expend in accomplishing tasks. Moreover, evidence indicates that inequitable rewards, especially underpayment inequity, lead to increased psychological tension, lower job satisfaction, and poor job performance. In times of economic retrenchment, when no one in the organization receives a salary increase, employees, for example, may perceive the situation as equitable if they believed it to be equitable prior to the retrenchment; thus, job satisfaction may not be adversely affected. However, simply distributing rewards equitably does not necessarily improve an otherwise poor motivational environment. In today's economic environment, with organizations being redesigned and reengineered and positions reduced, problems with perceived equity can be anticipated.

Unlike expectancy theory and equity theory, **goal-setting theory** suggests that it is not the rewards or outcomes of task performance per se that cause a person to expend effort, but rather the goal itself. There are three basic propositions in goal setting (Locke, 1968): (a) specific goals lead to higher performance than do general goals, such as "Do your best"; (b) specific, difficult goals lead to higher performance than specific, easy goals, provided that those involved accept the goals; and (c) incentives such as money, knowledge of results, praise and reproof, participation, competition, and time limits affect behavior only if they cause individuals to change their goals or to accept goals that have been assigned to them.

Timothy, for example, was new to a home care hospice program. An important skill in care with the terminally ill is therapeutic communication. Timothy and his manager recognized that he needed help to improve his skills in communicating with these patients and their families. His manager asked him to write two goals related to communication. Timothy expressed a desire to attend a communications workshop and also indicated he would try at least one new communication technique each week. Within a month, Timothy's therapeutic communication skills had already improved. As a result, Timothy was more satisfied with his position, his patients received more compassionate care, and Timothy found his work more rewarding.

According to goal-setting theory, the function of rewards is to help ensure that the individual will accept an assigned goal or to set a more specific, difficult personal goal. The specificity and difficulty of the goal mobilize energy and direct behavior toward goal accomplishment. If the person sees tasks and duties as reasonable and specific, difficult goals are likely to produce higher performance as long as such performance is rewarded and the individual is held accountable for the task.

Obviously there is no single approach to motivating staff members. Some methods work better than others with different people or in different settings. However, each theory of work motivation contributes something to our understanding of, and ultimately our ability to influence, employee motivation. Figure 19-2 illustrates a simple model of how the various motivational theories are related. First, there is a task to be accomplished. If this task is expressed in terms of a specific, difficult goal that is accepted by the staff member, a relatively high degree of performance may realistically be expected in most situations. How does

this happen? Goals, perceived ability, and perceived situational constraints all combine to form the perceived likelihood that effort will lead to a given level of performance or goal accomplishment. This expectancy, when combined with the belief that valued rewards will follow from goal attainment (instrumentality), prompts the expenditure of effort (motivation). Thus, goal-setting and expectancy theory suggest not only that staff members should know exactly what they should be doing, but also that they should perceive rewards as contingent on performance of their assigned tasks.

Managers who are effective leaders draw from their knowledge of various motivational theories to create the environment in which their staff derive needs satisfaction from the work itself. No motivation theory provides a complete description of the motivational process; each theory or technique brings a different perspective and contribution to understanding and influencing motivation. Effective staff motivation is best accomplished by judiciously combining theories and techniques so that their effects are complementary.

Employee Ability

Abilities and skills play a major role in individual behavior and performance. Some employees, even though highly motivated, simply do not have the abilities or skills to perform the job. Effective managers are proficient in matching each person's abilities and skills with the job requirements. (See Chapter 17.) The matching process is important because no amount of leadership, motivation, or organizational resources can make up for deficiencies in abilities or skills. Managers can also arrange for staff to participate in development programs that upgrade knowledge and skills of employees as job requirements change and in special programs, such as intensive workshops and continuing education. The nurse manager plays a crucial role in ongoing assessment and evaluation of employees, providing opportunities and encouragement for their advancement and maintenance of abilities. In addition, the nurse manager is in the best position to communicate the department's educational needs to the administration so that adequate resources are allocated for this function.

Employee Performance

A desired result of any employee's behavior is effective job performance. An important part of the manager's job is to define performance in advance and to state

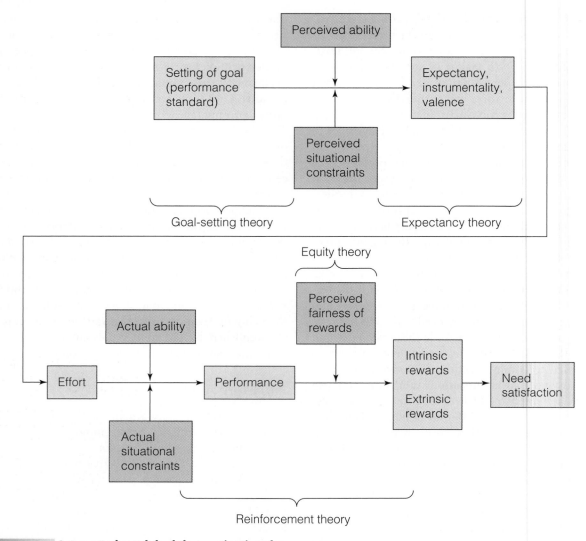

Figure 19-2 **Integrated model of the motivational process.**

desired results. Performance-related behaviors are directly associated with job tasks and need to be accomplished to achieve a job's objectives. From a manager's perspective, searching for ways to enhance performance includes such actions as identifying performance problems; integrating, facilitating, and coordinating the work of employees; and creating a motivational climate. Managers also may enhance an employee's performance by removing situational constraints, such as rotating shifts or providing assistance in overcoming constraints. Recognition also enhances performance. Cronin and Becherer (1999) found salary increases, release time for workshops, written commendations and feedback were the most meaningful ways to recognize staff behavior. Careful management of these factors helps ensure that a staff member's

effort or motivation is actively translated into effective job performance.

The Performance Appraisal

The **performance appraisal** process includes day-to-day manager–employee interactions (coaching, counseling, dealing with policy/procedure violations, and disciplining); written documentation (making notes about an employee's behavior, completing the performance appraisal form); the formal appraisal interview; and follow-up sessions that may involve coaching and/or discipline when needed.

Performance appraisals are conducted for a number of reasons. The primary reason is to give constructive feedback. Lilly (1997) states that a good appraisal system ensures that staff know what they are to do and how well they are doing it.

Performance appraisals often serve as the basis on which administrative decisions, such as the size of a salary increase or who gets promoted, are made. Ideally, accurate appraisal information allows the organization to tie rewards to performance. However, accuracy is a skill developed only with experience.

A final reason for doing performance reviews concerns fair employment practice law (e.g., Title VII of the 1964 Civil Rights Act, Age Discrimination in Employment Act). Performance appraisals and the decisions based on those appraisals, such as layoffs, are covered by several federal and state laws. In the past two decades, many employees have successfully sued their organizations over employment decisions that were based on questionable performance appraisal results.

Since the passage of Title VII of the Civil Rights Act of 1964, the courts have addressed numerous employment decisions in which performance appraisals have played an important role (Murphy & Cleveland, 1991). In many of these cases, the courts ruled the employment decisions illegal because the organization's appraisal system in some way was unsound. Although you can never be certain that your appraisal system is legally defensible, there are several steps to help ensure that an appraisal system is nondiscriminatory. (Also see Chapter 5.)

1. The appraisal should be in writing and carried out at least once a year.
2. The performance appraisal information should be shared with the employee.
3. The employee should have the opportunity to respond in writing to the appraisal.
4. Employees should have a mechanism to appeal the results of the performance appraisal.

5. The manager should have adequate opportunity to observe the employee's job performance during the course of the evaluation period. If adequate contact is lacking (e.g., the appraiser and the appraisee work different shifts), then appraisal information should be gathered from other sources.
6. Anecdotal notes on the employee's performance should be kept during the entire evaluation period (e.g., 3 months, 1 year). These notes, called critical incidents and discussed later, should be shared with the employee during the course of the evaluation period.
7. Evaluators should be trained to carry out the performance appraisal process (e.g., what is reasonable job performance, how to complete the form, how to carry out the feedback interview).
8. As far as possible, the performance appraisal should focus on employee behavior and results rather than on personal traits or characteristics (e.g., initiative, attitude, personality).

Regardless of how an organization uses performance appraisals, it is essential that they accurately reflect the employee's actual job performance. If performance ratings are inaccurate, an inferior employee may be promoted, another employee may not receive needed training, or there may not be a tie between performance and rewards (thus lessening employee motivation). For appraisal to be successful, the needs of the staff and requirements of the organization must be bridged (Wilson & Smith-Bodden, 1999).

Evaluation Philosophy

Although nurse managers may not have formal input into the type of appraisal instrument used in their organization, an understanding of the philosophy that underlies the appraisal system as well as the general focus of the system is important. First, one needs to consider whether evaluations are absolute or comparative. Most evaluation systems are based on **absolute judgment**: In appraising staff, the nurse manager evaluates performance against an internal standard. This internal standard reflects what the manager perceives as reasonable and acceptable performance for the employee. When evaluations are absolute in nature, it is possible for all employees to be evaluated as exceeding the standard for acceptable performance. Alternatively, it is possible that all employees are seen as barely meeting or as falling below the standard. In other words, the ratings received depend entirely on the judgment of the nurse manager.

Absolute judgment items

"Rate each staff nurse based on what you consider satisfactory performance."

	Fails to meet performance standard (1)	Does not quite meet performance standard (2)	Meets performance standard (3)	Exceeds performance standard (4)	Far exceeds performance standard (5)
1. Initiative					
2. Dependability					
3. Job knowledge					
4. Adherence to hospital policies					

Comparative judgment items

"Rate each staff nurse you supervise by comparing him/her with others you supervise."

	Bottom 10% of all staff nurses	Next 20%	Middle 40% of all staff nurses	Next 20%	Top 10% of all staff nurses
1. Initiative					
2. Dependability					
3. Appearance					
4. Proper utilization of time					

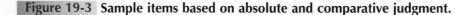

Figure 19-3 Sample items based on absolute and comparative judgment.

In contrast, evaluations based on **comparative judgment** require the nurse manager to rate employees by comparing them with one another: An employee's evaluation depends on the level of performance of his or her peers. A teacher who grades on a curve is making evaluations based on comparative judgment. Thus, comparative judgments are based on the relative standing among employees. Because comparative judgment evaluation systems call for the nurse manager to differentiate among those rated and because not all staff can receive high ratings, it is not surprising that most nurse managers prefer to make ratings based on absolute judgment. Examples of rating scales based on absolute judgment and comparative judgment are presented in Figure 19-3.

Components to Be Evaluated

Nurses engage in a variety of job-related activities. To reflect the multidimensional nature of the job, the performance appraisal form usually requires a nurse manager to rate several different performance dimensions, such as use of the nursing process, professionalism, safety, continuing education, and initiative. In developing an appraisal device, an organization can focus on employee traits, results, behaviors, and/or some combination thereof (Bernadin & Beatty, 1984). The specific focus of the form affects the whole appraisal process.

Traits and Personal Characteristics   Many appraisal systems focus on personal traits and characteristics, such as stability or ability to handle stress, because trait-oriented instruments are inexpensive to develop and can be used for a wide variety of positions (Murphy & Cleveland, 1991). In recent years, however, there has been a gradual shift away from trait-oriented systems, primarily because of charges that they discriminate against some groups. To satisfy legal requirements, the organization should be able to demonstrate the validity (job-relatedness) of the appraisal ratings. In most court cases, trait ratings have not been found to be job-related, and many organizations have been found guilty of discrimination (Bernardin & Beatty, 1984).

Organizations have also moved away from relying exclusively on trait ratings because they are not useful in helping to develop employees. In most health care organizations, a major reason for doing performance appraisals is to help employees improve. However, because most trait-rating dimensions are somewhat ambiguous (for example, what precisely is meant by "initiative"?), trait-oriented systems do not tell a staff nurse what to do differently in the future.

Results   All organizations, even nonprofit health care organizations, need to be concerned with the bottom line. If a hospital has a 35% occupancy rate or a 20% employee absenteeism rate, its future is in jeopardy. In recent years, therefore, top management has turned to appraising some employees at least partly on results. There are pros and cons to evaluating health care personnel on such a basis.

In theory, a results-oriented appraisal system is ideal. Employees know in advance what is expected. Objectives are quantifiable, objective, and easily measured. Unfortunately, in most health care jobs, it is not easy to identify measured, concrete objectives. For example, some aspects of a staff nurse's job, such as

providing quality patient care, are not easily quantified. Other aspects, such as the average number of minutes before answering a patient's call button, may be counted, but they are not worth the cost of measuring them. In addition, a results-oriented system is of little use for staff development; telling someone that he or she did not accomplish a goal does not tell the person how to accomplish it in the future. Although a results-oriented appraisal system has a number of positive attributes, total reliance on such a system for most health care jobs is often impractical.

Behavioral Criteria   In recent years, many health care organizations have adopted behavior-oriented performance appraisal systems rather than focusing on difficult-to-measure results or on vague traits that may cause legal problems. Behavior-oriented systems focus on what the employee actually does, as exemplified in Figure 19-4. Such a system gives new employees specific information on how they are expected to behave and is less likely to lead to legal problems. The behavioral focus facilitates employee development. The major drawbacks of a behavior-oriented appraisal system are that it is relatively time-consuming to develop and is tied to only one job or a narrow range of jobs. For example, the behavioral items presented in Figure 19-4 would be applicable only to staff nurses.

Combining Different Types of Criteria   As health care organizations have become more concerned with employee productivity in the last few years, some have developed appraisal systems that combine various types of criteria. In such a system, each employee may have a few major objectives he or she is expected to accomplish. In addition to being evaluated on whether these results were attained, individuals are also evaluated in terms of both general personal characteristics and behaviorally specific criteria.

Specific Evaluation Methods

Traditional Rating Scales   Many organizations use a **traditional rating scale** for all employees in a class (e.g., staff nurse, clinical nurse specialist), regardless of their specific job setting (e.g., outpatient surgery, neonatal intensive care). The traditional rating scale has the following characteristics (Heneman, Schwab, Fossum, & Dyer, 1989).

1. Several performance dimensions are generated. Normally these dimensions (e.g., dependability) are not based on a job analysis; instead, they are generated arbitrarily.

	Outstanding (5)	Above average (4)	Average (3)	Needs improvement (2)	Unacceptable (1)
1. Performs and documents physical assessment according to unit standard.					
2. Completes patient plan of care according to unit standard on each assigned patient within 24 hours of admission.					
3. Administers medications in a safe and timely manner.					
4. Participates in all mandatory inservice programs.					
5. Dresses according to unit dress code.					
6. Adheres to universal precautions with each patient.					

Figure 19-4 **Behavior-oriented performance appraisal items for the job of staff nurse.**

2. Performance dimensions are general in nature. Thus, they can be applied to a wide variety of jobs. In fact, an organization often uses the same rating scales for all of its employees.
3. Performance dimensions are equally weighted for an overall performance appraisal score. No dimension is seen as more important than any other dimension.
4. Absolute judgment standards are the basis on which ratings are made. Thus, identical behavior may get various appraisal ratings simply because different supervisors have different ideas of what satisfactory performance is.

In filling out a traditional rating scale, the appraiser is required to reflect on the appraisee's performance over the entire evaluation period (usually 12 months) and rate the individual against the rater's internal standard of performance. Individuals using trait-rating scales commonly complain either that the performance dimension (e.g., leadership) is irrelevant to the job in question or that they do not know exactly what is meant by the dimension. Such complaints arise because one appraisal form is being used across a variety of jobs and because the performance dimensions are not tied to concrete behaviors.

Essay Evaluation With the **essay evaluation** technique, the nurse manager is required to describe the employee's performance over the entire evaluation period by writing a narrative detailing the strengths and weaknesses of the appraisee. If done correctly, this approach can provide a good deal of valuable data for discussion in the appraisal interview. If used alone, however, an essay evaluation is subject to a number of constraints that can limit its effectiveness. For example, essay evaluations can be time-consuming to write, they depend on appraisers' abilities to express themselves in prose, and they can be difficult to defend in court because comments made by the manager may not be closely tied to actual job performance. Most organizations have found that essay evaluations are more useful when they are used in combination with other evaluation formats and when they are based on notes taken by the manager during the course of the evaluation period.

Forced Distribution Evaluation The **forced distribution evaluation** is similar to grading on a curve. The manager is required to rate employees in a fixed manner (see the comparative judgment items in Figure 19-3). If the rating scale has five categories, the manager may be required to spread employees' ratings equally over the five categories. Because this technique is constraining, most evaluators do not like it. One hears such complaints as, "I have two exceptional employees, but this system only allows me to put one of them in the highest category," or, "I don't have an employee who deserves to be rated in the lowest category." Because of the general dislike of forced distribution systems, they are not commonly used. In those instances where they are used, forced distribution systems were generally implemented because managers were giving all of their employees high ratings.

Behavior-Oriented Rating Scales   As noted earlier, focusing on specific behaviors in appraising performance has tremendous advantages. For example, new employees have specific information on how they should behave. Although there are several varieties of **behavior-oriented rating scales**, they all share a number of things in common. Behavior-oriented scales are developed as follows:

1. Groups of workers who are very familiar with the target job (generally, individuals doing the job and their immediate supervisors) provide written examples (*critical incidents*) of superior and inferior job behaviors.
2. These critical incidents are stated as measurable/quantifiable behaviors. (Examples are given in Figure 19-4.)
3. Critical incidents that are similar in theme are grouped together. These behavioral groupings (*performance dimensions*) are labeled, for example, *nursing process* or *communication*.
4. Statistical procedures are used to arrive at a subset of the original pool of critical incidents. These procedures eliminate items that do not clearly reflect the performance dimension into which they were grouped, overlap other critical incidents, or are poorly worded.

In view of the way that behavior-oriented rating scales are developed, it is apparent that such behavior-oriented appraisal measures can be used only for one job or a cluster of very similar jobs and that these scales are time-consuming and therefore expensive to develop. For these reasons, behavior-oriented systems are generally developed in which there are a large number of individuals doing the same job, such as staff nurses. Because employees and their managers actually develop the appraisal instrument, they have faith in the system and are motivated to use it.

Focus on Results   Whereas the other approaches to performance evaluation focus on an employee's personal characteristics (traits) or behavior, a focus on results requires setting objectives for what the employee is to accomplish. Although there are many variations of this technique, basically it involves two steps.

First, a set of work objectives is established at the start of the evaluation period for the employee to accomplish during some future time frame. These objectives can be developed by the employee's supervisor and given to the employee; however, it is better if the manager and employee work together to develop a set of objectives for the employee. Each performance objective should be defined in concrete, quantifiable terms and have a specific time frame. For example, one objective may need to be accomplished in 1 month (e.g., "Revise the unit orientation manual to reflect the new JCAHO standards"); another objective may not have to be met for 12 months (e.g., "Take and pass the CCRN examination within the next year"). In setting objectives, it is important that the employee perceive them as challenging yet attainable.

The second step involves the actual evaluation of the employee's performance. At this time, the supervisor and employee meet and focus on how well the employee has accomplished his or her objectives.

Although this system can be excellent for evaluating some jobs, such a system has not met with much success in health care, primarily because it is difficult to set challenging, clear, quantifiable goals for health care jobs, where tasks are based on variable patient needs. With increasing emphasis on outcomes, however, results-oriented assessments are becoming more commonly used in health care settings.

Potential Appraisal Problems

No matter what type of appraisal device is used, problems that lessen the accuracy of the performance rating can arise, such as leniency, recency, and halo errors; ambiguous evaluation standards; and written comments problems. These, in turn, limit the usefulness of the performance review. For example, if a performance rating can be shown to be inaccurate, it will be difficult to defend in court.

Leniency Error   Many nurse managers tend to overrate their staff's performance. This is called **leniency error**. For example, a manager may rate everyone on her or his staff as "above average." Although numerous reasons are given for inflated ratings (e.g., "I want my nurses to like me," "It's difficult to justify giving someone a low rating"), these reasons do not lessen the problems that leniency error can create for both the manager and the organization. For example, if you give a mediocre nurse lenient ratings, it is difficult to turn around and take some corrective action, such as demoting the person.

Leniency error can also be demoralizing to the best staff nurses, because they would have received high ratings without leniency. However, with leniency error, these outstanding nurses look less superior compared to their co-workers. Thus, leniency error tends to be welcomed by poorer performers and disliked by better ones.

Recency Error   Another difficulty with most appraisal systems is the length of time over which behavior is evaluated. In most organizations, employees are formally evaluated every 12 months. Evaluating employee performance over such an extended period of time, particularly if one supervises more than two or three individuals, is a difficult task. Typically, the evaluator recalls recent performance and tends to forget more distant events. Thus, the performance rating reflects what the employee has contributed lately rather than over the entire evaluation period. This tendency is called **recency error**; it too can create both legal and motivational problems.

Legally, if a disgruntled employee can demonstrate that an evaluation that supposedly reflects 12 months actually reflects performance over the last 2 or 3 months, an organization will have difficulty defending the validity of its appraisal system. In terms of motivation, recency error demonstrates to all employees that they only need to perform at a high level near the time of their performance review. In such situations, an employee is highly motivated (e.g., asking the supervisor for more work) just prior to appraisal but considerably less motivated as soon as it is completed.

As with leniency error, recency error benefits the poorly performing individual. Nurses who perform well year round may receive ratings similar to those mediocre nurses who spurt as their evaluation time

---

KEY TERMS

Leniency error   The tendency of a manager to overrate staff performance.

Recency error   The tendency of a manager to rate an employee based on recent events, rather than over the entire evaluation period.

Halo error   The failure to differentiate among the various performance dimensions when evaluating.

Ambiguous evaluation standards problem   The tendency of evaluators to place differing connotations on rating scale words.

Written comments problem   The tendency of evaluators not to include written comments on appraisal forms.

Peer review   A process by which other employees assess and judge the performance of professional peers against predetermined standards.

---

approaches. Fortunately, a simple procedure (recording critical incidents, discussed later in the chapter) greatly lessens the impact of recency error.

Halo Error   Sometimes an appraiser fails to differentiate among the various performance dimensions (e.g., nursing process, communication skills) when evaluating an employee and assigns ratings on the basis of an overall impression, positive or negative, of the employee. Thus, some employees are rated above average across dimensions, others are rated average, and a few are rated below average on all dimensions. This is referred to as **halo error**.

If a nurse is excellent, average, or poor on all performance dimensions, she or he deserves to be rated accordingly, but in most instances, employees have uneven strengths and weaknesses. Thus, it should be relatively uncommon for an employee to receive the same rating on all performance dimensions. Although halo error is less common and troublesome than leniency and recency error, it still is not an accurate assessment of performance.

Ambiguous Evaluation Standards   Most appraisal forms use rating scales that include words such as "outstanding," "above average," "satisfactory," or "needs improvement"; but different managers attach different meanings to these words, giving rise to what has been labeled the **ambiguous evaluation standards problem**. Organizations have attempted to address this problem in two ways. One approach is to have a group of nurse managers meet and discuss what each of them sees as outstanding performance, above average performance, and poor performance on each dimension. The goal is to arrive at a consensus on what level of performance is expected on each dimension. Thus, the group of nurse managers may decide that to be rated excellent on the dimension of self-development, a nurse must attend at least 10 inservice meetings in a year. When agreement is reached on the behavior that reflects each level of a dimension, this information should be communicated to those being evaluated.

A more formal approach to dealing with the ambiguous evaluation standards problem is to develop rating forms that have each gradation along the performance continuum (e.g., excellent, satisfactory) anchored by examples of behavior that is representative of that level of performance. Although a detailed discussion of the process an organization would use for developing such performance standards is too complex to go into here (usually, a consulting firm works with the organization), it involves groups of knowledgeable employees (e.g., job incumbents and their managers) meeting to discuss the important performance dimensions (e.g., nursing process) of a job. Then examples of different levels of performance are developed for each performance standard. For example, a rating of excellent on the performance standard of nursing process/assessment might be anchored by "assessment documented on >95% of charts reviewed," whereas a rating of poor on the same standard might be anchored by "assessment completed on <75% of charts reviewed."

Written Comments Problem   Almost all performance appraisal forms provide space for written comments by the appraiser. The wise manager uses this space to justify in detail the basis for the ratings, to discuss developmental activities for the employee in the coming year, to put the ratings in context (e.g., although the evaluation period is 12 months, the appraiser notes on the form that he or she has only been the nurse's manager for the past 3 months), or to discuss the employee's promotion potential. Unfortunately, few nurse managers use this valuable space appropriately; in fact, the spaces for written comments are often left blank. When there are comments, they tend to be few and general (e.g., "Joan is conscientious"), focus totally on what the individual did wrong, or reflect only recent performance.

The existence of the **written comments problem** should not be surprising. Most nurse managers wait until the end of the evaluation period to make written comments; thus, the manager is faced with a difficult, time-consuming task. Small wonder, then, that the few comments tend to be vague, negative in tone, and reflect recent events. Fortunately, regular note-taking can lessen the problems associated with written comments. (See Documenting Performance.)

The Appraiser

In most organizations, an employee's immediate manager is in charge of evaluating her or his performance. In many situations, this makes sense. The manager is familiar with the employee's work and thus is best able to evaluate it. If the immediate supervisor does not have enough information to evaluate an employee's performance accurately, alternatives are necessary. The manager can informally seek out performance-related information from other sources, such as the employee's co-workers, patients, or other managers who are familiar with the person being evaluated. The manager weighs this additional information, integrates it with his or her own judgment, and completes the evaluation.

Another alternative involves a formal use of other sources. Peer review or ratings are growing in use and are appropriate for professionals. **Peer review** is a process by which registered nurses assess and judge the performance of professional peers against predetermined standards. Peer review is designed to make performance appraisal more objective because multiple ratings give a more objective appraisal. Furthermore, peer review stimulates professionalism because it increases accountability and quality of performance and promotes self-regulation of practice (Mann, Barton, Presti, & Hirsch, 1990). It is used frequently in clinical ladder programs, self-governance models, and evaluation of advanced practice nurses. The steps for peer review follow:

1. The employee selects peers to conduct the evaluation. Usually, two to four peers are identified through a predetermined process.
2. The employee submits a self-evaluation portfolio. The portfolio might describe how he or she met objectives and/or predetermined standards during the past evaluation cycle. Supporting materials are included.
3. The peers evaluate the employee. This may be done individually or in a group. The individuals or group then submit a written evaluation to the manager.

4. The manager and employee meet to discuss the evaluation. The manager's evaluation is included, and objectives for the coming evaluation cycle are finalized.

Implementing a peer review involves several considerations. First, it is best to avoid selecting personal best friends for the review. Friends can provide poor ratings as well as inflated ratings, resulting in a negative experience. Second, consider how often to evaluate expert practitioners, for example, those nurses who have reached the top of a clinical ladder. The usual annual evaluations may not be necessary. Third, monitor the time needed for portfolio preparation. The object is to improve professionalism and quality of patient care, not to create more paperwork.

Another technique is **group evaluation**. In group evaluation, several managers are asked to rank employee performance based on job descriptions and performance standards. Usually, one manager facilitates the process. In addition to evaluating individual performance, performance of groups of nurses can also be evaluated in this way and group variances can be benchmarked and evaluated. Using group evaluation reduces personal bias, is timely, and can be effective (Huddleston, 1999).

Documenting Performance

Appraising an employee's performance can be a difficult job. A nurse manager is required to reflect on a staff member's performance over an extended period of time (usually 12 months) and then accurately evaluate it. Given that many nurse managers have several employees to evaluate, it is not surprising that they frequently forget what an individual did several months ago or that they may actually confuse what one employee did with what another worker did. A useful mechanism for fighting such memory problems is the use of **critical incidents**, which are reports of employee behaviors that are out of the ordinary, in either a positive or a negative direction. These critical incidents are recorded on a form or an index card with space for four items: name of employee, date and time of incident, a brief description of what occurred, and the nurse manager's comments on what transpired (Figure 19-5). Index cards are usually preferred to a page-size form because cards are more easily carried and are less likely to get torn.

Recording critical incidents as they occur is bound to increase the accuracy of the year-end performance appraisal ratings. Although this type of note taking may sound simple and straightforward, a manager can still run into problems; for instance, some managers feel sheepish about this kind of record keeping. Many managers are uncomfortable about recording behaviors; they see themselves as spies lurking around the work area attempting to catch someone. What they need to remember is that this note taking will enable them to evaluate the employee more accurately and makes recency error much less likely.

The best time to write critical incidents is just after the behavior occurred. The note should focus specifically on what took place, not on an interpretation of what happened. For example, instead of writing, "Ms. Hudson was rude," write, "Ms. Hudson referred to the patient as a slob." The nurse manager is responsible for deciding what are critical incidents. In some departments, coming to work on time may be noteworthy; in other departments, coming to work late is. Once a critical incident has been recorded, the manager should share it with the employee in private. If the behavior is positive, this provides a good opportunity for the nurse manager to praise the employee; if the behavior is considered in some way undesirable, the manager may need to coach the employee. (See Chapter 20.)

Because most nurse managers are extremely busy, they sometimes question whether note taking is a good use of their time. In fact, keeping notes is not a time-consuming process. The average note takes less than 2 minutes to write. If one writes notes during the gaps in the day (e.g., while waiting for a meeting to start), little, if any, productive time is used. In the long run, such note taking saves time. For example, keeping and sharing notes forces a manager to deal with problems when they are small and thus are more quickly addressed. In addition, completing the appraisal form at the end of the evaluation period takes less time when one has notes for reference.

A key factor in effectively using this note taking approach is how nurse managers introduce the technique

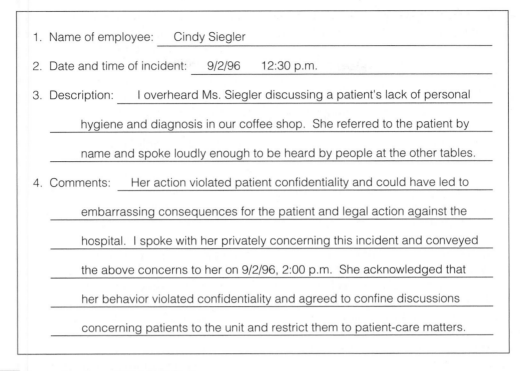

1. Name of employee: Cindy Siegler

2. Date and time of incident: 9/2/96   12:30 p.m.

3. Description: I overheard Ms. Siegler discussing a patient's lack of personal

   hygiene and diagnosis in our coffee shop. She referred to the patient by

   name and spoke loudly enough to be heard by people at the other tables.

4. Comments: Her action violated patient confidentiality and could have led to

   embarrassing consequences for the patient and legal action against the

   hospital. I spoke with her privately concerning this incident and conveyed

   the above concerns to her on 9/2/96, 2:00 p.m. She acknowledged that

   her behavior violated confidentiality and agreed to confine discussions

   concerning patients to the unit and restrict them to patient-care matters.

Figure 19-5 **Example of a critical incident.**

to their staff. To get maximum value out of note taking, nurse managers need to keep in mind two important facts: (a) the primary reason for taking notes is to improve the accuracy of the performance review, and (b) when something new is introduced, people tend to react negatively to it. Managers should be open and candid about the first fact, admitting that they cannot remember every event associated with every employee and telling employees that these notes will make more accurate evaluations possible. Even then, employees will still be suspicious about this new procedure. One way to get this note taking procedure off to a good start is for managers to make the first note they record on an employee a positive one, even if they have to stretch a bit to find one. By doing this, each employee's first contact with critical incidents is positive.

Based on the experience of organizations that have formally introduced the use of critical incidents, nurse managers tend to make three types of mistakes in using notes. Some managers fail to make them specific and behavior-oriented; rather, they record that a nurse was "careless" or "difficult to supervise." A second mistake concerns the tone of the notes. Some managers record only undesirable behavior. The third error is a nurse manager's failure to give performance feedback to the employee at the time that a note was written.

Each of these errors can undermine the effectiveness of the note taking process. If the notes are vague, the employee may not know specifically what was done wrong and therefore does not know how to improve. If only poor performance is documented, employees will resent the system and the nurse manager. If the nurse manager does not share notes as they are written, the employee will often react defensively when confronted with them at the end of the evaluation period. In sum, any nurse manager who is considering using this powerful note taking procedure needs to take the process seriously and to use it as it is designed.

By increasing the accuracy of the performance review, written notes also diminish the legal liability of lawsuits. If a lawsuit is brought, written notes are very persuasive evidence in court. Sharing the notes with employees throughout the evaluation period also improves the communication flow between the manager and the employee. Having written notes also gives the manager considerable confidence when it comes time to complete the evaluation form and to carry out the appraisal interview. The nurse manager will be less prone to leniency and recency error and will feel confident that the appraisal ratings are accurate. Not only does the nurse manager feel professional, but also the staff nurse shares that perception. In fact, it is typically found that with the use of notes, the performance appraisal interview focuses mainly on how the employee can improve next year rather than on how he or she was rated last year. Thus, the tone of the interview is constructive rather than argumentative.

One final issue needs to be addressed. Different employees react differently to the use of notes. Good employees react positively. Although the nurse manager records both what is done well and what is done poorly, good employees will have many more positive than negative notes and therefore will benefit from notes being taken. In contrast, poorer employees do not react well to notes being taken. Whereas once they could rely on the poor memory of the nurse manager as well as on a leniency tendency to produce inflated ratings, note taking is likely to result in more accurate (i.e., lower) ratings for poor employees. The negative reaction of poor employees, however, tends not to be a lasting one. Generally, the poor performers either leave the organization, or when they discover that they no longer can get away with mediocre performance, their performance actually improves.

Diagnosing Performance Problems

If the manager notes poor or inconsistent performance during the appraisal process, the manager must investigate and remedy the situation. Certain questions should be asked: Is the performance deficiency a problem? Will it go away if ignored? Is the deficiency due to a lack of skill or motivation? How do I know?

The first step is to begin with accepted standards of performance and an accurate assessment of the current performance of the staff member. This means job descriptions must be current and performance appraisal tools must be written in behavioral terms. It also implies that employee evaluations are regularly carried out and implemented according to recognized guidelines. Also, the employee must know what behavior is expected.

Second, the manager must decide whether the problem demands immediate attention and whether it is a skill-related or motivation-related problem. Skill-related problems can be solved through informal training, such as demonstration and coaching, whereas complex skills require formal training (e.g., inservice sessions or workshops). If there is a limit to the time an employee has to reach the desired level of skill, the manager must determine whether the job could be simplified or whether the better decision would be to

terminate or transfer the employee. In any deliberations, the manager must include budgetary considerations in the decision-making process. For example, would it be more cost-effective to hire an experienced nurse at a higher salary rather than to provide the necessary staff development to have the current employee reach a satisfactory performance level? Often, the resources of the organization determine which option the manager is able to exercise.

If the performance problem is due to motivation rather than ability, the manager must address a different set of questions. Specifically, the manager must determine whether the employee believes that there are obstacles to the expected behavior or that the behavior leads to punishment, reward, or inaction. For example, if the reward for conscientiously coming to work on holidays (rather than calling in sick) leads to always being scheduled for holiday work, then good performance is associated with punishment. Only when the employee sees a strong link between valued outcomes and meeting performance expectations will motivation strategies succeed. The manager plays a role in tailoring motivational efforts to meet the individual needs of the employee. Unfortunately, creating a performance–reward climate does not eliminate all problem behaviors. When the use of rewards proves ineffective, other strategies, such as coaching and discipline, are warranted. (See Chapter 20.)

To differentiate between lack of ability and lack of motivation, the manager can analyze past performance. If past performance has been acceptable and there has been little change in standards of performance, it is likely that the problem results from a lack of motivation. In contrast, if the nurse has never performed at an acceptable level, the problem may be primarily skill-related. Different intervention strategies should be used, depending on the source of the problem. The objective should be to enhance performance rather than to punish the employee. Figure 19-6 summarizes the steps to take.

The Performance Appraisal Interview

Once the manager completes an accurate evaluation of performance, he or she should arrange an appraisal interview. The appraisal interview is the first step in employee development.

Preparing for the Interview

The nurse manager must keep in mind what needs to be accomplished during the interview. If the appraisal

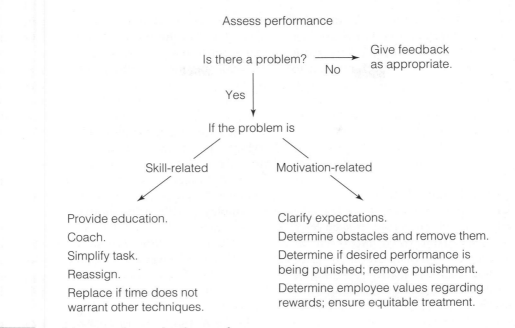

Figure 19-6 **Decision tree for evaluating performance.**

ratings are accurate, they are more likely to be perceived as so by the employee. This perception should, in turn, make the employee more likely to accept them as a basis for both rewards as well as developmental activities. More specifically, to motivate employees, rewards need to be seen as linked to performance. The performance appraisal interview is the key to this linkage. In the interview, the nurse manager needs to establish that performance has been carefully assessed and that, when merited, rewards will be forthcoming. Developmental activities also need to be derived from an accurate evaluation. If an employee is rated as "needs immediate improvement" on delegation skills, for example, any effort to remedy this deficiency must stem from the employee's acceptance of the need for improvement in delegation.

Even though they have tried to fill out the appraisal form accurately, nurse managers should still anticipate disagreement with some of their ratings. Most employees tend to see themselves as above-average performers. This tendency to exaggerate our own performance results from the fact that we tend to forget our mistakes and recall our accomplishments; we often rationalize away those instances where our performance was substandard (e.g., "I forgot, but with this heavy workload, what do you expect?"). Given this tendency to overevaluate one's own performance and the fact that most staff previously have had poor experiences with the evaluation process, nurse managers should expect that staff will lack confidence in the whole appraisal process.

A key step for making the appraisal interview go well is proper planning. The manager should set up the performance appraisal interview in advance, preferably giving at least 2 days' notice. The manager should schedule enough time: Most interviews last 20 to 30 minutes, although the time needed will vary considerably depending on the degree to which the nurse manager and the staff nurse have talked regularly during the year.

In preparing for the appraisal interview, the nurse manager should have specific examples of behavior to support the ratings. Such documentation is particularly important for performance areas in which an employee receives low ratings. In addition, the manager should try to anticipate how the staff member will react to the appraisal. For example, will the individual challenge the manager's ratings as being too low? Anticipating such a reaction, one can respond by saying, "Before I made my ratings, I talked with two other unit managers to make sure my standards were reasonable."

The setting also should be considered in planning the meeting. It is critical that the interview take place in a setting that is private and relatively free from interruptions. This allows a frank, in-depth conversation with the employee. Although it is difficult to limit interruptions in a health care setting, choosing the meeting time carefully will help. A nurse manager may be able to schedule the meeting when another manager can cover, or at a time when interruptions are least likely to occur. The most important point to remember is that a poor setting limits the usefulness of the interview. No one wants weaknesses discussed in public. Similarly, interruptions destroy the flow of the feedback session.

The Interview

The appraisal interview is most likely to go well if the nurse manager has written and shared critical incidents throughout the evaluation period. If such feedback has occurred, staff members go into the interview with a good idea of how they are likely to be rated, as well as what behaviors led to the rating. If the nurse manager has not kept notes throughout the year, it is very important to recall numerous, specific examples of behavior, both positive and negative, to support the ratings given.

The major focus of the feedback interview should be on how the nurse manager and the staff member can work together to improve performance in the coming year. However, establishing such an improvement-oriented climate is easier said than done. In giving feedback, a manager needs to be aware that every employee has a tolerance level for criticism beyond which defensiveness sets in. Thus, in reviewing an employee's performance, a manager should emphasize only a few areas—preferably, no more than two—that need immediate improvement. Unfortunately, evaluators often exceed an employee's tolerance level, particularly if performance has been mediocre. Typically, the manager will come up with an extensive list of areas needing improvement. Confronted with such a list, the staff member gradually moves from a constructive frame of mind ("I need to work on that") after one or two criticisms are raised to a destructive perspective ("She doesn't like me," "He's nitpicking," "How can I get even?") as the list of criticisms continues.

Key Behaviors for an Appraisal Interview

Key behaviors can greatly improve the way appraisal interviews are conducted. They are as follows:

1. *Put the employee at ease.* Many subordinates are nervous at the start of the appraisal interview, especially new employees who are facing their first evaluation or those who have not received frequent performance feedback from their manager over the

course of the evaluation period. To facilitate two-way communication during the interview, some managers rely on small talk, such as discussing the weather; others begin the interview by giving an overview of the type of information that was used in making the performance ratings, such as, "In preparing for this review, I relied heavily on the notes I have taken and shared with you throughout the year." Rather than trying to reduce the tension an employee may have at the start of the interview, it is better for a manager to ignore it. In many cases, if the manager has given the employee feedback throughout the evaluation period, the employee will not be unduly nervous at the start of the session.

2. *Clearly state the purpose of the appraisal interview.* This improvement-oriented theme should be conveyed at the beginning of the interview and will help the employee do the best possible job in the coming year.

3. *Go through the ratings one by one with the employee.* Provide a number of specific examples of behavior that led to each rating. Some nurse managers use only negative examples to support ratings, and this can cause problems. Employees are more likely to become defensive because the entire focus is on problem areas. If the manager pays no attention to good performance in certain areas, the employee will pay less attention to these behaviors in the future. In reviewing the ratings, the nurse manager should be careful not to rush. By systematically going through the ratings and providing behavioral examples, the nurse manager projects an image of being prepared and of being a professional. This is important for getting the staff nurse to accept the ratings and act on them.

4. *Draw out the employee's reactions to the ratings.* More specifically, the nurse manager needs to ask for the employee's reaction to the ratings and then listen, accept, and respond to them. Of the seven key behaviors for doing performance reviews, nurse managers have the most difficulty with this one. To carry out this phase of the interview effectively, the nurse manager must have confidence in the accuracy of the ratings.

When asked to express their reactions, individuals who have received low ratings will frequently question the rater's judgment ("Don't you think your standards are a little high?"). Not surprisingly, the manager whose judgment has been questioned then tends to get defensive, cutting off the employee's remarks and arguing for the rating in question. Being cut off sends a contradictory message to the employee. The individual was asked for reactions, but when given, the supervisor did not want to hear them. The nurse manager should anticipate that the ratings will be challenged and must truly want to hear the staff nurse's reaction to them.

After having listened to the employee's reactions, the nurse manager should accept and respond to them in a manner that conveys the manager has heard what the employee said (e.g., paraphrase some of the comments) and accepts the individual's opinion ("I understand your view"). In addition, the manager may want to clarify what has been said ("I do not understand why you feel your initiative rating is too low. Could you cite specific behavior to justify a higher rating?"). The nurse manager strives for a candid, two-way conversation and wants to know exactly how the employee feels.

5. *Decide on specific ways in which performance areas can be strengthened.* The focus of the interview should now shift to the future. If a thorough review of an employee's performance reveals deficiencies, the manager and employee may jointly develop action plans to help the individual improve. An action plan describes mutually agreed-on activities for improving performance. Such developmental activities may include formal training, academic course work, or on-the-job coaching. Together, the nurse manager and the staff nurse should write down the resulting plans. Because of the possibility of defensiveness, only one or two performance areas needing improvement should be addressed. The nurse manager should choose the area(s) that are most troublesome and focus attention on this (these). In arriving at plans for improving performance, the nurse manager should begin by asking the staff member for ideas on how to enhance personal performance. After the individual has offered suggestions, the nurse manager can offer additional suggestions. It is critical that such performance plans refer to specific behavior. In some cases, not only will the staff member be expected to do things in a different manner (e.g., "I will refer to a patient as Mr., Mrs., or Ms. unless specifically told otherwise"), but the manager may also be expected to change behavior ("I will post changes in hospital policy before enforcing them").

6. *Set a follow-up date.* After having agreed on specific ways to strengthen performance in problem areas, the nurse manager should schedule a subsequent meeting, usually 4 to 6 weeks after the appraisal interview. At this later meeting, the manager provides specific feedback on the nurse's recent performance. This meeting also gives the manager and the nurse an opportunity to discuss any problems they have encountered in attempting to carry out their agreed-on

performance/improvement plans. In most cases, this follow-up session is quite positive. With only one or two areas to work on and a specific date on which feedback will be given, the nurse's performance usually improves dramatically. Thus, the follow-up meeting is one in which the nurse manager has the opportunity to praise the employee.

7. *Express confidence in the employee.* The final key behavior is simple but often overlooked. It is nevertheless important that the manager indicate confidence that improvement will be forthcoming.

Since no more than two problem areas should be addressed in the appraisal interview, other problem areas may be considered later in the year. If the targeted performance areas continue to improve significantly, then 1 or 2 weeks after this follow-up session, the manager should meet again with the staff member, this time raising an additional area that needs attention. As before, specific ways to improve the performance deficiency are developed and written down, and another follow-up meeting is scheduled. In short, performance deficiencies are not ignored, they are merely temporarily overlooked.

Improving Appraisal Accuracy

For the manager and employee to get maximum benefit from an appraisal, it needs to encompass all facets of job performance and be free from rater error. Although attempting to get totally accurate evaluations is much like the search for the Holy Grail, there are ways to greatly improve the accuracy of appraisals.

Appraiser Ability

Accurately evaluating an employee's performance involves using the job description to identify behaviors required, observing the worker's performance over the course of the evaluation period and recalling it, and knowing how to use the appraisal form accurately (e.g., understanding what is meant by performance dimensions such as "initiative"). To the extent that any of these things are lacking, a manager's ability to rate accurately is limited.

Fortunately, a manager's ability to rate employees can be improved. An organization can develop detailed job descriptions and share them with the rater. Steps can be taken to give the rater greater opportunity to directly or indirectly observe an employee's behavior. For example, other supervisors can provide information on an employee's performance when the immediate supervisor is not present. Managers can be taught to take notes on an employee's behavior to facilitate recall. Also, managers can learn to use the appraisal form better through formal training.

Formal training programs help to increase appraiser ability by making raters aware of the various types of rating errors (the assumption being that awareness may reduce the error tendency), by improving raters' observational skills, and by improving raters' skill in carrying out the performance appraisal interview.

Appraiser Motivation

Although it is often assumed that managers are motivated to accurately appraise their employees, such an assumption is often fallacious (Murphy & Cleveland, 1991). Nurse managers have a multitude of tasks to perform, often immediately. Not surprisingly, then, they often view performance appraisals as something that can be done later. Furthermore, many managers do not see doing appraisals as a particularly important task, and some question the need for doing them at all. This is especially true if all employees receive the same percentage salary increase. Thus, if nurse managers are to be motivated to do appraisals well, they need to be rewarded for their efforts.

A nurse manager may spend little time on appraisals for several reasons: (a) the organization does not reward the person for doing a good job, (b) the manager's superior spends little time on the nurse manager's own appraisal (thus sending the message that doing appraisals is not important), and (c) if a nurse manager gives low ratings to a poor employee, a superior may overrule and raise the ratings. In short, in many health care organizations, the environment may actually dampen appraiser motivation rather than stimulate it.

Given these reasons for not spending time on appraisals, it is fairly obvious how an organization can enhance appraiser motivation. First, the nurse manager needs to be rewarded for conscientiously doing performance reviews. Second, the nurse manager's superior needs to present a good model of how an appraisal should be carried out. Finally, as far as possible, the nurse manager should be able to reward the highly rated staff. This becomes more likely as outcomes are used as the basis for reimbursement to the organization and, subsequently, the organization bases rewards on productivity. For the organization and its employees to benefit from the performance appraisal system, pay increases should not be across-the-board,

layoffs should not be based on seniority, and promotions should be tied to superior performance.

Rules of Thumb

For approximately 5% of employees, the prescriptions given in this chapter will not work, for reasons yet unknown. Additional suggestions or "rules of thumb" derived from practical experience include the following.

- *Go beyond the form.* Too often, people doing evaluations cite an inadequate form as an excuse for doing a poor job of evaluating their employees. No matter how inadequate an appraisal form is, managers can go beyond it. They can focus on behavior even if the form does not require it. They can set goals even if other supervisors do not. They can use critical incidents. In short, nurse managers should do the best job of managing that they can and not let the form handicap them.
- *Postpone the appraisal interview if necessary.* Once the appraisal interview begins, there appears to be some natural law of management that the session must be completed in the time allotted, whether the session is going well or has degenerated into name calling. Managers forget the goal of the appraisal interview is not merely to get an employee's signature on the form but also to get the employee to improve performance in the coming year. Therefore, if the interview is not going well, a manager should discontinue it until a later time. Such a postponement allows both the manager and the employee some time to reflect on what has transpired as well as some time to calm down.

  In postponing the meeting, the manager should not assign blame ("If you're going to act like a child, let's postpone the meeting"), but should adopt a more positive approach ("This meeting isn't going as I hoped it would; I'd like to postpone it to give us some time to collect our thoughts"). Most managers who have used this technique find the second session, which generally takes place 1 to 2 days later, goes much better.
- Don't be afraid to change an inaccurate rating. New managers often ask whether they should change a rating if an employee challenges it. They fear that by changing a rating, they will be admitting an error. They also fear that changing a rating will lead to other ratings being challenged. A

practical rule of thumb for this situation is if the rating is inaccurate, change it, but never change it during the appraisal interview. Rather, if an employee challenges a rating and the manager believes the employee has a case, the manager should tell the person that some time is needed to think about the rating before getting back to the employee.

The logic behind this rule of thumb is as follows: If a manager does a careful job of evaluating performance, few inaccurate ratings will be made. But no one is perfect, and on occasion, managers will err. When such an error occurs, the manager should correct it. Most employees respect a manager who admits a mistake and corrects it. By allowing for time to reflect on the ratings, a manager eliminates the pressure to make a snap judgment.

Summary

- Job performance is determined by motivation and ability. Motivation factors include compensation, benefits, job design, leadership style, recruitment and retention, and employee needs and goals. Ability factors include responsibilities, education, skills, and abilities.

- Managers can motivate staff effectively by judiciously combining the theories and techniques so that their effects are complementary.

- Motivational theories are classified as content theories or process theories. Content theories emphasize individual needs or the rewards that may satisfy those needs. Examples are Maslow's hierarchy of needs, Alderfer's existence–relatedness–growth theory, and Herzberg's two-factor theory.

- Process theories emphasize how the motivation process itself directs individual performance. Examples are behavior modification, expectancy theory, equity theory, and goal-setting theory.

- Doing performance appraisals is one of the most difficult and most important management activities. Accurate appraisals provide a sound basis for both administrative decisions (e.g., salary increases) and employee development.

- Absolute judgment or comparative judgment may be used to evaluate employees.

- Criteria to be evaluated may include individual traits, outcome results, behavioral criteria, or a combination.

- Evaluation methods include rating scales, essays, forced distribution categories, behavior rating scales, and evaluation of results.

- To enhance the accuracy of the performance appraisal, the manager should use critical incidents throughout the evaluation period. Critical incidents minimize the influence of errors and increase the quality of the review.

- Problems with employee appraisal include leniency error, recency error, halo error, ambiguous standards, and the inadequate use of written comments.

- To improve the value of the appraisal interview, the manager can try several techniques: putting the employee at ease, clearly stating the purpose of the appraisal, reviewing the ratings one by one while providing specific examples, seeking the employee's reactions, mutually determining ways to improve performance, setting a follow-up date, and expressing confidence in the employee.

LEADERSHIP AND MANAGEMENT in Action

1. Describe three different techniques used to motivate staff.
2. Identify and describe the various methods of appraisal. What are the strengths and weaknesses of each?
3. List three common appraisal errors. How can managers minimize errors in performance evaluations?

References

Adams, J. S. (1963). Toward an understanding of inequity. *Journal of Abnormal and Social Psychology, 67*, 422.

Adams, J. S. (1965). Injustice in social exchange. In L. Berkowitz (Ed.), *Advances in experimental social psychology*, vol. 2. New York: Academic Press.

Alderfer, C. P. (1972). *Existence, relatedness, and growth*. New York: Free Press.

Behling, O., Schreisheim, C., & Tolliver, J. Present theories and new directions in theories of work effort. *Journal Supplement Abstract Service* of the American Psychological Corporation.

Bernardin, H. J., & Beatty, R. W. (1984). *Performance appraisal: Assessing human behavior at work*. Boston: Kent-Wadsworth.

Cronin, S.N., & Becherer, D. (1999). Recognition of staff nurse job performance and achievements: Staff and manager perceptions. *Journal of Nursing Administration, 29*(1), 26–31.

Heneman, H. G., Schwab, D. P., Fossum, J. A., & Dyer, L. D. (1989). *Personnel/human resource management.* Homewood, IL: Richard D. Irwin.

Hersey, P., & Blanchard, K. (1988). *Management of organizational behavior: Utilizing human resources,* 5th ed. Englewood Cliffs, NJ: Prentice-Hall.

Herzberg, F. (1966). *Work and the nature of man.* Cleveland, OH: World.

Herzberg, F., Mausner, B., & Snyderman, B. (1959). *The motivation to work.* New York: Wiley.

Huddleston, D. (1999). Empowerment of nursing staff for optional performance. *Journal of Nursing Administration, 29*(12), 5, 16.

Lilly, R. (1997). Individual performance review. *Nursing Management, 4*(3), 20–21.

Locke, E. A. (1968). Toward a theory of task motives and incentives. *Organizational behavior and human performance, 3,* 157.

Mann, L. M., Barton, C. F., Presti, M. T., & Hirsch, J. E. (1990). Peer review in performance appraisal. *Nursing Administration Quarterly, 14*(4), 9–14.

Maslow, A. H. (1943). A theory of human motivation. *Psychological Review, 50,* 370.

Maslow, A. H. (1954). *Motivation and personality.* New York: Harper.

Murphy, K. R., & Cleveland, J. N. (1991). *Performance appraisal.* Boston: Allyn & Bacon.

Skinner, B. F. (1953). *Science and human behavior.* New York: Free Press.

Vroom, V. H. (1964). *Work and motivation.* New York: Wiley.

Wilson, P., & Smith-Bodden, J. (1999). Does your appraisal system measure up? *Nursing Managaement, 6*(1), 27–30.

 Additional on-line resources for this chapter can be found on the World Wide Web at http://www.prenhall.com/sullivan_decker. Select Chapter 19 from the drop-down menu.

Enhancing Employee Performance

Looking Ahead

The level of employee performance determines how successfully an organization operates. A key factor influencing performance is the manager's ability to help develop the skills and knowledge of the staff so they can perform the job better. Assessing the needs of employees, planning educational programs, and implementing those programs are important steps managers can take to improve organizational operations. This chapter provides an overview of day-to-day and long-term actions that can be used to develop and maintain employees as well as steps to discipline employees when necessary.

Objectives

After reading this chapter, you will be able to:

- Discuss underlying considerations in staff development.
- Describe the social learning theory, relapse prevention, and adult education theory.
- Describe different methods used in staff development.
- Discuss successful coaching techniques.
- Describe key behaviors to use when confronting an employee about procedural violations.
- Discuss effective guidelines for disciplining or terminating an employee.

The essence of management is getting things done through other people. Skillful nurse managers recognize the importance of directing their energies toward enhancing the performance of all employees. Though cost effective and worthwhile, pursuing the satisfaction and productivity of employees is often difficult, especially when the manager must deal with employee problems. Each employee situation is different. The individual situation, as well as organizational goals and objectives, determines the type of intervention strategy the manager can use to assist in employee development. This chapter discusses general strategies for staff development and for coaching, disciplining, and terminating employees. Chapter 21 focuses on selected personnel problems in more detail.

Staff Development

Every individual is unique and, therefore, will vary in education, skills, and ability. There are a few common denominators; for example, all new staff nurses will have passed state board examinations. Yet educational preparation will vary, and some people will not have developed all of the skills and knowledge necessary to perform at the expected level. Furthermore, new nursing practice and technology call for ongoing staff education. One of the nurse manager's major responsibilities is to enhance staff performance, an activity usually referred to as **staff development**.

Most early educational theories were based on the belief that the fundamental purpose of education was the transmission of the totality of human knowledge from one generation to the next. This is a workable assumption, provided that the quantity of knowledge is small enough to be managed collectively by the educational system and that the rate of change is small enough to allow the increase of knowledge to be packaged and delivered. Today, however, these conditions do not exist. Instead, we live in a period of knowledge explosion in which cultural and technological change is rapid. For example, from the time a student enters nursing school to a few years after completing the educational program some of the early learning already is out of date. The implications of this are twofold. First, education must be viewed as a lifelong continuous process. Second, education must become a partnership between the learner and experts so that it occurs every day in an unstructured manner.

The process of education operates constantly during conscious human activity. How people learn, the content of what they need to learn, the processes of

> ### KEY TERMS
>
> ***Staff development*** The process of enhancing staff performance with specific learning activities.
>
> ***Needs assessment*** An evaluation of learning needs in a select population.
>
> ***Planning*** The preparation for learning including obtaining materials and matching learner needs with educational methods.
>
> ***Social learning theory*** A behavioral theory based on reinforcement theory that proposes new behaviors are learned through direct experience or observation that can result in positive or negative outcomes.
>
> ***Relapse prevention*** A model that emphasizes learning a set of self-control and coping strategies in order to increase the retention of newly learned behavior.

learning, and how to teach all are important to education. People even need to be taught how to learn so they can do their learning efficiently and are prepared to learn new information as it becomes available.

Every health care organization has specific goals, and their attainment requires trained personnel. Therefore, most organizations have specialized educational personnel, either assigned directly to nursing service or as part of an education department. Such departments administer ongoing employee development and orientation programs; nonetheless, the nurse manager remains extensively involved in the instructional process. A new employee, for example, must be taught specific work rules and tasks as well as new nursing or medical practices at the unit level. Trained personnel are the key to success in a work group and in the organization itself. Properly educating employees usually results in higher productivity, fewer accidents or mistakes, better morale, greater pride in work, and better nursing care.

Needs Assessment

The first step in staff development is a **needs assessment** for an educational program. Too often, staff development programs are initiated simply because they have been advertised and marketed, because they have been done in the past, or because other organizations have offered them. Because only educational institutions can legitimately view education as an end in itself, health care organizations must justify how an educational activity can achieve an organizational goal, such as better patient care, reduced operating costs, or more efficient or satisfied personnel. Systematic determination of educational needs based on organizational goals can be used as a basis for developing specific content. In this way, staff development programs are used in the most cost-effective and efficient manner.

The decision to offer educational programs should be based on teaching behaviors that (a) can be made more effective and efficient by educational efforts (e.g., a streamlined dressing technique), (b) need maintenance (e.g., cardiopulmonary resuscitation, infection control), (c) new employees need to learn (e.g., required documentation), (d) employees who are transferred or promoted need to learn (e.g., a nurse who transfers to intensive care and needs education about thermodilution catheters), and (e) are needed as a result of new knowledge or new technology (e.g., a new chemotherapeutic agent). Staff development specialists and managers can identify learning needs through a variety of strategies: checklists, advisory groups, quality improvement data, professional standards, and group brainstorming.

Some educational programs are dictated by federal, state, or local regulations. Among these mandatory classes are the following:

- Infection control
- Employee fire and patient safety
- Quality assurance/quality improvement (QA/QI)
- Cardiopulmonary resuscitation (CPR)
- Handling of hazardous materials

Additional requirements may be established through professional organization standards. The Joint Commission on Accreditation of Healthcare Organizations (JCAHO) has delineated standards for orientation, training, and education of hospital staff (1993). These standards are summarized in Table 20-1.

Planning

After needs have been determined, the next step is to plan staff development programs. **Planning** entails identifying learner objectives and matching them with educational methods. Learner objectives, like client outcomes, should be specific, measurable statements about desired behaviors, skills, or knowledge to be acquired within a specific time frame. The strategy used to affect the desired outcome should be based on learning needs, the employee, and available resources.

Nurse managers have a variety of resources at their disposal. The staff development or education department may use a variety of media, such as closed-circuit television, online computer instruction, satellite programs, competency-based programs, self-study, and traditional didactic programs. Other alternatives are using experienced staff members as teachers, preceptors, or mentors; unit-based educators; or off-site continuing education programs.

Three main questions should be considered in assessment and planning: Can the learner do what is required? How should the staff development program be arranged to facilitate learning? What can be done to ensure that what is learned will be transferred to the job? Educators must rely on principles of learning and basic knowledge about educational materials to develop instructional interventions. Also, theories of motivation can be applied to build the individual's desire to learn and to apply skills and concepts learned. Three learning theories help guide what we know about staff development. They are social learning theory, relapse prevention, and adult education theory.

Social Learning Theory   Bandura described **social learning theory** in 1977. It is a behavioral theory based on reinforcement. Bandura believed people learn new behaviors through direct experience or by observing other people performing the behaviors, which result in positive and negative outcomes. The observer learns that successful behaviors should be retained and behavior that is punished or not rewarded should be abandoned. According to social learning theory, the anticipation of reinforcement influences what the person does or does not observe. This response suggests that observational learning is more effective when the observer is informed in advance about the benefits of adopting a certain behavior than when the observer is rewarded for imitative behavior. Knowing the benefits in advance also increases the observer's attentiveness to the model's actions. After observing the model, the observer formulates how and in what sequence certain response components must be combined in order to produce the desired, new behavior. In other words, behavior is learned through cognitive processes before it is performed. Information is commonly conveyed by physical demonstrations, pictorial representations, verbal or written descriptions, and different media sources. Figure 20-1 illustrates this theory.

Relapse Prevention   **Relapse prevention** emphasizes learning a set of self-control and coping strategies in order to increase retention of newly learned behaviors;

Table 20-1	JCAHO Standards for Orientation, Training, and Education of Staff

Orientation	• Organization-wide orientation to include:
	    Mission, governance, policies, and procedures
	    Infection control plan and individual's role
	    Available employee health services
	    Safety management program and individual's role
	    Emergency procedures and individual's role
	• Department/unit orientation to include:
	    Job description
	    Performance expectations
	    Department/unit policies and procedures
	    Equipment/utility systems
	    Special procedures
	    Safety responsibilities
	    Roles in preventing infection
	    Role in QA-QI activities
	    How employee's job relates to others
	• Additional orientation is required for special areas, such as the operating room and intensive care areas.

Education and Training	• The organization plans education and training for all staff and dedicates resources on annual basis.
	• A written description of in-house education and training for staff includes target audience, learning objectives, and methods employed.
	• Education and training are based on:
	    Patient population
	    Type and nature of care/service provided
	    Needs of individual staff as related to their job
	    Health care advances
	    Findings from performance appraisal
	    Peer review
	    General safety issues
	    Update of infection control practice

Quality Assurance/ Quality Improvement	• Process to evaluate the effectiveness of orientation, education, and training activities exists. • Evaluation of education is a part of the organization's quality improvement strategies.
Competence	• Plan for competence assessment and privileging includes the mechanism for demonstrating who, how, and when competencies are delineated and demonstrated. • Each department/service/unit identifies equipment that requires expertise for safe and effective use and identifies policies and procedures that describe tasks required to use this equipment safely and effectively. • Competence assessment includes education, experience, certification, and validation of performance. • An annual summary, by category, of the performance results of patient care providers is submitted to the governing body as a part of the hospital's program to assess and improve quality.

Note: Adapted from "JCAHO unveils new standards for orientation, education, and training," 1993, *Nursing Staff Development Insider,* 2(2), p. 4. Mosby-Year Book, Inc.

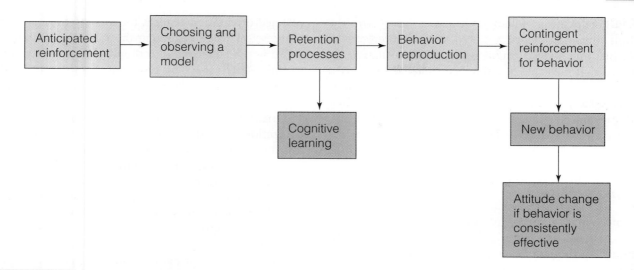

Figure 20-1 **Social learning theory.**

it is illustrated in Figure 20-2. The premise behind this model is that learners are (a) taught to anticipate high-risk situations, (b) taught coping strategies for avoiding high-risk situations, and (c) taught that slight slips or relapses are predictable and need not become failures. As a result, learner self-efficacy increases because the learner anticipates potential problems and is confident in using coping strategies. In addition, this model minimizes the possibility of small relapses turning into absolute failure due to a violation of abstinence. Based on this model, learners should be encouraged to identify possible failure situations and ways to cope with them and practice such situations using new skills in the neutral environment of education.

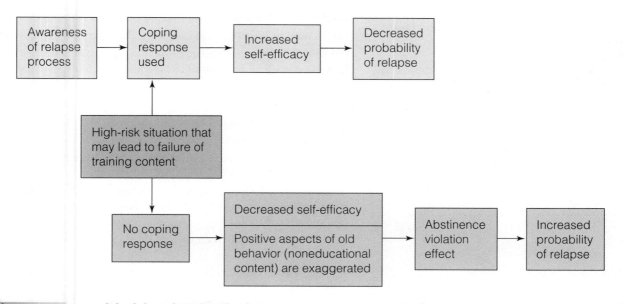

Figure 20-2 **A model of the educational relapse process.** *Note:* **From "Relapse prevention for managerial training: A model for maintenance of behavior change," by R. D. Marx, 1982,** *Academy of Management Review, 7*(3), **pp. 433–441. Used by permission.**

Adult Education Theory Knowles proposed the **adult education theory**, which described differences in the learning styles of adults and children; it was assumed that the same teaching principles could be used for both children and adults. Knowles suggests four basic conceptual differences between adult and child education: self-concept, experience, readiness to learn, and time perspective. These characteristics are described in Table 20-2.

Implementation

Implementation is the gathering together of educators, learners, and the materials and methods needed. Although most staff development is carried out by the staff development or education department, staff development is also a unit responsibility. Two areas, orientation and on-the-job training, involve the nurse manager.

Orientation Getting an employee started in the right way is very important. Among other things, a well-planned **orientation** reduces the anxiety that new employees feel when beginning the job. In addition, socializing the employee into the workplace contributes to unit effectiveness by reducing dissatisfaction, absenteeism, and turnover. (Also see Chapters 18 and 20.)

Orientation is a joint responsibility of both the organization's staff development personnel and the nursing manager. In most organizations, the new staff nurse completes the orientation program, whereupon the nurse manager (or someone appointed to do this) provides an on-site orientation. Staff development personnel and unit staff should have a clear understanding of their respective, specific responsibilities so that nothing is left to chance. The development staff should provide information involving matters that are organization-wide in nature and relevant to all new employees, such as benefits, mission, governance, general policies and procedures, safety, quality improvement, infection control, and common equipment. The nurse manager should concentrate on those items unique to the employee's specific job.

Table 20-2 Characteristics of Adult Learners and Educational Implications

Characteristics of Adult Learners	Implications for Adult Learning
Self-concept: The adult learner sees himself as capable of self-direction and desires others to see him the same way. In fact, one definition of maturity is the capability to be self-directing.	A climate of openness and respect is helpful in identifying what the learners want and need to learn. Adults enjoy planning and carrying out their own learning exercises. Adults need to be involved in evaluating their own progress toward self-chosen goals.
Experience: Adults bring a lifetime of experience to the learning situation. Youths tend to regard experience as something that has happened to them, while to an adult, his experience is him. The adult defines who he is in terms of his experience.	Less use is made of transmittal techniques; more of experiential techniques. Discovery of how to learn from experience is key to self-actualization. Mistakes are opportunities for learning. To reject adult experience is to reject the adult.
Readiness to learn: Adult developmental tasks increasingly move toward social and occupational role competence and away from the more physical developmental tasks of childhood.	Adults need opportunities to identify the competence requirements of their occupational and social roles. Adult readiness-to-learn and teachable moments peak at those points where a learning opportunity is coordinated with a recognition of the need to know. Adults can best identify their own readiness to learn and teachable moments.
A problem-centered time perspective: Youths think of education as the accumulation of knowledge for use in the future. Adults tend to think of learning as a way to be more effective in problem solving today.	Adult education needs to be problem-centered rather than theoretically oriented. Formal curriculum development is less valuable than finding out what the learners need to learn. Adults need the opportunity to apply and try out learning quickly.

Note: Taken from *The modern practice of adult education* by M. S. Knowles, 1970, New York: Association Press. Used by permission.

KEY TERMS

Adult education theory A theory, described by Knowles, that children and adults learn differently.

Implementation The gathering together of resources (e.g., learning materials) and actualization of a plan.

Orientation A process by which staff development personnel and managers ease a new employee into the organization by providing relevant information.

Preceptor An experienced individual who assists new employees in acquiring the necessary knowledge and skills to function effectively in a new environment.

As discussed in Chapter 17, new employees often have unrealistically high expectations about the amount of challenge and responsibility they will find in their first job. If they are assigned fairly undemanding, entry-level tasks, they feel discouraged and disillusioned. The result is job dissatisfaction, turnover, and low productivity. So one function of orientation is to correct any unrealistic expectations. The nurse manager needs to outline very specifically what is expected of new employees and assure them that they will eventually be able to progress to more challenging tasks. Such realistic job previews should cover the informal aspects of the job, about which an employee could possibly have more unrealistic expectations than about such concrete areas as the pay scale or hours.

Socializing new employees can sometimes be difficult because of the anxiety people feel when they first come on the job. They simply do not hear all of the information they are given. They spend a lot of energy attempting to integrate and interpret the information presented, and consequently they miss some of it. So repetition may be necessary the first few days or weeks on the job.

Because nurse managers are an extremely important part of the socialization process, they should discuss everything that they expect of the new employee openly and specifically. The new employee adapts more rapidly if this is done. The manager should address everything from standards of performance, attendance, and treatment of patients to the feedback the employee should expect in performance appraisals.

One method of orientation is the **preceptor** model, which can be used to assist new employees and to reward experienced staff nurses. The preceptor model provides a means for orienting and socializing the new nurse as well as providing a mechanism to recognize exceptionally competent staff nurses. Staff nurses who serve as preceptors are selected based on their clinical competence, organizational skills, ability to guide and direct others, and concern for the effective orientation of new nurses. The primary goal is for preceptors to assist new nurses to acquire the necessary knowledge and skills so that they can function effectively on the job.

Preceptorships offer new nurses the advantage of an on-the-job instruction program tailored specifically to their needs. Staff nurses (preceptors) benefit by having an opportunity to sharpen their clinical skills, and increasing their personal and professional satisfaction. The new nurse works closely with the preceptor for approximately 3 weeks, although the duration of the preceptorship may vary according to the nurse's individual learning needs or the organization's policies.

The primary function of the preceptor is to orient the new nurse to the unit. This includes proper socialization of the new nurse within the group as well as familiarizing her or him with unit functions. The preceptor teaches any unfamiliar procedures and helps the new nurse develop any necessary skills. The preceptor acts as a resource person on matters of unit functions as well as policies and procedures.

New nurses may need to use their preceptors as counselors as they make their transition to the unit. If new nurses experience discrepancy between their educational preparation or their expectations and the realities of working in the unit, the preceptor's role as counselor can prove invaluable in helping them cope with "reality shock."

The preceptor also serves as a staff nurse role model demonstrating work-related tasks, how to set priorities, solve problems and make decisions, manage time, delegate tasks, and interact with others. In addition, the preceptor evaluates the new nurse's performance and provides both verbal and written feedback to encourage development.

The staff development department plays an integral role in the preceptor arrangement by providing the initial orientation, familiarizing the new employee with the organization and general policies and procedures before he or she begins work with the preceptor. The staff development department's function is to teach the experienced nurse the role of a preceptor, principles of adult education applicable to learning needs, how to teach necessary skills, how to plan teaching, how to evaluate teaching and learning objectives, and how to provide both formal and informal feedback.

Mentors Mentors take a greater role than preceptors in developing staff. Precepting usually is associated with orientation of staff, whereas mentoring occurs over a much longer period and involves a bigger investment of personal energy. A **mentor** is a wiser and more experienced person who guides, supports, and nurtures a less experienced person. Mentors tell you what you need to know and show you how to get it. Preceptors and preceptees are assigned to each other, whereas the mentor and mentee find one another, generally outside formal development programs. Mentors trust you with a job by giving assignments that are important; they test your limits and provide opportunities for learning. Mentors help by talking to you. They introduce you to people who may be helpful to your career development. Having a mentor instills a sense of greater personal satisfaction, increased self-confidence, and enhanced self-esteem. The relationship usually is intensely personal and rarely is hidden.

Mentors are usually the same sex as the protégé, 8 to 15 years older, highly placed in the organization, powerful, and willing to share their experiences. They are not threatened by the protégé's potential for equaling or exceeding them. Protégés are selected by mentors for several reasons: good performance, loyalty to people and the organization, a similar social background or a social acquaintance with each other, appropriate appearance, opportunity to demonstrate the extraordinary, and high visibility.

Mentor/protégé relationships seem to advance through several stages. The initiation stage usually lasts 6 months to a year, during which the relationship gets started. The *protégé* stage is that in which the protégé's work is not yet recognized for its own merit, but rather as a byproduct of the mentor's instruction, support, and encouragement. The mentor thus buffers the protégé from criticism. A *breakup*

stage may occur from 6 months to 2 years after a significant change in the relationship, usually resulting from the protégé's taking a job in another department or organization so that there is a physical separation of the two individuals. It also can occur if the mentor refuses to accept the protégé as a peer or when the relationship becomes dysfunctional for some reason. The *lasting friendship* stage is the final phase and will occur if the mentor accepts the protégé as a peer or if the relationship is reestablished after a significant separation. The complete mentor process usually includes the last stage.

Nurse managers can serve as mentors to their employees through some of the strategies already discussed in this chapter (e.g., coaching, giving positive feedback). Managers also can support their more senior staff to take on mentoring roles with newer staff.

Staff Development Methods Staff development can be divided into internal (on the unit) and external (off the unit) sources. Internal sources include on-the-job instruction, workshops for staff, and inservice programs. External sources are formal workshops presented by an education department within the hospital and educational activities outside the hospital, including college courses, conferences, and continuing education workshops.

For effective adult education, the student needs, at a minimum, (a) material to be presented, (b) practice using the new knowledge and/or skill, and (c) feedback about performance. Box 20-1 lists the key behaviors for on-the-job instruction, which include presenting the material, allowing the employee to practice the skill, and providing feedback about that practice. These behaviors also incorporate most of the elements of learning theory discussed earlier in this chapter.

There must be opportunity for practice of the desired behaviors and feedback about it. For instance, if

---

Box 20-1 Key Behaviors in On-the-Job Instruction

1. In writing, outline each step of the task to be taught.
2. Explain the objectives of the task to the employee.
3. Show the employee how to do it (without talking).
4. Explain key points. (Write them down if they are complex.)
5. Let the employee watch you do it again.
6. Let the employee do the simple parts of the task (optional).
7. Help the employee do the whole task. (Watch, and give feedback.)
8. Let the employee do the whole task. (Give feedback when task is finished.)
9. Praise the employee for doing the task correctly.

Note: Adapted from *Health care management microtraining* by P. J. Decker, 1983, St. Louis: Decker & Associates. Used by permission.

KEY TERMS

KEY TERMS

Mentor   A more experienced person who guides, supports, and nurtures a less experienced person.

On-the-job instruction   An educational method using observation and practice that involves the employees learning new skills after being employed.

Evaluation   The investigative process to determine whether outcomes were achieved and to what extent.

an individual is shown how to perform CPR, practices it, and is given feedback on his or her success, the person could be expected to be able to perform CPR. Reading about or listening to a lecture about how to do cardiopulmonary resuscitation provides no assurance that the recipient actually could resuscitate an individual in an emergency.

The most widely used educational method is **on-the-job instruction**. This often involves assigning new employees to experienced nurses, preceptors, or the nurse manager. The learner is expected to learn the job by observing the experienced employee and by performing the actual tasks under supervision.

On-the-job instruction has several positive features, one of which is its cost-effectiveness. Learners learn effectively at the same time they are providing necessary nursing services. Moreover, this method reduces the need for outside instructional facilities and reliance on professional educators. Transfer of learning is not an issue because the learning occurs on the actual job. However, on-the-job instruction often fails because there is no assurance that accurate and complete information is presented, and the on-the-job instructor may not know learning principles. As a result, presentation, practice, or feedback may be inadequate or omitted.

On-the-job instruction fulfills an important function; however, staff members involved may not view it as having equal value to more standardized and formal classroom instruction.

To implement effective on-the-job instruction, the following are suggested:

1. Employees who function as educators must be convinced that educating new employees in no way jeopardizes their own job security, pay level, seniority, or status.

2. Individuals serving as educators should realize that this added responsibility will be instrumental in attaining other rewards for them.

3. The manager should carefully pair teachers and learners to minimize any differences in background, language, personality, attitudes, or age that may inhibit communication and understanding.

4. The manager should select teachers on the basis of their ability to teach and their desire to take on this added responsibility.

5. Staff nurses chosen as teachers should be carefully educated in the proper methods of instruction.

6. The manager should formalize assignments so that nurses do not view on-the-job instruction as happenstance or second-class instruction.

7. The manager should rotate learners to expose each learner to the specific know-how of various staff nurses or education department teachers.

8. The manager must make it clear to employees serving as teachers that their new assignment is by no means a chance to get away from their own jobs but that they must build instructional time into their workload.

9. The nurse manager must realize that the efficiency of the unit may be reduced when on-the-job instruction occurs.

10. The teacher and nurse manager must supervise the learner closely to prevent him or her from making any major mistakes and carrying out procedures incorrectly.

Other Educational Techniques   As technology continues to advance rapidly and the number of people requiring instruction increases, teaching is becoming more efficient and the learning process accelerating. Many organizations are using self-learning modules, such as online computer classes, closed-circuit television, computerized clinical simulations, interactive video instruction, satellite broadcasts (some of which are interactive), audiotapes, videotapes, and long-distance learning via cable television. These methods allow an instructor to convey information in a uniform manner on several occasions or at several locations at one time; many lessons can be repeated. These methods can enhance the instructor's presentation as well as reduce the need for an instructor to present every detail in person.

Evaluation

Few issues in education create as much controversy or discussion as evaluation. **Evaluation** is an investigative process to determine whether the education was cost-effective, the objective was achieved, and learning was applied to the job. Educators usually agree on the need for sound appraisal of educational programs, but they seldom agree on the best method to do evaluation and rarely do empirical evaluation. Typically, a program is initially reviewed at the corporate level before its implementation. The same program is used over and over until someone in authority decides the program is no longer useful or no longer effective, or, more commonly, until attendance decreases.

The purpose of evaluation is to determine whether the educational program has a positive effect on day-to-day operating problems and to identify elements of the program that need improvement. Designing sound evaluation tools is difficult and costly, though necessary. Four evaluation criteria should be used: learner reaction, learning, behavior change, and organizational impact. *Learner reaction* is usually ascertained through a questionnaire completed at the end of a program. The questionnaire may ask about the program's content, the educator, the educator's objectives, the methods used, physical facilities, and meals. Only required questions should be asked; irrelevant data should not be gathered. Learner reactions are important because (a) positive reactions ensure organizational support for a program, (b) reactions can be used to assess the program, and (c) reactions indicate whether the learners liked the program.

Learning criteria assess the knowledge—the facts and figures—learned in the educational program. Knowledge is typically measured by paper-and-pencil tests that can include true–false, multiple choice, fill-in-the-blank, matching, and essay questions.

But the acquisition of knowledge is not enough. Was that knowledge converted into *behavioral change*? One of the biggest problems in education is that instruction does not necessarily transfer from the classroom to the job—often because learners are taught the theory and the technique but never learn how to translate these into behavior on the job. There is a big difference between learning and doing; if behavior is not measured after the program (or on the job), it cannot be determined whether the instructional program has affected behavior or helped the employee transfer the new behavior to the job. Transfer from the classroom to the job is critical to the success of the educational program.

The objective of many staff development programs can be expressed in terms of *organizational impact*, such as reduced turnover, fewer grievances, reduced absenteeism, improved quality of care, and fewer accidents.

These are usually expressed in quantified data and can be easily tied to dollars.

It is often difficult to determine whether changes in such areas can be unequivocally attributed to the staff development program or to other variables in the organization, such as changes in management, increased pay, new equipment, better selection, or changes of some other kind. To rule out the effect of these variables, those who establish the program must take particular care in deciding the length of time for data collection, the unit of analysis, randomization, and other experimental design issues. The most important criteria for measuring results are those that are closely related to the key training behaviors. Despite all of the difficulties in collecting and analyzing such data, cost-related data should be collected because they can provide evidence to higher administration that educational efforts do affect organizational effectiveness.

Designing Staff Development Programs for a Multicultural Staff

Addressing cultural differences, particularly those of the foreign-born nurse, is an important consideration in planning staff development programs. Some cultures outside the United States are more group-oriented than Americans are and often place group needs over individual needs in an attempt to promote harmony and solidarity. In addition, some cultures avoid confrontation and emphasize commitment, cooperation, and gentleness (Martin, Wimberley, & O'Keefe, 1994).

The goal of designing culturally sensitive programs is to eliminate stereotypes, remove barriers, prevent misinterpretations, and promote functioning. Common social barriers are language and cultural expectations. In some countries, nurses defer to physicians for all decision making, whereas in the United States such behavior would be viewed as inappropriate and inefficient. Therefore it is important to include during the orientation period information about the role of the nurse, including interdependent and independent functions, management expectations, and effective communication skills.

Cultural barriers also may exist. In many developing countries, needles and other disposable items are reused, families provide personal care, certain types of technology may not be available, or views on using technology to sustain life may differ. In addition, many foreign nursing programs do not incorporate psychosocial skills into their educational programs. Therefore, special programs may need to be developed to ensure a level of competence in this area. Basic nursing skills may need to be reviewed as well as safety procedures. Several such programs have been described in the literature. Common components include (a) socialization into the nursing role, (b) how to understand and be understood, (c) the development of social skills, and (d) the use of preceptors (Baj, 1995; Burner, Cunningham, & Hattar, 1990; Martin, Wimberley, & O'Keefe, 1994; Thiederman, 1989).

Day-to-Day Coaching

Coaching, the day-to-day process of helping employees improve their performance, is an important tool for effective nurse managers. Yet coaching is probably the most difficult task in management and often is neglected. In one short interaction, it encompasses needs analysis, staff development, interviewing, decision making, problem solving, analytical thinking, active listening, motivation, mentoring, and communication skills. Intervening immediately in performance problems on a day-to-day basis usually eliminates small problems before they become larger ones and the subject of discussion in performance appraisal interviews or disciplinary actions. Coaching also should be used when performance meets the standard but improvement can still be obtained.

Before entering into a coaching session, the nurse manager (coach) should prepare for the interaction. The goal of the meeting is to eliminate or improve performance problems such as incorrect flow sheet documentation, excessive absenteeism, or frequent personal phone calls. The manager should try to anticipate how the employee will react ("Everybody gets personal phone calls") in order to formulate an appropriate response ("I am here to talk about the number of personal phone calls you receive"). In general, coaching sessions should last no more than 5 to 10 minutes. The steps in successful coaching follow:

1. *State the targeted performance in behavioral terms:* "For the past two days, the physical assessment portions of your flow sheets have not been filled out."

2. *Tie the problem to consequences for patient care, functioning of the organization, or to the person's self-interest:* "It's difficult for other nurses and physicians to know whether the patient's status is changing, and therefore it's hard to know how to treat the patient. Physical assessments are a standard of practice in our unit. Failure to document assessments could lead to legal problems should the patient's record go

before a court of law." This is an important but often overlooked step because it cannot be taken for granted that the employee knows why the behavior is a problem. If employees are expected to act in a certain way, they need to understand why the behavior is important and be rewarded when it has improved. Also, avoid threatening language, such as "if you want to stay in this unit, you had better complete your documentation." This puts the employee on the defensive and makes the person less receptive to change.

3. *Having stated the problem behavior, avoid jumping to conclusions but instead explore reasons for the problem with the employee.* Listen openly as the employee describes the problem and the reasons for it. If the problem was caused by ignorance—for instance, lack of familiarity with the standard of care on performing and documenting assessments—simply inform the nurse of the appropriate behavior and end the coaching session.

4. *Ask the employee for his or her suggestions and discuss ideas on how to solve the problem.* In many cases, the employee knows best how to solve the problem and is more likely to be committed to the solution if it is his or her own. It is better to encourage employees to solve their own problems, but this does not mean that managers cannot add suggestions for improvement. It is essential to listen openly to understand the employee's perspectives.

5. *How formal should the coaching session be?* If the problem is minor and a first-time occurrence, you may simply state what actions will be taken to solve the problem and end the meeting. In most cases, however, you and the employee should agree on specific behavioral steps each will take to solve the problem; write down these steps for later reference.

6. *Arrange for a follow-up meeting, at which time the employee will receive performance feedback.* It is possible that an employee may bring up personal problems as a cause for the work problems. The coaching session then verges on becoming a counseling session. When the employee brings up personal problems, nurse managers should convey their concern and willingness to work with the employee to get help for the problems. In most cases, nurse managers will not be the direct source of the help but rather will help the

employee seek out other, more appropriate, sources. It is important that nurse managers not delve into potential personal problems ("Are there problems at home that I should know about?") unless staff raise them. The employee's personal life is not the manager's business.

Dealing with a Policy or Procedure Violation

As with day-to-day coaching, the nurse manager should prepare to **confront** an employee about a policy or procedure violation. The leadership style of the manager is important in determining whether the employee perceives he or she is being told what to do versus being sold on the idea that she or he is an important contributor to the staff. The steps involved in confrontation are similar to coaching. These steps are outlined in Table 20-3.

The first key behavior is to determine whether the employee is aware of the policy. The employee should have received policy information at orientation, and an updated policy manual should be readily accessible to all employees. It is also important to know whether the policy has been enforced consistently. If policies regarding tardiness are not applied to everyone on a daily basis, efforts to change this behavior in one individual predictably will be unsuccessful. It is better to

identify policies and procedures that the majority of staff accept and to determine which employee(s) need direction in compliance.

Second, the nurse manager should describe the behavior that violated the policy in a manner that conveys concern to the employee regarding the outcome. By focusing on the employee's behavior, the manager avoids making the interaction a personal issue.

After stating that the policy has been violated, the nurse manager should have documents stating the policy so that interpretation issues can be clarified. For example, if the policy being violated is the requirement that nurses report to a peer about their patients when leaving the unit, the nurse manager should have a copy of the policy in hand.

The next step is to solicit the employee's reason for the behavior (e.g., what is preventing the person from informing a peer about patients when leaving the unit). Allow sufficient time for the employee to respond while at the same time guarding against the pursuit of extraneous, unrelated issues. In the latter event, redirect the employee's attention to the policy violation and suggest dealing with other issues at another time.

The nurse manager also must convey to the employee that she or he cannot continue breaking an established policy. In the previous example, the manager could discuss the effects of the behavior, such as medications not given, IVs running dry, and patients being left unattended, as reasons for the policy.

Table 20-3 Key Behaviors in Confrontation

Behavior	Example
1. Prepare before the meeting.	Is the employee aware of the policy and procedure? Desired behavior? Has the policy/procedure been consistently enforced? How will the employee react?
2. Without attacking the person, describe the undesired behavior. Tie that behavior to its consequences for the patients, organization, or employee.	Jane, were you aware that it is clinic policy to notify *both* the clinic manager and the hospital supervisor when you will be absent from work? Not only were we worried about you, but we had to reschedule patient procedures because we did not have the staff to attend to both clinic appointments and special procedures.
3. Solicit and openly listen with empathy to the employee's reasons for the behavior.	Why didn't you notify someone about your absence?
4. Explain why the behavior cannot continue, and ask for suggestions in solving the problem. If none are offered, suggest solutions. Agree on steps each will take to solve the problem.	In the future, you will need to notify both the clinic manager and the hospital supervisor if you cannot come in. How do you suppose you might do this since you do not have a phone?
5. Set and record a specific follow-up date.	Can we meet again in 1 month to review this plan?

Next, the manager should explore alternative solutions so that negative outcomes will be avoided. Ask the employee for suggestions for solving the problem, and discuss each of the suggestions. Offer help if it is appropriate. Decide and agree on a course of action. The last step in the process is to set up a reasonable date to follow up with the employee on adherence to the established policy.

Although it is not always possible to deal with policy or procedure violations in a distinct step-by-step sequence, it is beneficial for the nurse manager to proceed in an orderly manner. Many policy violations require early and decisive interventions, and these must be handled in an immediate, forthright manner. Positive results will emerge when the manager addresses policy violations within the context of a formalized plan of action.

Disciplining Employees

Most managers, including those in nursing, dread having to **discipline** an employee. Nevertheless, there will be occasions where discipline is necessary (e.g., when a regulation has been violated, jeopardizing patient safety). In the discipline process, the nurse manager must never lose sight of the reason for discipline. The primary function of discipline is not to punish the guilty party, but to teach new skills and encourage that person and others to behave appropriately in the future.

When faced with a disciplinary situation, the nurse manager should maintain close contact with the organization's human resource department and administration. Before taking any disciplinary action, the manager should discuss the action he or she intends to take and seek approval for it. This close coordination between the nurse manager and administration is essential to guarantee that any disciplinary action is administered in a fair and legally defensible manner.

KEY TERMS

Confrontation   A communication technique used to address specific issues such as policy violations.

Discipline   The action taken when a regulation has been violated.

Terminate   To fire an employee.

To further ensure fairness, rules and regulations must be clearly communicated, a system of progressive penalties must be established, and an appeals process must be available. To enforce rules or regulations, employees need to be informed of them ahead of time, preferably in writing.

If a rule is violated, penalties should be progressive. For minor violations (e.g., smoking in an unauthorized area), penalties may progress from an oral warning, to a written warning placed in the employee's personnel folder, to a suspension, and ultimately to termination. For major rule violations (e.g., theft of property), initial penalties should be more severe (e.g., immediate suspension). An appeals process should be built into an organization's disciplinary procedures to ensure that discipline is carried out in a fair, consistent manner. Guidelines for effective discipline can be found in Box 20-2.

Terminating Employees

Unfortunately, some employees do not respond to techniques to enhance performance, and nurse managers will face the day when they must **terminate**, or fire, an employee. As with a disciplinary action, the nurse manager should maintain close contact with the organization's human resource department and

Box 20-2   Guidelines for Effective Discipline

1. Get the facts before acting.
2. Do not act while you are angry.
3. Do not suddenly tighten your enforcement of rules.
4. Do not apply penalties inconsistently.
5. Discipline in private.
6. Make the offense clear. Specify what is appropriate behavior.
7. Get the other side of the story.
8. Do not let the disciplining become personal.
9. Do not back down when you are right.
10. Inform the human resource department and administration of the outcome and other pertinent details.

Box 20-3   Steps in Employee Termination

1. *Calmly state the facts of the situation and explain the reasons for termination.* Use behavioral terms, and be prepared to give examples of the behavior in question. Do not get angry or defensive.
2. *Explain the termination process.* State the date of the termination and the employee's and organization's role in the process.
3. *Ask for employee comment, and respond calmly and openly.* Listen with empathy, but do not be drawn into the employee's emotion. Focus on the facts of the case.
4. *End the meeting on a positive note.* Wish the employee success in the future, and express confidence in this. Inform the employee what, if any, references will be provided to prospective employers. Have the employee leave immediately so that other employees will not be demoralized.

Note: Adapted from Health Care Education Associates, 1987, *Models of excellence for nurse managers.* St. Louis: Mosby.

nursing administration. Again, the manager must discuss the termination and seek approval for it.

Preparation before terminating an employee is essential. To prepare, answer the following questions:

1. Did you set your expectations clearly from the beginning? Did you review the job description, performance appraisal criteria, and pertinent policies and procedures with the employee? These expectations should have been in writing.
2. Did you document the employee's performance on a continuing basis using the critical incident or a similar method?
3. Did you keep the employee informed about his or her performance on a regular basis?
4. Did you conduct coaching sessions or deal with policy or procedure violations in a timely manner? Were the sessions and the agreed-on actions in these meetings documented?
5. Were you honest with the employee about the poor performance or the policy that was violated? Were you specific about behaviors that failed to meet expected standards? Was the expected performance stated in behavioral terms?
6. Were you consistent among employees in how you dealt with performance issues and policy or procedure violations?
7. Did you follow up? Did you deliver the actions you agreed to in the coaching sessions?
8. Did you document everything in writing? The importance of this cannot be overstated.

This checklist applies to almost every instance of termination. The few exceptions might be theft or physical abuse of a patient. Even in the latter instances, observation and documentation are crucial to avoid legal challenges.

The steps in terminating an employee are similar to those for disciplining, except there are no plans to correct the behavior and no follow-up. Box 20-3 outlines the steps in employee termination.

Even with careful documentation and the most conscientious adherence to organizational policies regarding termination, firing an employee may be followed by legal action, grievance procedures, and stressful and time-consuming hearings. A preferable alternative is that the employee voluntarily resign. Careful documentation may allow the manager to suggest that the employee voluntarily leave the organization. This allows the employee to leave without a record of termination.

Summary

- Staff development is used to enhance employee performance through development of specific job skills using orientation, formalized education, and on-the-job instruction.
- The functions of staff development include assessment of educational needs, planning and implementation based on principles of learning and cultural needs, and evaluation.
- The most important aspect of staff development programs is transferring knowledge in order to change work behavior.
- Educational programs should enhance the organization's effectiveness.
- Coaching is the day-to-day process of helping employees improve their performance or eliminate a performance problem.
- When a policy or procedure violation occurs, confrontation is necessary. The manager should make

the employee aware of the violation and its consequences. The manager should elicit reasons for the behavior and agree on steps to prevent future recurrence.

- When rule violations occur, disciplinary action is need. Penalties should be progressive.
- When staff members do not respond to discipline, managers must terminate their employment. At this time, the manager must stay in close contact with the human resource department and administration when planning and carrying out a termination.

■ LEADERSHIP AND MANAGEMENT ___ *in Action*

1. Describe the principles of learning that should be considered in staff development.
2. As a manager, how would you go about confronting an employee who has violated a procedure?
3. Describe the principles to consider while disciplining an employee.

References

Baj, P. A. (1995). Integrating the Russian emigré nurse into U.S. nursing. *Journal of Nursing Administration, 25*(3), 43–47.

Bandura, A. (1977). *Social learning theory.* Englewood Cliffs, NJ: Prentice-Hall.

Burner, O. Y., Cunningham, P., & Hattar, H. S. (1990). Managing a multicultural nurse staff in a multicultural environment. *Journal of Nursing Administration, 20*(6), 30–34.

Decker, P. J. (1983). *Healthcare management microtraining.* St. Louis: Decker and Associates.

Joint Commission on Accreditation of Healthcare Organizations (JCAHO). (1993). *Accreditation manual for hospitals.* Oakbrook Terrace, IL: Author.

Knowles, M. S. (1970). *The modern practice of adult education.* New York: Association Press.

Martin, K., Wimberley, D., & O'Keefe, K. (1994). Resolving conflict in a multicultural nursing department. *Nursing Management, 25*(1), 49–51.

Marx, R. D. (1982). Relapse prevention for management training. *Academy of Management Review, 7,* 433–441.

Thiederman, S. (1989). Managing the foreign-born nurse. [Letter]. *Nursing Management, 20*(7), 13.

Managing Selected Personnel Problems

Employees with Problems

Overachievers or Super-Achievers
Disgruntled Employees
Overstressed Employees
The Employee with a Substance
  Abuse Problem

Absenteeism

A Model of Employee Attendance
Managing Employee Absenteeism
Absenteeism Policies
A Systems Perspective
Family and Medical Leave

Workplace Violence

Looking Ahead

Chapter 21 addresses specific problems nurse managers face when interacting with a group of employees as a whole and with the individuals that make up that group. Difficulties ranging from overachievement to excessive stress to substance abuse to absenteeism begin with specific individuals and, in turn, affect group dynamics. This chapter presents these issues and attempts to define strategies you can employ to help manage them.

Objectives

After reading this chapter, you will be able to:

- Discuss how super-achievers, disgruntled employees, and staff with substance abuse problems affect work-group functioning.
- Describe methods to use with these selected personnel problems.
- Identify signs of substance abuse in employees.
- Discuss the Americans with Disabilities Act and substance abuse.
- Describe methods for managing employee absenteeism.
- Identify potential sources of violence and recognize steps needed to ensure employee safety.

A major challenge confronting managers today is not only improving individual performance and productivity, but enhancing the efforts of the entire work group. Some of the general techniques for enhancing performance described in Chapter 20 are ineffective because individual problems affect group functioning. Problems with overachievers, disgruntled employees, overstressed employees, or employees abusing alcohol or drugs are addressed in this chapter. Excessive absenteeism is discussed as well. There are no proven methods for managing these problems; the strategies presented here are a starting point. Assistance from the human resource department often is needed.

Employees with Problems

Overachievers or Super-Achievers

Even though super-achievers are exceptionally productive, are technically proficient, and account for a large part of the organization's output, they can present management problems that equal or exceed their productivity.

Russell (1989) classified these super-achiever nurses as the Bull or A-Bomb, Killer Angel, or the Know-It-All. Bulls or A-Bombs, the most common type, are grouped together because the individual may show both characteristics. Bulls believe that their ideas, ways of doing things, and beliefs are the only way. Their main weapon is abusive, intimidating, and overwhelming behavior. The A-Bomb displays tantrum-like behaviors as a substitute for the direct attack. The tantrums can be physically dangerous. Strategies for managing Bulls and A-bombs follow:

1. Let them run their course if no physical danger is involved. Give them time to cool off.
2. Present your position, which will require standing up to them. You may need to raise your voice to get their attention.
3. Do not argue, but continue to state your view firmly.
4. Outside of these confrontations, ask them for advice.
5. You will not change their behavior by yourself; professional help may be needed.

Killer Angels achieve their goals by digs and cutting remarks. Killer Angels feel the need to be right at the expense of others and take deliberate efforts to make other employees look less competent. They have a need to appear superior to all around them. Management strategies follow:

1. Confront the employee directly with the behavior. Confrontation lets the person know you know what she or he is doing.
2. Provide Killer Angels with a forum in which they can air their views, such as problem-solving meetings. Always set ground rules in these meetings, and do not let the Killer Angel dominate.
3. Seek the Killer Angel's advice.

The Know-It-All truly is an expert, and wants everyone to know this. The Know-It-All is the least dangerous super-achiever. He or she wants to be admired and thus gives advice on anything and everything. The best strategy is to mentally filter out the expert advice. However, if the Know-It-All causes problems with co-workers, confront the behavior in private. Coaching techniques often work with these employees.

In spite of the problems they pose to the manager and co-workers, super-achievers are your best technical nurses. Carefully examine your strategy with each individual and seek appropriate help as needed.

Disgruntled Employees

Disgruntled employees are ones who are always complaining, behavior that affects morale on the unit. They complain about anything and everything, but they direct most complaints against the organization and may air them in public, which can affect how others view the organization. Although the temptation is to label this as an attitude problem, complaining is a behavior and as such can be addressed by the following:

1. Remember to set standards of performance and communicate them to the employee.
2. Keep notes about incidents of complaining in behavioral terms.
3. Take action early, and be consistent among employees.
4. Use key behaviors for coaching found in Chapter 18.
5. Follow up as scheduled.

Overstressed Employees

Stress, burnout, and lack of time management are major concerns in the nursing profession. Nurses daily confront pain, grief, dying, and death. In addition, they must often deal with the stress of having inadequate staff to care for high-acuity patients. Chapter 13 includes a model of stress and specific strategies for time management and stress reduction.

The Employee with a Substance Abuse Problem

As substance abuse has become increasingly prevalent in society, nursing has not remained immune. Estimates of the problem among nurses range from 2 percent to 18 percent (Sullivan, 1991). Substance abuse is the primary cause of disciplinary action against nurses by state boards of nursing (Chesney, 1988). Substance abuse not only is detrimental to the impaired nurse but also jeopardizes patients' care, thereby also exposing the employing agency to greater liability.

Early recognition of alcohol or drug dependency and prompt referral for treatment are generally recognized as responsibilities of the nurse manager, although the role of the nurse manager varies according to organizational policy.

Identifying the Employee with a Substance Abuse Problem   It is not easy to identify anyone who is abusing substances. The primary symptom is denial, which is present in the sufferer as well as in those around him or her. The person in denial really does not believe what seems obvious. Furthermore, alcohol or drug problems in women in general, as well as in nurses in particular, are stigmatized in today's society. This stigma, added to the profession's own negative attitudes regarding the disorder, encourages nurses—even those who break through their own denial—to continue to conceal their problem. The result is that nurses dependent on alcohol or drugs may continue practicing nursing, endangering both patients' and their own lives. Before obvious serious consequences take place, some general signs and symptoms may become evident as a nurse's dependency progresses (Boxes 21-1 and 21-2).

In addition to the signs and symptoms listed in Boxes 21-1 and 21-2, the nurse manager should be alert for frequently incorrect narcotics counts, alteration of narcotics vials, patient reports that their pain medications are ineffective, inaccurate recording of pain medication administration, discrepancies in narcotics records, large amounts of narcotic wastage, and marked shift variations in the quantity of drugs required on a unit.

If the manager discovers signs or symptoms in an employee or becomes aware of the unit changes described, further investigation is warranted, and administration should be informed. Often, with unit discrepancies, that simply means checking the schedule to see who was working when most of the errors occurred. Usually, one or two people emerge as those most likely to have been available during the time of the discrepancies. Further checking and observation may reveal individual behaviors suggesting a person has a substance abuse problem.

Even if the manager is unsure of her or his perceptions or if the actions are so vague that the manager has many doubts about the identity of the person, the situation will be clarified in time. Untreated, addiction continues; as tolerance increases, use will increase, and the person will become increasingly careless about covering up actions. Thus, the manager will become more certain about a person's abuse problem. However, the longer it takes to identify the problem, the longer the nurse may continue to practice, jeopardizing both patients and self. Thus, the manager should carefully assess information about possible dependency problems but not wait too long. How long is a matter of judgment for the manager and administration.

Box 21-1   Signs of Alcohol or Drug Dependency

- Family history of alcoholism or drug abuse
- Frequent change of work site (same or other institution)
- Prior medical history requiring pain control
- Conscientious worker with recent decrease in performance
- Decreased attention to personal appearance
- Frequent complaints of marital and family problems
- Reports of illness, minor accidents, and emergencies
- Complaints from co-workers
- Mood swings/depression/suicide attempts
- Strong interest in patients' pain control
- Frequent trips to the bathroom
- Increasing isolation (night shift request; eating alone)
- Elaborate excuses for tardiness
- Difficulty in meeting schedules/deadlines
- Inadequate explanation for missing work

Note: From *Chemical dependency in nursing: The deadly diversion* by E. J. Sullivan, L. Bissell, and E. Williams, 1988, Menlo Park, CA: Addison-Wesley Nursing.

Box 21-2 | Physical Symptoms of Alcohol or Drug Dependency

- Shakiness, tremors of hands, jitteriness
- Slurred speech
- Watery eyes, dilated or constricted pupils
- Diaphoresis
- Unsteady gait
- Runny nose
- Nausea, vomiting, diarrhea
- Weight loss or gain
- Blackouts (memory losses while conscious)
- Wears long-sleeved clothing continuously

Note: From *Chemical dependency in nursing: The deadly diversion* by E. J. Sullivan, L. Bissell, and E. Williams, 1988, Menlo Park, CA: Addison-Wesley Nursing.

Strategies for Intervention   Once the manager has identified a nurse with a substance abuse problem, intervention with that nurse must be planned. With the assistance of a superior, the manager should examine the organization's policies and procedures and licensure laws and prepare for the intervention. Reporting laws vary from state to state, as do consequences. Diversion programs offering referral, assistance, and monitoring may be offered in lieu of disciplinary action in some states. Whether these programs or disciplinary action is used, however, identifying and assisting substance-dependent nurses to return to work have been found to be cost effective (LaGodna & Hendrix, 1989; Sullivan, 1986).

Before intervening, the manager should collect all documentation or information about the nurse's behavior that would suggest an abuse problem. Documentation includes records of absenteeism and tardiness (especially recent changes), records of patient complaints about ineffective medications or poor care, staff complaints about job performance, records of controlled substances, and physical signs and symptoms noticed at different times. Dates, times, and behaviors should be carefully noted. Any one behavior means very little; it is the composite pattern that identifies the problem.

Next, the manager should identify appropriate resources to help the nurse. Internal resources include an employee assistance program (EAP) counselor, if the organization has one, or other nurses recovering from alcohol or drug dependency who have offered to help. External resources include the names and phone numbers of treatment center staff, other recovering nurses (if known), and Alcoholics Anonymous or Narcotics Anonymous. It is absolutely essential that several sources be provided so that the nurse knows that help from someone who knows how he or she feels is available and how to get it. This support cannot be emphasized enough. Failing to offer this assistance

is like telling the diabetic he has diabetes and failing to tell him where he can get insulin.

In addition to assistance for the nurse, the manager should check on health insurance provisions for substance abuse treatment. Many insurance carriers have recognized that successful treatment reduces the use of other health care services and, thus, reduces the cost of health care. Accordingly, they offer coverage for treatment to encourage participants to enter recovery programs. Others, unfortunately, do not. Because many of an organization's employees may be covered under the same health care plan, the manager should be able to check these provisions. If the policy does not cover inpatient care, the nurse may be able to afford outpatient care, which is considerably less expensive. So, the nurse manager should not assume treatment is unavailable even when there is little or no insurance coverage. Alcoholics Anonymous and Narcotics Anonymous are effective alternatives, and both are free.

Before initiating the intervention, the manager must examine his or her own attitudes about the abuse problem. Probably, the drug or alcohol abuse has gone on for some time, and both the manager and the staff may have lost patience with the person whose performance and attendance may have forced others to do more than their fair share of the work. If substance abuse was suspected, others may have felt that the person should just "pull herself together," "stop doing it," and, as a last resort, should "know better." Once they understand that alcohol or drug dependency is an illness, however, they realize that none of these behaviors are possible; willpower and education have not prevented others from becoming addicted. The manager will need to deal with the staff's feelings later, but at this time it is enough to be certain that his or her own attitudes will not imperil the intervention. It is important that the message be clearly one of help and hope.

The goal of the intervention is to get the nurse to an appropriate place for an evaluation of the possible problem. Treatment centers or therapists who specialize in substance abuse are recommended to conduct the evaluation. They have the necessary experience for diagnosing and, if indicated, treating the disease.

The manager must also decide beforehand what action on the part of the nurse will be acceptable. If the nurse refuses to go for an evaluation, what will be the consequences? The organization's policies and the state board of nursing regulations must be met, and the manager must be clear about the consequences (e.g., discipline, termination) and willing to carry them out. Most experts in treating addictions in nurses recommend that the nurse be offered the option of substance abuse evaluation and, if needed, treatment. If she or he does not agree to that, then the manager should follow the usual disciplinary process and make a report to the state board of nursing, if indicated.

Once preparations have been made, the intervention should be scheduled as soon as possible. Others may be asked to join the manager, but the group should be small and restricted to only those involved in past problems, a substance abuse or human resource staff person, or the manager's supervisor. In some organizations, the top nursing administrator conducts all substance abuse interventions and, in that case, the nurse manager must fully inform the administrator of all circumstances leading to the intervention and provide all the documentation needed. Also, the manager should participate in the intervention so that all relevant information is presented and denial is kept to a minimum.

The intervention should be scheduled at a time and place when interruptions can be avoided. It is best to surprise the nurse with a request to come to the office. Denial can build, rationalizations can be developed, and defensiveness can increase if the nurse is given time to consider the problem.

The manager should present the nurse with the collected evidence showing a pattern of behaviors that suggests an abuse problem might be occurring and that an evaluation must be undertaken to know for sure. It is important to focus on the problem behaviors, not on the inadequacy of the person. The individual has already experienced shame and guilt about the use. The manager has an opportunity to help the nurse recognize that substance abuse is an illness that needs treatment; then the nurse will be better able to accept that a problem exists.

In the best-case scenario, the nurse admits the problem, is grateful to be getting help, and goes willingly to treatment. It is best to go directly to treatment from the worksite if this can be arranged beforehand. It is important to move quickly before denial resurfaces.

Some nurses, of course, will continue to deny the obvious, in which case the manager must continue to confront the nurse with the reality of the circumstances. If the nurse refuses to go for an evaluation, the manager must follow the organization's disciplinary process. If the nurse is using alcohol or drugs at the time, immediate removal from patient care is necessary. The manager should arrange to have someone (either a family member or another staff member) drive the nurse home, whether the nurse is going to treatment or not. Not only do alcohol or drugs make the nurse an unsafe driver, but the stress of the intervention may distract the nurse even more.

If the nurse agrees to go for an evaluation and/or treatment, specific plans must be made. It should be clear to all parties when the nurse will contact the treatment center (the sooner the better, even if mood-altering chemicals are not being used at the time) and when the nurse will report back to the manager the recommended course of action. It is possible to arrange with a treatment facility for reports to be made directly to the manager, but federal regulations regarding confidentiality prohibit treatment staff from reporting a patient's status to anyone without that person's written consent. Because the goal of treatment is recovery, which includes returning to work, most facilities request that the nurse give this consent.

Treatment As with other forms of medical treatment, treatment for substance abuse has moved from the inpatient to the outpatient setting. Whereas a few years ago a patient could be expected to be admitted to a month-long hospitalization for substance abuse, today treatment is offered in several different formats along a continuum of care. These include inpatient treatment for detoxification (3 to 5 days), partial hospitalization (day treatment for 1 to 2 weeks), intensive outpatient treatment (e.g., 3 nights a week for 3 hours each night), traditional outpatient treatment (e.g., 4 hours a week, including some group therapy and one-to-one sessions), and weekly aftercare group sessions for 3 months. The choices of treatments and their order ideally are based on the patient's status, environmental supports, and potential for relapse. Unfortunately, the decision is usually based on insurance coverage, which varies considerably among insurers.

The decision to allow an employee to return to work or even to require the employee to avoid returning for any period of time will be based on the recommended treatment. Withdrawal from narcotics very likely will require inpatient detoxification; partial hospitalization also may be recommended. If the employee needs time off for these treatments, sick leave can be used, or the employee may be given an unpaid leave of absence (see the section on the Americans with Disabilities Act and substance abuse).

Reentry Reentry to the workplace must be carefully planned, whether the employee has been absent for any length of time or not. It is especially important for the manager and administration to recognize the threat that access to the category of drugs the nurse was addicted to (e.g., narcotics) poses to recovery. Return to work is usually recommended, but not all treatment staff are familiar enough with nursing to be aware of the danger of putting the nurse in constant, daily contact with the drugs that may have been abused in the past. However, it is vitally important to the nurse's recovery that he or she return to work, preferably in the same setting. This dilemma has often been dealt with in two ways. One method is to reassign the nurse for a period of time (possibly as long as 2 years) to a job or a unit where few mood-altering drugs are given, such as the nursery, department of education, rehabilitation, home care, or patient care audits. Although reassignment presents a problem for the organization and may be disappointing to the nurse, it is far better to make this accommodation than to jeopardize the nurse's recovery by providing access to drugs too soon. This is less a concern with nurses who abused only alcohol.

Another method is to retain the nurse on the unit but not allow administration of mood-altering medications. In fact, state law or organizational policy may require that recovering nurses in the early posttreatment period be restricted from handling controlled substances, carrying narcotic keys, being in charge, or working overtime. This method requires that other staff not only know about the nurse's problem but also be willing to give pain and sleep medications to that nurse's patients. Because this involves disclosing the nurse's addiction, management and staff must decide whether this is reasonable, and the nurse must agree.

Recovering nurses may be discouraged from working evening or night shifts. A reentry contract may be used to specify these restrictions. The contract also may require documentation of participation in recovery groups and random urine drug tests. Ideally, the reentering nurse should have an identified support person available at work.

These restrictions are usually necessary only for the nurse who was addicted to narcotics, but each case should be individually decided based on the amount of stress in the job, the need for rotating shifts, and other factors that may inhibit recovery.

Health care today requires that every employee function at peak efficiency and effectiveness. Health care organizations cannot afford to protect an employee whose professional functioning is impaired by substance abuse. Discharging the employee and allowing the person to go to another institution to continue practicing and endangering patients, as well as himself or herself, cannot be allowed. The nurse manager is the front-line contact with staff. He or she can be alert to the signs and symptoms of substance abuse problems, learn intervention techniques and skills, and help recovering nurses return to the workplace. Concern for patients' safety requires intervention, and humane concern for nurse colleagues mandates that such assistance be made available.

The Americans with Disabilities Act and Substance Abuse The Americans with Disabilities Act (ADA) went into effect July 26, 1990, and applies to employers of 15 or more people. This law prohibits discrimination in personnel policies (such as hiring and firing) and other employment-related issues if an individual has a qualifying disability. Because alcohol or drug dependency limits one or more of the nurse's activities (see Chapters 5 and 17), it is considered a disability under the ADA. Only those who have been identified with substance-abuse disorders, either diagnosed or self-reported, are protected under the law. A person using drugs or who is under the influence of alcohol in the workplace is not protected from the job-related consequences of that use.

The same consideration must be given to the nurse addict as to a nurse with a hearing impairment. This means providing sick leave and treatment opportunity, as well as making reasonable job accommodations. Several reasonable job accommodations have been mentioned previously: assignment to a unit where narcotics and sedatives are not given or are given infrequently, exemption from shift rotation, exemption from charge duties, and the like. Furthermore, the employee's drug-abuse history must be kept private. The ADA confidentiality provisions require the employer to keep records on employee substance abuse (i.e., disability) in separate, locked files with access limited to a need-to-know basis.

As with other chronic diseases, alcohol and drug dependency is a disorder prone to relapse. How relapses will be treated under this law is not clear. As with many other personnel issues, it is wise for the nurse manager to consult with human resources and administration about ADA requirements.

Absenteeism

Although it is difficult to determine the extent or the cost of nurse absenteeism, it is well established that absenteeism in health care organizations is both pervasive and expensive (Bureau of National Affairs, 1988; Taunton, Krampitz, & Woods, 1989). The costs of absenteeism, however, go beyond its effects on patient care and dollar costs. Absenteeism can have a detrimental effect on the work lives of the other staff nurses. In some cases, they may have to work shorthanded; they are expected to cover the unit despite their missing colleagues. Working shorthanded, especially for an extended period of time, can create both physical and mental strain. These nurses may be forced to skip breaks, hurry through meals, work extended hours, abbreviate their interactions with patients, cancel scheduled nonwork activities, and so on. Even if temporary replacements are called in, the work flow of the unit will still be disrupted. For example, standard organizational procedure may need to be explained to replacement nurses.

Given the undesirable effects of absenteeism, it is not surprising that absenteeism has drawn a good deal of attention in the health care field. For the nurse manager, the question is what she or he can do to lessen the unit's recurrent absenteeism problem. But before considering ways to manage absenteeism, the manager must understand its causes. The following section presents a useful model for understanding nurse absenteeism or, conversely, nurse attendance.

A Model of Employee Attendance

To understand employee absenteeism, it is important to distinguish voluntary from involuntary absenteeism. For example, not coming to work in order to finish one's income taxes would be seen as **voluntary absenteeism** (i.e., absenteeism under the employee's control). In contrast, taking a sick day because of food poisoning would be considered **involuntary absenteeism** (i.e., largely outside of the employee's control). Although this distinction seems reasonable in theory, in practice it is often difficult to distinguish these two

---

KEY TERMS

Voluntary absenteeism Absenteeism that is under the employee's control.

Involuntary absenteeism Absenteeism that is not under the employee's control.

Total time lost The number of scheduled days an employee misses.

Absence frequency The total number of distinct absence periods, regardless of their duration.

Attendance barriers The events that affect an employee's ability to attend, e.g. illness, family responsibilities.

Absence culture The informal norms within a work unit that determine how employees of that unit view absenteeism.

---

categories because of a lack of accurate information (few employees will admit to abusing sick leave).

Some organizations try to distinguish voluntary from involuntary absenteeism by the way they measure absenteeism. Traditionally, health care organizations have measured absenteeism in terms of **total time lost** (i.e., the number of scheduled days an employee misses). Given that one long illness can drastically affect this absenteeism index, total time lost is clearly not a perfect measure of voluntary absenteeism. In contrast, **absence frequency** (i.e., the total number of distinct absence periods, regardless of their duration) is somewhat insensitive to one long illness. Therefore, absence frequency has been used as an indirect estimate of voluntary absenteeism.

This distinction between absence frequency and total time lost should make sense to nurse managers. For example, an employee who missed nine Mondays in a row would have nine absence frequency periods as well as nine total days absent. In contrast, a person who missed nine consecutive days of work would have nine total days lost but only one absence frequency period. Intuitively, it seems likely that the first individual was much more prone to being absent voluntarily than the second.

Although there are many models of attendance/absenteeism behavior, a revised version of one developed by Rhodes and Steers (1990) is the basis of discussion in this chapter. According to this model (Figure 21-1), an employee's attendance at work is largely

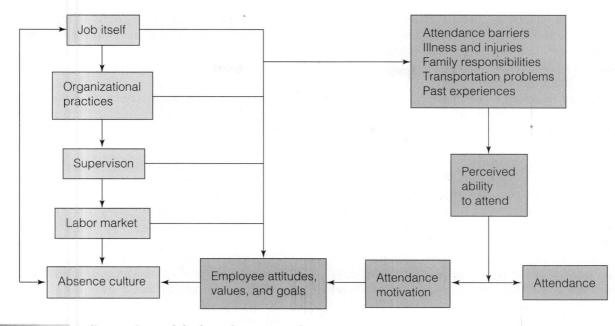

Figure 21-1 **A diagnostic model of employee attendance.**

a function of two variables: the individual's ability to attend and motivation to attend.

As seen in Figure 21-1, an employee's ability to attend can be affected by such **attendance barriers** as personal illness or injury, family responsibilities (e.g., a sick child), or transportation problems (e.g., an unreliable automobile). Although it is natural for a manager to view such barriers as resulting in involuntary absenteeism, sometimes this is too simplistic a judgment. For example, an employee whose car was not running may consciously have not made alternative arrangements to get to work the next day because he or she was not motivated to attend. From this example, it should be apparent that some of the distinctions portrayed in Figure 21-1 are not always clear-cut. It should also be obvious that in trying to understand employee absenteeism, a manager will have to make assumptions about why the behavior is occurring (e.g., a manager cannot be certain that a person was actually ill).

According to the attendance model, an employee's motivation to attend is affected by several factors: the job itself, organizational practices, the absence culture, supervision, the labor market, and the employee's attitudes, values, goals, and past experiences.

In assessing the *job itself*, employees holding more enriched jobs are less likely to be absent than those with more mundane jobs. Enriched jobs may increase attendance motivation because employees believe that

what they are doing is important and because they know that other employees are depending on the job holder (i.e., if the job holder doesn't do his or her job, other employees can't do theirs).

The nature of a job influences attendance through its effect on attendance motivation as well as on illness and injuries (i.e., attendance barriers). For example, a job that requires heavy lifting (e.g., moving patients from beds to stretchers) may increase the likelihood that a staff nurse will be injured. Similarly, a job that exposes a nurse to individuals with highly contagious conditions, such as in an outpatient clinic, may increase the likelihood of illness.

As portrayed in Figure 21-1, *organizational practices* also can influence attendance motivation. Some health care organizations have absence control policies that reward employees for good attendance and/or punish them for excessive absenteeism. An organization also may be able to increase attendance motivation by carefully recruiting and selecting employees. (See Chapter 17.) In addition to affecting attendance motivation, organizational practices may influence an employee's ability to attend. Organizational activities, such as offering wellness programs, employee assistance programs, van pools, on-site child care, or coordinating car pools could influence an employee's ability to attend work.

The **absence culture** of a work unit (or an organization) can also influence employee attendance motivation.

Some work units have an absence culture that reflects a tolerance for excessive absenteeism. Other units have a culture in which being absent is frowned upon. Although an organization's absence culture can be affected by organizational practices (e.g., attendance policies) and the nature of the jobs involved (e.g., people in higher-level jobs tend to be less accepting of co-workers calling in sick), it is also affected by informal norms that develop among work group members. For example, people in a cohesive work group may develop an understanding that missing work, except for an emergency or a serious illness, is unacceptable. Such an attendance culture is likely to emerge if the employees work in jobs that they see as important (e.g., providing direct patient care) and if an employee being absent causes a hardship for co-workers (e.g., forced overtime, being called in on a day off).

Supervision also influences attendance motivation (Rhodes & Steers, 1990; Taunton, Hope, Woods, & Bott, 1995). A nurse manager can influence the nature of a staff nurse's job (e.g., the degree of responsibility given and participation in decision making), decisions about personnel, the consistency with which organizational practices are applied (e.g., whether sanctions are enforced for abuse of sick leave), and a work unit's absence culture by stressing the importance of good attendance.

Another factor that influences attendance is the *labor market*. To the extent that the local employment market for nurses leads an employee to perceive it would be easy to find an equivalent job if she or he lost or disliked the current one, one would expect a lower level of attendance motivation than if market conditions were less favorable. This might happen during a nursing shortage.

Although features of the job itself, organizational practices, absence culture, supervision, and the labor market can all have a direct effect on employee attendance motivation, these factors also can interact with an *employee's attitudes* (e.g., job satisfaction), *values* (e.g., personal work ethic), or *goals* (e.g., desire to get promoted). If a person who seeks variety works in a job that does not provide it, the employee may become dissatisfied and thus more likely to abuse sick leave. Employee attitudes, values, and goals also can have a direct effect on attendance motivation. For example, a staff nurse with a high personal work ethic or who has a goal of getting promoted should be more highly motivated to attend work than a nurse who lacks such a work ethic.

An employee's attendance behavior also is influenced by past experiences. For example, if an employee's

perfect attendance in the previous year was not rewarded, we might expect the employee's attendance motivation to decrease in the coming year. Conversely, if a co-worker with an outstanding attendance record received a promotion, peers who value a promotion and who witnessed this linkage between performance and reward would be more motivated to attend work in the upcoming year.

Managing Employee Absenteeism

The attendance model in Figure 21-1 is useful not only for understanding why absenteeism occurs but also for developing strategies to control it. Some causes of absenteeism, such as transportation difficulties or child care problems, may be beyond the direct control of nurse managers. The manager, however, should try to do what is possible, either in interactions with staff nurses or by attempting to get the organization to change policies that may be interfering with a nurse's ability or motivation to attend work. On the other hand, a manager must be careful that the steps taken do not go so far as to discourage the legitimate use of sick leave. Clearly, one does not want sick nurses coming to work and exposing patients and co-workers.

To diagnose the key factors leading to absenteeism, the manager needs information from several sources, including staff, the human resources department, other nurse managers, and administration. Absence patterns can answer such questions as these: (a) Is absenteeism equally distributed across staff nurses? (b) In comparison to other units, does your area of responsibility have a high absenteeism rate? (c) Are most absences of short or long duration? (d) Does the absenteeism have a consistent pattern (e.g., occur predominantly on weekends or shortly before a person quits)? Although there may be little that a manager can do directly to affect the staff's ability to attend, there may be several actions the organization can take. For example, to lessen child care problems, the organization could set up or sponsor a child care center. To reduce transportation problems, an organization could provide shuttle buses or coordinate car pools. Health fairs, exercise programs, and stress-reduction classes could be offered to promote health. Given that alcoholism and drug abuse are widely recognized as important causes of absenteeism (Rhodes & Steers, 1990), it may be prudent for an organization to offer access to an employee assistance plan. In addition to these organizational actions, a nurse manager, through coaching, may be able to influence a staff nurse's attendance. (See Chapter 20 for information on how to coach staff.)

Clearly, the best way for nurse managers to control absenteeism is by encouraging their staff's motivation to attend, but there are other absenteeism management strategies that a nurse manager might consider. These include

- Enriching the staff nurse's job by increasing its responsibility, variety, or challenge
- Reducing job stress (e.g., by providing more timely and more concrete information)
- Creating a norm of excellent attendance (e.g., by emphasizing the negative impact of a nurse not coming to work)
- Enhancing advancement opportunities (e.g., by providing developmental experiences so that the best employees are promotable)
- Improving co-worker relations (e.g., by considering co-worker compatibility when scheduling work and/or creating work teams)
- Trying to select employees who will be satisfied with and committed to their jobs
- Being a good role model by rarely taking sick days
- Discussing the employee's attendance during the performance appraisal interview
- Rewarding good attendance with salary increases and other rewards
- Enforcing absenteeism control policies (e.g., carrying through on employee discipline when there is an attendance problem)

Absenteeism Policies

Most organizational policies allow employees to accrue paid sick days—typically, 1 sick day for every month employed. Unused sick days accrue across time to some maximum number (e.g., 60 days). Typically, if an employee leaves the organization with accumulated sick leave or days above the maximum, the person simply loses it. Although such a policy may seem reasonable, it may actually encourage unwanted behavior. For example, once a nurse has reached the maximum limit for accrued sick days, the person may see no reason for not using sick days that would otherwise be lost. Such a policy also encourages employees who know they will be leaving the organization (e.g., those about to retire or change jobs) to use accumulated sick leave.

An innovative approach for managing absenteeism is substituting personal days for unused sick days. Two problems arise if personal days are not given: Employees are forced to lie (i.e., say they are sick when they are not) to carry out what they see as legitimate

activities (e.g., attending a conference with their child's teacher), and their manager has no warning and therefore may have difficulty covering for the absent employee. By substituting personal days for sick days, the employee no longer has to lie, and the nurse manager may have time to plan for a replacement. In moving to a policy that incorporates the use of personal days, an organization typically allocates fewer paid sick days but adds personal days. For example, instead of 12 sick days, an employee may annually receive 9 sick days and 3 personal days. With the availability of personal days, a staff nurse can inform the nurse manager in advance of the need for a personal day off. In many cases, the two of them can arrive at a day off that is optimal for both of them.

Realizing that they have not been motivating good attendance, some progressive organizations have allowed sick days to accumulate without an upper limit. Then, when an employee leaves the organization, she or he is paid for unused sick days (e.g., one-half day's pay for each unused sick day). Other organizations allow retiring employees to add unused sick days to days worked. Still, other organizations have paid employees for their sick days, allowed the conversion of sick days to vacation days or additional pay. Although uncommon, a few organizations have experimented with special financial incentives such as cash bonuses or other prizes as a reward for good attendance. Taunton et al. (1995) found low absence among staff nurses in a hospital with (a) incentives for attendance (an extra earned holiday for perfect attendance for 6 months), (b) deterrents for absence (no pay for first day of an absence episode), and (c) a clearly established policy with progressive discipline for infractions.

Obviously, changing an organization's paid sick leave policy is beyond the control of the nurse manager. However, a concerted effort by an organized group of nurse managers can be effective in getting the human resource department and the administration to initiate such changes. Considering the high costs of absenteeism, these changes can be quite cost effective.

Most health care organizations have formal policies concerning how much absenteeism is allowed. Once this limit is reached, disciplinary steps are prescribed. In disciplining an employee, it is important that the nurse manager follow the discipline policy carefully. The effectiveness of discipline as a strategy for reducing absenteeism is limited. Most discipline policies only take effect after excessive absenteeism. Not surprisingly, most employees know what this is and are careful not to exceed it. In effect, the nurse manager is left with an absenteeism problem but not one that she or he is able to address through the use of discipline.

A Systems Perspective

Many of the managerial actions addressed in other chapters of this book are relevant to the control of absenteeism. For example, in recruiting employees, the use of a realistic job preview should increase the congruence between job characteristics and employee values and expectations. Similarly, basing merit pay and advancement opportunities on an employee's overall performance appraisal rating (which is partly based on attendance) will motivate better attendance. Also, leadership skills are important in getting the organization to change policy to lessen absenteeism (e.g., providing payment for unused sick days).

Two specific issues are relevant to employee selection: the use of personal characteristics and past behavior. Although personal characteristics (e.g., marital status, child care responsibility) have been linked to higher absenteeism rates, for legal reasons a nurse manager should not base a hiring decision on such personal characteristics. On the one hand, it is difficult to argue that every person within a category (e.g., married females with children) is likely to be prone to absenteeism. On the other hand, the past behavior of a specific job candidate is potentially valuable information because absenteeism tendencies tend to be consistent from job to job (Breaugh, 1981). Although the reasons why some individuals have a higher level of absenteeism year after year are unclear (e.g., some people may be more susceptible to illness, others may have less of a work ethic), past behavior can be used as a predictor of future behavior. An applicant's previous absenteeism record may be acquired by written or telephone reference checks.

In a practical sense, nurse managers want strategies for dealing with employees with excessive absences. Several steps can be taken.

1. Set expectations with each new employee. Give her or him the attendance policy in writing, and clarify any questions.
2. Monitor each individual's attendance, and document it.
3. Intervene early and consistently, coaching and dealing with policy or procedure violations as appropriate.
4. If discipline is called for, use the key behaviors for disciplining in Chapter 20.

5. Be sure to reward staff who have good attendance. Ensure that any organizational rewards are delivered, and give your personal reward through feedback in performance appraisals.
6. Be a role model for good attendance yourself.

These steps will set a tone of intolerance for poor attendance.

Family and Medical Leave

The federal **Family and Medical Leave Act (FMLA)** took effect in August 1993 and has a significant impact on employers. Under this act, all public employers (federal, state, and local) and all private employers employing 50 or more individuals must provide their eligible employees with leave of up to 12 weeks during any 12-month period for the employee's own serious illness, the birth or adoption of a child, the placement of a foster child into the household, or the care of a seriously ill child, spouse, or parent. The FMLA also allows eligible employees to maintain health insurance coverage while on leave and allows them to return to the same or equivalent position at the end of the leave period. The leave may be taken all at once, periodically (if the employer agrees) or by working part-time, such as after the birth of a child. The employee must be allowed to take leave for qualified purposes without pressure or discouragement by the employer or manager. More generous collective-bargaining agreements or state laws supersede the FMLA, but the FMLA supersedes any inconsistent or less generous provisions.

Employees are eligible to take leave if they

- have worked for the employer for at least 12 months;
- have worked at least 1250 hours during the previous 12 months; and
- are at a work site with 50 or more employees, or at a site where 50 workers are employed within 75 miles of the work site (50 employees/75 miles rule).

The FMLA is quite complex. There are multiple employee and employer responsibilities of which managers must be aware. State law and collective-bargaining agreements may make the organization's leave policy unique. Furthermore, the overlap and interaction between the Americans with Disabilities Act and the FMLA is complicated and largely unaddressed by federal regulation at this point. Only a fraction of the FMLA leave is disability related. It is important for the manager to work closely with the human resource department in executing the provisions of this law.

Workplace Violence

Workplace violence is on the rise. According to the 1994 U.S. Bureau of Labor Statistics, 38 percent of all workplace violence occurs in health care settings. Studies suggest that employees in emergency departments and psychiatric settings are most at risk (Rogers, 1997). However, the National Institute of Occupational Safety and Health (1996) reports that 27 percent of nonfatal assaults occur in nursing homes. In an ANA study, one-third of the nurses disclosed that they were victims of workplace violence (Carroll & Goldsmith, 1999).

By definition, **workplace violence** is any violent act, including physical assaults and threats of assault, directed toward persons at work or on duty (NIOSH, 1996). Most nurses indicate that patients were their assailants. (Carroll & Goldsmith, 1999). NIOSH confirms that 45 percent of assaults are by patients, but assaults are also made by disgruntled family members, co-workers, employers, and employees. Some assaults are episodes of domestic violence that occur at work.

In the ANA study, nurses identified incidents of verbal abuse, sexual assaults and physical violence (Carroll & Goldsmith, 1999). NIOSH reports that the types of violence experienced in health care settings include biting, kicking, beating, squeezing, pinching, scratching, twisting, hitting, stabbing, shooting, rapes, and threats.

A manager should make an effort to identify potential sources of violence and take whatever steps necessary to ensure employee safety. This includes instituting policies regarding assessing and reporting threats, supplying adequate staffing, providing training about recognizing potential assailants or agitators, conflict resolution and de-escalation tactics, and instituting environmental controls (adequate lighting, security devices, bullet-resistant barriers in the emergency department, etc.) and safe work practices (escort services; judicious use of restraints or seclusion; alerting staff about patients with histories of violent behavior, dementia, or intoxication; and, not wearing health instruments [stethoscopes, hemostats, scissors] that could be used as a weapon) (ANA, 1994; Carroll & Goldsmith, 1999; NIOSH, 1996).

Summary

- The behaviors of employees who are overachievers, are disgruntled, are overstressed, abuse substances, or are frequently absent affect work-group functioning. Nurse managers need to identify problems early and intervene if necessary.

- Identifying, intervening, and returning nurses with substance abuse problems to the workplace help the organization, the manager, and the affected nurse.

- Substance abuse not only is detrimental to the impaired nurse but also jeopardizes patient care and places the organization at increased liability.

- Employee attendance is affected by the job, organizational practices, supervision, absence culture, labor market, and the employee's values, goals, and past experiences.

- An organization can improve employee attendance by addressing specific barriers, such as adding a child care center, coordinating car pools, or offering health promotion and employee assistance.

- Innovative solutions to absenteeism problems include substituting personal days for sick days, allowing sick days to accrue and unused days to be paid to the employee, or converting unused sick days to paid days at retirement.

- An effort should be made to identify potential sources of violence in the workplace and steps should be taken to ensure employee safety.

■ LEADERSHIP AND MANAGEMENT
in Action

1. What are the common signs of substance abuse in employees?

2. How do problem employees affect work-group functioning?

3. What is the difference between voluntary and involuntary absenteeism? How can a manager decrease absenteeism?

References

American Nurses Association [ANA] (1994). *Workplace violence: Can you close the door on it?* Washington, DC: Author.

Breaugh, J. A. (1981). Predicting absenteeism from prior absenteeism and work attitudes. *Journal of Applied Psychology, 66,* 555–560.

Bureau of National Affairs. (1988, March 10). *Bulletin to management.* Washington, DC: Bureau of National Affairs.

Carroll, V., & Goldsmith, J. (1999). Abused in the workplace. *Reflections, 25*(3), 24–27, 46.

Chesney, A. (1988). State board of nursing licensure violations and actions—1985. In E. Sullivan, L. Bissell, & E. Williams (Eds.), *Chemical dependency in nursing: The deadly diversion* (pp. 171–174). Menlo Park, CA: Addison-Wesley Nursing.

LaGodna, G. E., & Hendrix, M. J. (1989). Impaired nurses: A cost analysis. *Journal of Nursing Administration, 19*(9), 13–18.

National Institute for Occupational Safety and Health [NIOSH] (1996). *Violence in the workplace: Risk factors and prevention strategies.* Washington, DC: Government Printing Office.

Rhodes, S., & Steers, R. (1990). *Managing employee absenteeism.* Reading, MA: Addison-Wesley.

Rogers, B. (November/December 1997). Is health care a risky business? *The American Nurse, 29*(5), 5.

Russell, L. N. (1989). Managing the "super-achiever" nurse. *Nursing Management, 20*(2), 38–39.

Sullivan, E. J. (1986). Cost savings of retaining chemically-dependent nurses. *Nursing Economics, 4,* 179–200.

Sullivan, E. J. (1991). Impaired health care professionals. In E. G. Bennett & D. Woolf (Eds.), *Substance abuse,* 2nd ed. (pp. 293–304). Albany, NY: Delmar.

Taunton, R. L., Hope, K., Woods, C., & Bott, M. J. (1995). Predictors of absenteeism among hospital staff nurses. *Nursing Economic$, 13,* 217–229.

Taunton, R. L., Krampitz, S. D., & Woods, C. Q. (1989). Absenteeism-retention links. *Journal of Nursing Administration, 19,* 13–21.

CHAPTER 22

Collective Bargaining

Federal Legal Structure for Labor–Management Relations

Early Federal Regulation of
Collective Bargaining
National Labor Relations Act
(Wagner Act)
The Labor Management Relations
Act (Taft–Hartley Act)
Labor Management Reporting and
Disclosure Act
Federal Sector Collective
Bargaining
1974 Health Care Amendments
to Taft–Hartley

Process of Unionization

Selection of a Bargaining Agent
Certification to Contract
Contract Administration
The Nurse Manager's Role
The Grievance Process:
An Example
Decertification

Major Issues in Collective Bargaining for Nurses

Unit Determination
Labor-Management Committees
Definition of Supervisor

Nurses, Unions, and Professional Associations

Future of Collective Bargaining

Looking Ahead

What position do you take on the issue of collective bargaining? It is, after all, one of the most controversial issues facing us as nurses. This chapter focuses on the history of, process of, and various issues surrounding collective bargaining. To help you better appreciate the complexities involved in this divisive topic, an in-depth look at the history and legal structure of labor relations, unionization, and collective bargaining is provided. Further examination of the process of unionization, as well as issues in collective bargaining that are specific to nurses, rounds out the discussion.

Objectives

After reading this chapter, you will be able to:

- Discuss the history of collective bargaining.
- Describe the process of unionization.
- Discuss the standards used in unit determination.
- Describe the role of labor-management committees.
- Define supervisor and professional employee.
- Describe the role of the ANA in collective bargaining.

Other than the continuing argument about the appropriate education for nurses, collective bargaining is the most controversial and divisive issue in nursing. Some believe that collective bargaining reduces the professionalism of nursing; others view it as a mechanism to prevent employers from exploiting nurses. It has been seen as a complex legal issue, best dealt with by attorneys and other experts specifically trained to handle the problems it presents. It has been seen as creating a barrier between the nurse manager and the staff nurse. It has been characterized as separating the manager from the staff by limiting courses of action and interfering with the manager's ability to make decisions and implement changes. All of these reasons, and many others, have divided the nursing population into opposing sides, each vigorously defending its position.

Regardless, increasing numbers of nurses are joining unions. They are motivated by low wages, poor benefits, increased workloads, lack of job security, lack of input into organizational decision making, and discrimination to gain control over their work environment (Briles, 1998; Buerhaus & Staiger, 1997; Gruenberg, 2000; Ponte et al., 1998).

The purpose of this chapter is to clarify labor relations involving nurses in the health care setting. The legal structure of collective bargaining is explained primarily by the federal laws pertaining to it. The chapter also discusses the processes of achieving and losing union representation in a health care setting. In addition, the chapter addresses major issues regarding health care collective bargaining, explains the role of the American Nurses Association in collective bargaining, and discusses the future of collective bargaining for nurses.

Federal Legal Structure for Labor–Management Relations

Early Federal Regulation of Collective Bargaining

Before federal laws governing labor relations in this country were enacted, disputes between the owners or managers of a company and the company's labor force were settled by the judiciary branch of government. During this period of American history, the courts often ruled that **collective bargaining**, collective action taken by workers to secure better wages or working conditions, was illegal. Reynolds, Masters, & Moser (1986, p. 387) note that "this long period of judicial

control was repressive and negative in character. Judges for the most part concluded that unionism was an undesirable activity that, if it could not be prevented altogether, should be held within narrow limits." During this period, judges enforced their orders through the use of **injunction**, an order issued by a judge at the request of one party against another party directing it to refrain from a certain act. In labor disputes, it was usually issued at the request of a business to prevent a strike or other form of work stoppage.

In 1890, the United States Congress passed the Sherman Antitrust Act. This act was intended to limit the ability of industry to engage in acts designed to lessen competition. One consequence of the act was to prevent the growth of organized labor by declaring illegal "any contract, combination . . . or conspiracy in the restraint of trade" (Balliet, 1981, p. 47). Its application to unions was upheld by the Supreme Court in 1908.

In 1914, Congress passed the Clayton Antitrust Act in hopes of ending the application of the Sherman Act to unions by limiting the right of federal courts to issue injunctions. Because of its vague language, the act was interpreted by the court system as actually increasing the power of employers to obtain injunctions against unions (Balliet, 1981).

Several violent strikes in the late 1800s, the most significant of which was the Pullman Strike of 1884, prompted Congress to begin to take a more active role by intervening in disputes between labor and management, beginning with the Railway Labor Act of 1926. Although the jurisdiction of this act was limited to the railway industry, it marked the first time the government declared the right of private employees to join or not join unions without the interference of their employers. According to Herman and Kuhn (1981), this legislation marked a reversal of the legal status of unions.

The Norris–LaGuardia Act of 1932 was the first national policy in labor relations (Reynolds et al., 1986). This act denied the federal courts the right to issue injunctions in ordinary labor disputes. It also limited the jurisdiction of federal courts in boycotts, picketing, and strikes. It recognized the right of employees to have full freedom of association and to choose representatives to negotiate terms and conditions of employment (Balliet, 1981).

National Labor Relations Act (Wagner Act)

The **National Labor Relations Act** (1935), more popularly known as the **Wagner Act**, is the major statute

Collective bargaining   The negotiations that occur between unions and an organization.

Injunction   An order issued by a judge at the request of one party against another party directing it to refrain from a certain act.

National Labor Relations Act (Wagner Act)   A federal statute that established the right of employees to organize unions and bargain collectively.

Labor Management Relations Act (Taft–Hartley Act)   A federal act that addresses unfair labor practices, the rights of employees as individuals, the rights of employers, and national emergency strikes.

regulating private industry labor-management relations in the United States. It was passed during an anti-business period of American history because of the belief that collective bargaining should be used to regulate the terms and conditions of employment and that workers should be able to organize strong and stable unions without bitter strikes (Reynolds et al., 1986).

The National Labor Relations Act firmly established the right of employees to bargain collectively and to organize unions for this purpose. It established a process for the selection of a bargaining agent by secret ballot and established the National Labor Relations Board (NLRB) to administer elections and to prosecute unfair labor practices by employers. The Wagner Act defined five employer unfair labor practices (Sloane & Witney, 1988):

1. An employer could not interfere, restrain, or coerce employees in exercising their right of self-organization.
2. An employer could not dominate or interfere with the formation, administration, or finances of labor organizations.
3. An employer could not discriminate between union and nonunion employees in regard to hire or tenure of employment in any labor organization.
4. Employers could not discriminate against anyone filing unfair labor practice charges or giving testimony.
5. Employers could not refuse to bargain with their employees' representatives.

The Wagner Act had its critics. Passed by a Democratic House of Representatives and Senate with the full support of President Roosevelt, the act would seem to have settled disputes in labor relations. Herman and Kuhn (1981, p. 44) noted that this act "protected unions from employers but not employers from unions." Thus, while employers had restrictions placed on their activities, unions could operate without restrictions and with the support of government.

Two other criticisms are often leveled against this act. The first was that it applied only to businesses engaged in interstate commerce. This was overcome by a number of states passing similar laws known as "little Wagner Acts." Some of these states—Connecticut, Hawaii, Idaho, Massachusetts, Michigan, Minnesota, Montana, New York, Oregon, Pennsylvania, Utah, and Wisconsin—passed laws that allowed nurses to bargain collectively (Flannigan, 1983).

The second criticism was that the rights of individual employees within the union were not protected. These shortcomings, along with changing public sentiment against unions, led to the passage of the next major piece of federal labor relations legislation: the Taft–Hartley Act.

The Labor Management Relations Act (Taft–Hartley Act)

Formally known as the **Labor Management Relations Act (LMRA)**, the **Taft–Hartley Act** was passed in 1947 over the veto of President Truman and sought to address the problems created by the Wagner Act. Whereas the Wagner Act protected individuals and unions from employers, the Taft–Hartley Act addressed unfair union labor practices, the rights of employees as individuals, the rights of employers, and national emergency strikes. This was done while keeping the major components of the Wagner Act intact.

The Taft–Hartley Act specified the following six unfair labor practices for unions:

1. Unions could not restrain or coerce employees while exercising their collective bargaining rights.
2. Unions could not cause employers to discriminate against employees in order to encourage or discourage union membership.
3. Unions could not refuse to bargain in good faith with employers about wages, hours, and other employment conditions.
4. Certain types of strikes and boycotts were outlawed.
5. Unions could not charge excessive or discriminatory initiation dues and fees.

6. Employers could not be required to pay for work not performed, a concept known as **featherbedding**.

Additional sections of this act clarified management rights regarding freedom of speech; allowed the president and the attorney general of the United States, and the courts and special boards to outlaw strikes in cases of public emergency; forbade labor unions from making contributions to federal elections; set legal restrictions on union disputes; and made it unlawful for government employees to strike.

As federal law, Taft–Hartley applied only to businesses doing interstate commerce. The act did not apply to government employees, agricultural workers, domestic employees, or supervisors. Thus, coverage for employees in not-for-profit health care institutions, which was previously available under the Wagner Act, was withdrawn under Taft–Hartley. From 1947 to 1974, the only nurses eligible for collective bargaining were those who worked in for-profit health care institutions or for health care facilities operated by a state government that recognized nurses' rights to collective bargaining.

Labor Management Reporting and Disclosure Act

The next major piece of federal legislation to deal with labor relations was the Labor Management Reporting and Disclosure Act. Signed in September 1959 by President Eisenhower, it is also known as the Landrum–Griffin Act. This legislation was adopted because "there was continued complaint of corruption and high-handed procedures in trade union government" (Reynolds et al., 1986, p. 399). This act amended Taft–Hartley by enacting further protection for union members and the public against arbitrary action by union officials. The act gave equal rights and privileges to every member of a labor organization, established procedures for union and employee financial disclosure, established guidelines for dealing with union trusteeships, outlined union election procedures, and established that union funds must be used for union purposes.

Federal Sector Collective Bargaining

In 1962, President John Kennedy issued Executive Order 10988. This order extended to employees of the executive branch of government the rights of collective bargaining enjoyed by private-sector employees, but with some major differences. One difference was a prohibition on the right to strike. Another difference was that arbitration over contract negotiations was not permitted.

Executive Order 10988 also limited the scope of bargaining. Bargaining between the federal government and its employees did not include salaries and wages set by congressional act, assignment of personnel, or updating due to technical changes.

Executive Order 11491 (1970) made additional changes to labor–management relations in the federal sector. This order created the Federal Labor Relations Council to oversee federal government collective bargaining. It also required government employee unions to follow the same election and financial disclosure regulations as expected in the private sector.

1974 Health Care Amendments to Taft–Hartley

Probably the most significant piece of legislation involving collective bargaining and nurses occurred in 1974, when Congress passed amendments to the Taft–Hartley Act making employees of private nonprofit hospitals and nursing homes eligible for collective bargaining. Originally, under the Wagner Act, employees of hospitals and nursing homes had been eligible for collective bargaining. The passage of Taft–Hartley in 1947 changed this status and excluded employees of nonprofit health care institutions from coverage because of the potential for harm to the public if health care was not available. In extending this coverage, Congress "sought to balance the rights of employees to bargain against the right of the public to uninterrupted health care" (Herman & Kuhn, 1981, p. 58). The amendments did not cover employees of government-operated facilities. Although nurses working in state, county, or city hospitals were not affected by this legislation, they often were covered by the laws of their applicable jurisdiction.

To ensure the balance between the rights of employees and the rights of the public to health care, Congress passed a special set of dispute-settling procedures to be applied in the health care industry:

1. Before changing or terminating a contract, one party must notify the other of its intent to do so 90 days prior to the contract expiration date. This is 30 days more than specified for other industries.
2. If after 30 days of this notification both sides cannot agree, then the Federal Mediation and Conciliation Service (FMCS) must be notified.

3. The FMCS will appoint either a mediator or an inquiry board within 30 days.
4. The mediator or board must make recommendations within 15 days.
5. If after 15 more days both sides cannot agree, then a strike vote can be conducted and a strike scheduled.
6. If a strike vote is affirmed, then a 10-day written notice must be given to management indicating the date, time, and place of the strike (Guido, 1988). This is to ensure that a hospital has adequate time to provide for continuity of patient care in the event of a strike.

To enforce these amendments, the National Labor Relations Board (NLRB) established separate provisions for the health care industry. These provisions include (a) recognition of appropriate bargaining units for health care employees so that the hospital would not have to conduct separate contract negotiations with many different unions, a concept called **undue unit proliferation** (explained later in the chapter) and (b) the determination of locations where unions could solicit members and distribute literature in the hospital without disrupting patient care or interfering with work time. Currently, solicitation of members can occur in hospital cafeterias, gift shops, and main lobbies (Sloane & Witney, 1988).

Process of Unionization

Selection of a Bargaining Agent

The process of establishing a union in any setting begins with the selection of a bargaining agent certified to conduct labor negotiations for a group of individuals. This process is known as a **representation election** and is presided over by the National Labor Relations Board (NLRB). For an election to occur, the union must demonstrate that interest is shown by at least 30 percent of the employees affected by this action. In this process, the union will ask eligible employees to sign a card authorizing an election. Once the 30 percent level is reached, the union can petition the NLRB to conduct an election. The NLRB then meets with both the union and the employer. At the conclusion of this meeting the NLRB will have determined three things:

1. Who is eligible to participate in the union. This is a problematic issue and not easily resolved, be-

cause registered nurses employed as staff nurses are eligible for collective bargaining but registered nurses employed as management are not. Registered nurses who work for an organization, but in a capacity outside the traditional nursing department, such as a clinic, home health care, or in education, may or may not be eligible for membership. This issue alone can take many days or weeks to resolve.
2. Whether the signatories are employees of the organization.
3. A date for union election.

The election is conducted by the NLRB within 45 days, using a secret ballot. All individuals eligible for representation by the union are notified of the election time and date. On election day, eligible employees are asked to choose not only whether they wish to be represented by a union but also which union they want to represent them.

Many unions represent RNs in collective bargaining; therefore, the ballot may contain several choices for the **bargaining agent**. In addition to various state nurses associations (SNAs), other major unions representing nurses include the American Federation of State, County, and Municipal Employees (AFSCME), and the Service Employees International Union (SEIU) (Lundy, 1997). To place its name on the ballot, a union needs to show that at least one person eligible to vote in the election has signed an authorization card requesting that this union be a choice in the election.

The election outcome is determined by the group receiving a simple majority of the votes cast. Thus, if 500 people are eligible for coverage by the contract but only 100 people vote and union A receives 51 votes, union A wins. If no group receives a simple majority on the first ballot, a runoff election is held between the top two vote recipients. The union winning this election is certified to enter into contract negotiations with the employer.

The process of selecting a bargaining agent produces a tense, emotional climate that affects everyone in the organization. It is important for both nurse managers and staff nurses to remember that during this period, the rules of unfair labor practice apply. Nurse managers must refrain from any action that could be seen as interfering with the employees' right to determine their collective-bargaining representative. Such actions include individually questioning staff nurses about their knowledge of collective-bargaining activities and making promises or threats to individual staff members based on the outcome of the election. Promising raises or promotions if the union is defeated or promising pay cuts and demotions if the union succeeds are examples of unfair practices. Staff nurses also must be careful that their discussions regarding collective bargaining take place away from the work site and not on work time.

Certification to Contract

Certification by the NLRB of a union to be the bargaining agent does not automatically mean employees have a contract. It does mean that a group of people have the right to enter into a contract with an employer, a concept known as **certification to contract**. The actual contract and its provisions must be written and voted on by the union membership, a process that may take some time. Issues considered mandatory subjects of bargaining are rates of pay, wages, hours of employment, conditions of employment, and grievance procedures (NLRA, Sec. 9a). In addition, the contract may specify other areas provided that both parties agree they should be included. These can include a union security clause, a management rights clause, seniority, fringe benefits, layoff and reduction in work language, floating procedures, insurance, retirement, and professional issues. The contract is considered to be in effect when both management of the organization and employees agree on its content. The final agreement is subject to a ratification vote by

> ### KEY TERMS
>
> *Certification to contract*   A process by which a union, certified by the NLRB as a bargaining agent, can enter into a contract with an employer that has been voted on by the union membership.
>
> *Ratification*   Passage of the contract by a simple majority vote of the union membership.
>
> *Decertification*   The process of changing union affiliation or removing the union altogether.
>
> *Grievances*   Formal expressions of complaints, generally classified as misunderstandings, contract violations, or an inadequate labor agreement.

the affected employees. Passage of the contract, or **ratification**, is obtained by a simple majority of eligible members who vote.

Contract Administration

The role of administering the contract then falls to an individual designated as the union representative. This individual may be an employee of the union or a member of the nursing staff. It is the duty of the union representative to provide fair and equal representation to all members of the unit. The role of the union representative is to explain the provisions of the contract to the union membership and be available to help in the grievance process.

Decertification

Occasionally, members of a particular unit may decide that the union they have chosen to represent them may not be the union they want or that no union at all is needed. In such a case, the members of the bargaining unit have the right to either change their union affiliation or remove the union by using a process known as **decertification**. This process is essentially the same as that followed by the NLRB for a representation election. Once again, an employee who is a member of the bargaining unit must submit to the NLRB signed documents showing that at least 30 percent of the bargaining unit membership request an election to remove a union as their representative. Then the NLRB will review the signatures for authenticity, set a date and time, and conduct an election by secret ballot. The winner is determined by a majority of the cast ballots. Once an election has been conducted, the NLRB will not return to the same work site for a vote by the same group for a period of 1 year (NLRA, Sec 9[e]2).

The Nurse Manager's Role

The nurse manager in a health care organization where nurses are organized into a collective-bargaining unit needs to be aware of the five categories of unfair labor practices described in the NLRA (Sec. 8A). They are: (a) interference with the right to organize, (b) domination, (c) encouraging or discouraging union membership, (d) discharging an employee for giving testimony or filing a charge with the NLRB and (e) refusal to bargain collectively. Another responsibility of the nurse manager is to participate in resolving **grievances**, using the agreed-upon grievance procedure. Grievances can usually be classified as (a) contract violations, (b) violations of federal or state law, (c) failure of management to meet its responsibilities, and (d) violation of agency rules (ANA, 1985). Grievances may be caused by misunderstandings that usually stem from circumstances surrounding the grievance, a lack of familiarity with the contract, or an inadequate labor agreement.

The grievance procedure used will be negotiated and clearly described in the labor agreement. Most likely, it will contain a series of progressive steps and time limits for submission/resolution of grievances.

The Grievance Process: An Example

The following steps comprise the typical grievance process.

Step 1. The employee talks informally with her or his direct supervisor, usually as soon as possible after the incident has occurred. A representative of the bargaining agent is allowed to be present. If the grievance is not adjusted in the informal discussion, a written request for the next step is given to the immediate supervisor within 10 work days. A written response must be received within 5 work days. The employee, supervisor, and agent will be present for any discussion.

Step 2. If the response to step 1 is not satisfactory, a written appeal may be submitted within 10 work days to the director of nursing or her or his designee. The employee, agent, grievance chairperson, and the top nursing administrator or designee can be present for discussion. Again, written response will be provided in 5 work days subsequent to these meetings. In most bargaining units, the positions of agent and

grievance chairperson are separated. Generally, the grievance chairperson is an officer in the bargaining unit.

Step 3. The employee, agent, grievance chairperson, nursing administrator, and director of human resources meet for discussions. The 10- and 5-day time limits for appeal and answer are again observed.

Step 4. This final step is arbitration, which is invoked when no solution suggested is acceptable. An arbitrator who is a neutral third party is selected and is present at these meetings. The submission of a grievance may be required within 15 days after step 3 is completed.

Often, a statement included in each of the steps states that if the time limits are not observed by one party, the grievance may be considered resolved and further action barred. The contract also usually specifies how an arbitrator is selected.

Here are some suggestions that may be helpful in handling grievances (Beletz, 1977):

1. The objective of the grievance procedure is not to achieve conquest. You have to work with one another after resolution of the grievance, so treat each other with courtesy and respect. Don't threaten or bluff. Don't withhold facts or information relating to the grievance.

2. *Do not*, whatever your position, allow disagreements or disputes among members of your team (e.g., management) to be public. Both the bargaining unit and the management team must present a solid front when faced with one another.

3. Expedience is a must; delaying tactics serve only to heighten emotions. However, allow time to consider all of the facts.

4. Stay objective. Emotionalism usually leads to further problems. If discussions escalate into angry exchanges, adjourn and reschedule later.

5. Implementing decisions or filing grievances requires planning. Get all the facts and information, witnesses, and documentation. Evaluate and anticipate the other party's position and possible response. Know the strengths and weaknesses of the issue for both sides. Find out whether any similar situations occurred and what decision was reached. Use all the resources available. Seek guidance from those higher in administrative positions.

6. Never refuse to meet with the grievant's representatives. The right to representation is one of the advantages of being under the auspices of a collective-bargaining unit.

7. The bargaining unit representative, though in a unique position, is not immune from reprimand

or discipline. When not involved in bargaining unit activities, the agent is an employee who must observe the rules and regulations of the organization, and the employer has the right to a full day's work and an acceptable level of performance. However, while handling grievances, the employee/agent is not really considered an employee. She or he is considered the representative and advocate of the employee who filed the grievance.

8. Integral to bargaining are solutions that may also accommodate future changes and needs. Therefore, think ahead. Once a grievance is filed, a chain reaction may occur, and almost any imaginable outcome may end up as the solution. However, a carefully written grievance procedure should obviate this possibility.

9. Be prepared to give or take acceptable compromises and alternative solutions within the framework of the contract, no matter which party suggests them. Know your bottom line for compromise. Do not submit to emotional appeals as to what is fair. The contract is the sole determinant of what is fair; if necessary, a neutral third party will be called on to interpret the contract. What one person considers fair may not necessarily be seen in the same light by the other.

10. Pat formulas do not settle grievances or solve problems. A formula would negate the needed judgment and flexibility that are so necessary to grievance handling.

11. Observe the time limits. If you do not, the bargaining unit may lose the right to continue the grievance to the next level, or both the bargaining unit and management may lose in an eventual arbitration.

12. In adjusting a grievance, knowledge is very important. As with any interaction between people, your statement is colored by your temperament and is interpreted by the other party in accordance with his or her own temperament.

13. Gloating over a win is human, but remember that you may lose the next one; don't become overconfident. Similarly, don't blame the other side for taking advantage of your mistakes. Learn from them, and don't repeat them the next time.

The Grievance Hearing   In the grievance hearing, remember these key behaviors (Trotta, 1976):

1. Put the grievant at ease. Do not interrupt or disagree. Let the grievant have her or his say.

2. Listen openly and carefully. Search for what the employee is trying to say. Take notes.

3. Discuss the problem calmly and with an open mind. Avoid arguments, avoid antagonizing others, and avoid the urge to win. Negotiate.

4. Get the story straight. Get all the facts. Ask logical questions to clarify doubtful points. Distinguish fact from opinion.

5. Consider the grievant's viewpoint. Do not assume she or he is automatically wrong.

6. Avoid snap judgments. Do not jump to conclusions. But be willing to admit mistakes.

7. Make an equitable decision, then give it to the grievant promptly. Do not pass the buck.

Strikes

When an agreement cannot be reached through collective bargaining, employees usually strike. A **strike** is an organized stoppage of work by employees within the union. Striking is not commonly used by nurses. By law, a 10-day notice must be given to allow hospitals the opportunity to prepare for striking nurses' absences. Also, employers have the right to permanently replace striking employees.

Major Issues in Collective Bargaining for Nurses

Since the passage of the 1974 health care amendments to Taft–Hartley, which extended collective bargaining privileges to employees of health care institutions, three major issues have emerged of particular interest to nurses: unit determination, labor–management committees, and the determination of who is a supervisor.

Unit Determination

The term **unit determination** refers to the decision-making process the NLRB uses to determine the composition of a given group for collective bargaining. In this process, the NLRB could use their discretion in determining unit composition because the guidelines given by Congress in the 1974 amendments instructed that there be no undue unit proliferation. This was done "to discourage frequent disruption of patient services caused by seemingly endless rounds of bargaining between a hospital and multiple unions" (Gullett & Kroll, 1990, p. 62). Such disruptions could be a potential nightmare, because many hospitals have more than 200 different job categories that could result in 200 different unions.

Following passage of the 1974 amendments, the NLRB determined the composition of each bargaining unit on a case-by-case basis. To meet the congressional mandate that there be no undue unit proliferation, the NLRB adopted a standard to determine unit composition called community of interest. In this standard, the NLRB did not try to structure the best unit possible. Instead, it allowed the interests of the various employee groups seeking representation to devise their own bargaining unit.

In 1984, the NLRB changed from a community of interest standard to a **disparity of interest standard**. This new standard required that employee groups seeking representation would have to show a greater difference between their job and those of others in the institution to allow them separate representation (Gullett & Kroll, 1990). Under the community of interest standard, the NLRB accepted any of six existing units. These were registered nurses, other professionals, technical employees, service and maintenance workers, business-office-clerical, and guards. (By law, guards must be in separate units.) Under the new disparity of interests standard, the NLRB recognized only four units: professionals, technical employees, service-maintenance employees, and guards. This was a source of concern for labor unions. Hospital management groups wanted to recognize only those unions composed of all professionals, all nonprofessionals, and guards. Unions wanted the interpretation changed to include all separate job classifications in the hospital.

This dispute resulted in the NLRB on September 1, 1988, proposing a rule identifying eight separate eligible bargaining units in health care:

1. Registered nurses
2. Physicians
3. All professionals, except registered nurses
4. Technical employees
5. Skilled maintenance employees
6. Business, office, and clerical employees
7. Guards
8. Nonprofessional employees

After a number of legal challenges, these rules were eventually upheld by the U.S. Supreme Court in April 1991.

Labor–Management Committees

A second, popular, development during the past two decades is the formation of labor–management committees. Labor–management committees allow staff nurses and nursing managers to communicate on a less formal basis to help resolve potential or actual problems. Their emergence has been seen as valuable. One outcome of these committees has been the development of shared governance by many nursing departments, which allows for a more formalized approach to interactions among staff nurses, nurse managers, and administrators. Porter-O'Grady (1989, p. 351) notes that "through these key groups clinical staff define, delineate, create, approve, and evaluate all nursing practice activities."

However, institutions that use labor–management committees may be in violation of federal labor law. The National Labor Relations Act defines a labor organization as "any organization of any kind, or any agency or employee representation committee in which employees participate and which exists for the purpose . . . of dealing with employers concerning grievances, labor disputes, wages, rates of pay, hours of employment, or conditions of work" (Sec. 2[5]). Furthermore, the law defines one unfair labor practice by the employer as being "to dominate or interfere with the formation or administration of any labor organization or contribute financial or other support to it" (Sec. 8[a]2).

According to Sherer (1994), the NLRB has found that such committees are a violation of federal labor law because the committees created by the employer served the purpose of dealing with conditions of employment. Although it remains to be seen exactly how much of an impact these rulings have on the creation of labor-management committees in the health care industry, it must be remembered that the committees, in many cases, have been created by management as advisory groups, not as decision-making groups. Hence the recommendations made by the committee may or may not be implemented by the organization and may be subject to change in the future by the

KEY TERMS

Supervisor Any individual having authority in the interest of the employer to hire, transfer, suspend, lay off, recall, promote, discharge, assign, reward, or discipline other employees.

Professional employee Any employee engaged in work predominantly intellectual and varied in character.

organization without the consent or consultation of the committee.

Definition of Supervisor

A third issue of interest to nurses involved in collective bargaining is the definitions of supervisor and professional employee. A **supervisor** is defined as "any individual having authority in the interest of the employer to hire, transfer, suspend, lay off, recall, promote, discharge, assign, reward, or discipline other employees" (NLRA, Sec. 2[11]). A **professional employee** is defined as "any employee engaged in work predominantly intellectual and varied in character as opposed to routine, menial, manual, mechanical or physical work; involving the consistent exercise of discretion and judgement in its performance" (NLRA, Sec. 2[12]). Because registered nurses are employed at both professional and supervisory levels in an organization, the NLRB must determine what RN positions are eligible to be in collective-bargaining units. The NLRB has consistently allowed RNs in nonsupervisory positions to be eligible for collective bargaining because they were seen as professional employees. The positions of nurse manager, clinical director, and chief nurse executive have often been designated as not eligible for collective bargaining because they fit the definition of supervisor.

This designation was challenged in 1994 in the Supreme Court case of *National Labor Relations Board v. Health Care & Retirement Corporation of America*. In this case, three LPNs filed unfair labor practice charges with the NLRB after being discharged by an Ohio nursing home. The NLRB ruled in favor of the LPNs believing that they did not fit the definition of supervisor and ordered them reinstated. The case was appealed to the Sixth Circuit Court, which found that the LPNs did meet the definition of supervisor because in the course of their normal duties they directed the work of nursing assistants, thus removing them from protection by the NLRA. The Supreme Court agreed with the reasoning of the Sixth Circuit Court.

This case has significance because it broadens the definition of supervisor while limiting the definition of a professional employee. More recently, however, the NLRB ruled that charge nurses could not be considered supervisors even though their work includes direction of other workers. The board noted that charge nurses' supervisory work is to coordinate team work, not to hire, fire, decide salaries, and administer discipline. This ruling is significant because it upholds the designation of a professional employee used prior to the 1994 Supreme Court decision. Alaska's Providence Medical Center, whose administration refused to bargain with a unit that included nurses who rotated to charge duties, appealed the case, but the ruling that charge nurses are not supervisors was upheld by the Supreme Court.

Nurses, Unions, and Professional Associations

Since its inception, the American Nurses Association has had an active interest in the economic security of nurses. One of the purposes of ANA was "to promote the usefulness and honor, the financial and other interests of the nursing profession" (Flannigan, 1976, p. 169). Although this statement was useful in helping to shape the role of the profession in supporting collective bargaining for nurses, the ANA did not officially adopt an economic security program that included collective bargaining until 1946 (Flannigan, 1976). Since that time, the ANA has actively promoted collective bargaining for nurses through the Economic and General Welfare Program, which now is called the Department of Labor Relations and Work Place Advocacy.

The American Nurses Association is a registered labor organization, but it does not engage in direct collective bargaining. The actual certification of units, negotiation of contracts, and administration of contracts is conducted by the state nurses associations (SNAs). Although the ANA supports collective bargaining and takes an active role in promoting collective bargaining, the SNAs have the freedom to independently decide their own level of participation regarding collective bargaining. All of the SNAs have a labor relations program as a part of their purpose and conduct programs to address the needs of the nurses in their state regarding financial and job security.

Many people believe that collective bargaining is a new movement in nursing, but the fact is that nurses have been concerned with their economic and general welfare for some time. In 1893, nursing leaders established their first organization, the American Society of Superintendents of Training Schools for Nurses, one of whose purposes was a commitment to promote the general welfare of nurses (Miller, 1980). The Nurses' Associated Alumnae of the United States and Canada was formed 4 years later to provide a national association for all nurses rather than just those interested in education. This association became the American Nurses Association (ANA) in 1911.

In the early 1900s, working conditions and salaries for nurses were extremely poor. The nation was in a general economic depression, and the health care system reflected the lack of growth found in other sectors of the economy. Nurses' working conditions were abysmal: long hours, no fringe benefits, and substandard wages. Just prior to the collapse of the economy in 1929, some nurses began to recognize that protest and collective action were necessary if the conditions of the nurse were to improve. In 1928, ANA incorporated into its legislative policy specific references to the general welfare, health, and education of nurses.

In 1945, Shirley Titus, then the executive director of the California Nurses Association, chaired a committee to study the employment conditions of nurses; as a result of the findings of this committee, ANA adopted what was called the Economic Security Program. However, just as this program began to make progress, ANA adopted a no-strike policy in 1950—a policy that was rescinded some years later. At the time, though, this position, along with the passage of the Taft–Hartley Act in 1947, which excluded nonprofit hospitals from any legal obligation to bargain with their employees, left the nurses with virtually no power to bring about change in their working conditions or salaries. The only options available were work stoppages, mass resignations, informational picketing, or individually leaving a work situation. None of these activities, however, was very influential in bettering the situation of the nurse in general.

In 1974, the health care amendments referred to earlier made it possible for nurses to use legal sanctions if necessary to ensure bargaining related to conditions of employment. Since the passage of these amendments, many state nurses associations (SNAs) have qualified as legal bargaining agents for nurses. In addition, ANA changed its structure in 1982 to become a federation of state nurses' associations. This change has rendered the state associations more direct

representation of their member nurses. It remains to be seen how this structure change will affect nurses' collective bargaining activities.

Collective bargaining looks increasingly attractive to nurses because of their growing frustration about the inability to practice nursing as they believe it should be practiced, to influence their working conditions, or to bring about improved personnel policies and benefits. Nurses are meeting this frustration in several ways: they leave nursing, they seek another position in the same or different health care agency, they endure their present position, or they seek some form of collective action by joining a union or seeking to have a state nurses association represent them. Historically, the use of the SNA as a bargaining agent has been a divisive issue among nurses within the professional organization and among employing agencies. Some nurses believe that the professional organization should not serve as a labor organization—that this dualism represents a conflict of professional purposes and standards. Others believe that there is no conflict—that the promotion of nurses' economic security and general welfare is a major responsibility of the organization.

Another major difficulty in the representation of nurses by SNAs is the conflict regarding membership of supervisory personnel in the association. How can a nurse manager or supervisor who is helping administer a union contract belong to the same organization that serves as bargaining agent for the nurses who are her subordinates? An apparent conflict exists over the nurse manager's divided loyalty. Proponents of SNAs as collective bargaining agents suggest that collective bargaining is only one responsibility of the professional organization and that nurses in administration can belong to the same organization. Opponents of SNAs argue otherwise.

A few SNAs have been charged with violating federal labor laws because association board members have held hospital administrative positions. However, the NLRB has consistently ruled that associations are *not* in violation of labor law when these board members are insulated from labor relations activities. When they are not insulated, and thus control finances of the organization and give local units collective bargaining advice, federal appeals courts have ruled that those associations *are* in violation of federal labor law (Lorenz, 1982). Furthermore, where there is a clear conflict of interest the NLRB has revoked the SNA's certification as sole agent (*NLRB v. North Shore University Hospital*, 1983). This created a dilemma for SNAs, which, in following this NLRB ruling, may be in violation of ANA membership rules when they changed their bylaws excluding administrators from holding office in the organization.

In 1999 the ANA House of Delegates changed its bylaws to create the United American Nurses (UAN) as the labor arm of the ANA. UAN held its first National Labor Assembly (NLA) in June 2000. Under the UAN bylaws, state nurses associations or their collective bargaining units are members of the UAN, which is designed to provide national support to nurses' collective bargaining efforts.

Complicating the collective bargaining issue today are numerous other efforts to organize nurses. Established unions in a variety of fields (e.g., steelworkers, textile workers, food workers, UAW Teamsters, AFL/CIO) are attempting to recruit nurses. Employees of individual health care organizations are forming their own collective bargaining organization and include nurses. In other cases, nurses of a health care institution are establishing their own collective bargaining organization. So collective bargaining in nursing runs the gamut from national collaboration of state organizations to coordination with other employees in health care to individual units of nurses.

Future of Collective Bargaining

The use of collective bargaining as a method of nurses to influence the practice environment and to ensure their economic security holds both concerns and promises, especially with the radical changes occurring in health care today. The concerns are that the very processes of collective bargaining separate rather than unite nurses, notably between staff nurses and those in management. What the future holds for collective bargaining in nursing is uncertain and unknown.

Summary

- Major federal legislation addressing collective bargaining includes the Wagner Act (1935), the Taft–Hartley Act (1947), the Landrum–Griffin Act (1959), and the 1974 amendments to the Taft–Hartley Act to include health care employees.

- The process of achieving unionization involves selecting a bargaining agent, developing a contract between the employer and the employees, and ratifying the contract.

- Major issues involving the continuation of collective bargaining for nurses include determining who can

be in the union, the role of labor–management committees, and the definition of the supervisor.

- The American Nurses Association, through its state nurses associations and its recently-established labor arm, the United American Nurses, provides collective bargaining services to nurses, but the ANA is not the only union that represents nurses.

- Poor employment conditions for nurses spurred development of unionization in nursing.

- A recent Supreme Court ruling determined that charge nurses are not supervisors and thus may be members of the collective-bargaining unit.

- The future of collective bargaining for nurses is uncertain and unknown.

■ LEADERSHIP AND MANAGEMENT
in Action

1. What does the process of unionization encompass?
2. Describe the grievance process.
3. How is the ANA involved in collective bargaining?

References

American Nurses Association (1985). *The grievance procedure.* Kansas City, MO: Author.

Balliet, L. (1981). *Survey of labor relations.* Washington, DC: Bureau of National Affairs.

Beletz, E. (1977, August). Some pointers for grievance handlers. *Supervisory Nurse, 8,* 56.

Briles, J. (1998). Gender traps in today's workplace. *Revolution: Journal of Nurse Empowerment, 8*(2), 31–38.

Buerhaus, P. I., & Staiger, D. O. (1997). Future of the nurse labor market according to health executives in high managed-care areas of the United States. *Image: Journal of Nursing Scholarships, 29*(4), 313–318.

Clayton Antitrust Act, c. 647, 26 Stat. 209 (1890).

Executive Order 10988. 3 C.F.R. 1959–1963 Comp. p. 521 (1962).

Executive Order 11491. 5 C.F.R. 1970 Comp. p. 888 (1970).

Flannigan, L. (1976). *One strong voice: The history of the American Nurses Association.* Kansas City, MO: American Nurses Association.

Flannigan, L. (1983). *Collective bargaining and the nursing profession*. Kansas City, MO: American Nurses Association.

Gruenberg, G. (February 21, 2000). Why more nurses find unionization attractive. *St. Louis Post-Dispatch*.

Guido, G. W. (1988). *Legal issues in nursing: A source book for practice*. Norwalk, CT: Appleton & Lange.

Gullett, C. R., & Kroll, M. J. (1990). Rule making and the National Labor Relations Board: Implications for the health care industry. *Health Care Management Review, 15*(2), 61–65.

Herman, E. E., & Kuhn, A. (1981). *Collective bargaining and labor relations*. Englewood Cliffs, NJ: Prentice-Hall.

Labor Management Relations Act (Taft–Hartley), c. 120, 61 Stat. 136 (1947).

Labor Management Reporting and Disclosure Act, P.L. 86–257, Title VII, Stat. 542 (1959).

Lorenz, F. J. (1982). Nursing administration and undivided loyalty. *Nursing Administrative Quarterly, 6*(2), 67.

Lundy, M. C. (1997). How nurses can organize for the purposes of collective bargaining. *Revolution, 7*(4), 38.

Miller, R. U. (1980). Collective bargaining: A nurse dilemma. *American Operating Room Nurse Journal, 31*(7), 1195.

National Labor Relations Act (Wagner Act), c. 120, 61 Stat. 136 (1947).

National Labor Relations Board v. Health Care & Retirement Corporation of America, U.S., 1124 S.Ct. 1778 (1994).

National Labor Relations Board v. North Shore University Hospital, 724 f.2nd, 269, 2nd Cir., 1983, 259 NLRB 852.

Norris–LaGuardia Act, c. 90, 47 Stat. 70 (1932).

Porter-O'Grady, T. (1989). Shared governance: Reality or sham? *American Journal of Nursing, 89*(3), 350–351.

Ponte, P. R., Fay, M. S., Brown, P., Doyle, M., Peron, J., Zizzi, L. & Barrett, C. (1998). Factors leading to a strike vote and strategies for reestablishing relationships. *Journal of Nursing Administration, 28*(2), 35–43.

Railway Labor Act, c. 347, 44 Stat. 577, sec.7 (1926).

Reynolds, L. G., Masters, S. H., & Moser C. H. (1986). *Labor economics and labor relations*, 9th ed. Englewood Cliffs, NJ: Prentice-Hall.

Sherer, J. (1994, May 20). Controversial committees. *Hospital & Health Networks, 64*, 66–67.

Sherman Antitrust Act, c. 647, 26 Stat. 209 (1890).

Sloane, A. A., & Witney, F. (1988). *Labor relations*, 6th ed. Englewood Cliffs, NJ: Prentice-Hall.

Trotta, M. S. (1976). *Handling grievances: A guide for management and labor*. Washington, DC: Bureau of National Affairs.

Index

Page numbers in *italics* denote figures; those followed by "t" denote tables.